Familial Fitness

Familial Fitness

*Disability, Adoption, and
Family in Modern America*

SANDRA M. SUFIAN

THE UNIVERSITY OF CHICAGO PRESS   CHICAGO AND LONDON

The University of Chicago Press, Chicago 60637
The University of Chicago Press, Ltd., London
© 2022 by The University of Chicago
Published 2022
Printed in the United States of America

31 30 29 28 27 26 25 24 23 22   1 2 3 4 5

ISBN-13: 978-0-226-80853-6 (cloth)
ISBN-13: 978-0-226-80870-3 (paper)
ISBN-13: 978-0-226-80867-3 (e-book)
DOI: https://doi.org/10.7208/chicago/9780226808673.001.0001

Library of Congress Cataloging-in-Publication Data

Names: Sufian, Sandra M. (Sandra Marlene), author.
Title: Familial fitness : disability, adoption, and family in modern America /
    Sandra M. Sufian.
Description: Chicago : The University of Chicago Press, 2022. |
    Includes bibliographical references and index.
Identifiers: LCCN 2021031076 | ISBN 9780226808536 (cloth) |
    ISBN 9780226808703 (paperback) | ISBN 9780226808673 (ebook)
Subjects: LCSH: Special needs adoption—United States—History—20th century. |
    Adoption—United States—History—20th century. | Children with disabilities—
    Psychological testing—United States. | Foster parents—United States.
Classification: LCC HV875.55 .S84 2022 | DDC 362.4083/0973—dc23
LC record available at https://lccn.loc.gov/2021031076

FOR PAUL

Contents

The bibliography can be found at https://press.uchicago.edu/sites/sufian/.

Figures

Abbreviations

ADA   Americans with Disabilities Act
ADC   Aid to Dependent Children
AFCARS   Adoption and Foster Care Analysis and Reporting System
AFDC   Aid to Families of Dependent Children
ASFA   Adoption and Safe Families Act
ARENA   Adoption Resource Exchange of North America
ART   assisted reproductive technologies
CAPTA   Child Abuse Prevention and Treatment Act
CWLA   Child Welfare League of America
DD ACT   Developmental Disabilities Act
DDAP   Developmental Disabilities Adoption Project
FAS   fetal alcohol syndrome
HHS   United States Department of Health and Human Services
HIV/AIDS human immunodeficiency virus/acquired immunodeficiency
         syndrome
ICWA   Indian Child Welfare Act
MEPA   Multiethnic Placement Act
NACA   North American Center on Adoption
NACAC   North American Council on Adoptable Children
NAIES   National Adoption Information Exchange System

A Note on Language

This book uses historical terminology about disability that contemporary readers may find problematic and objectionable, including *defective, feebleminded, idiot, imbecile, moron, normal, mentality, deficient, pathological backgrounds, handicapped*, and *mental retardation*. These are terms I use to reference the language used by my historical subjects. I invoke the term *intellectual disability*, where relevant, when using my voice. At first mention, I put these terms in quotes but do not thereafter.

Although I am mindful of person-first language, I use the term *children with disabilities* and *disabled children* interchangeably for variety. I use *disability* and *disabled* here as denoting a product of corporeal-environmental (social world) interaction.

I use the term *children labeled disabled* to more specifically connote the classification social workers made that socially discredited certain children based on presumed physical or mental states, whether or not the children had an impairment. *Children labeled disabled*, with or without impairments, were stigmatized as such. By employing this term, I want to emphasize that what Erving Goffman has described as a spoiled identity is what counted for children's futures; the attribution of disability is what mattered.[1] These children were subject to certain policies and procedures as a function of disability (potential or diagnosed) and had different outcomes and options in adoption than those whom social workers did not categorize this way.

I also use the terms *social workers, adoption professionals*, and *adoption workers* interchangeably.

I use the term *adoption leaders* to refer to those professionals who held leadership positions in the Child Welfare League of America or in adoption agencies, or who were leading commentators about adoption practices and policies. These were the people who influenced adoption practice.

Parent disability advocates and *parent adoption advocates* refer to parent advocates who fought for the rights of their disabled or adopted children, respectively. These advocates appear as historical actors when I discuss the emergence of the term "special needs."

Disability and Belonging in Adoption History

In 2010, a Tennessee nurse, Torry Ann Hansen, put her seven-year-old adopted son, Artyom Savelyev/Justin Hansen, on a plane alone back to Russia with a note in his backpack that said she could no longer parent him. Hansen expected that his orphanage would take him back. The note said:

> This child is mentally unstable. He is violent and has severe psychopathic issues. I was lied to and misled by the Russian orphanage workers and director regarding his mental stability and other issues. . . . After giving my best to this child, I am sorry to say that for the safety of my family, friends, and myself, I no longer wish to parent this child.[1]

The incident sparked national and international fury because of the shocking way Hansen's decision unfolded, with critics arguing that she had committed child abandonment. The US government was deeply worried about the potential long-term political and diplomatic reverberations of Hansen's move to sever the relationship with her son. It had prompted then–Russian President Dmitry Medvedev and Foreign Minister Sergei Lavrov to condemn the act and call for a halt to US-Russian adoptions, many of which involved children with disabilities. In 2012, Vladimir Putin banned US adoptions from Russia altogether as a response to US sanctions against Russia imposed by the Magnitsky Act.[2] And in a weird twist in 2017, President Trump and his son used the topic of Russian adoptions as the cover for an illicit campaign meeting with Russian officials with known ties to the Kremlin on June 9, 2016.[3]

The cascade of events in the Hansen case reveals how adoption can become a flash point in global politics, and, closer to home, how this form of family is bound up with major societal and political concerns about child welfare and family. Hansen's decision to annul her adoption, and especially the note she attached to her son's backpack, raised profound questions at the time about the lifelong commitments adoptive parents make to their children, the obligation to seek and access help before "returning" a "troubled" child, the nature of motherhood, and whether, in fact, love could conquer all.[4] For adoption specialists, it also raised service-based questions, such as: " 'Did the mother get accurate information about the boy before adopting, as well as training and education, so she would be prepared for the challenges of parenting a child who had been institutionalized [in a Russian orphanage]?' and, most pointedly: 'Were post-adoption services readily available to her so that she could help her son, and herself, rather than giving up?' "[5]

Hansen's case seems extreme, but at the time it happened it resonated for me because I was in the midst of doing research for a project on the historical confluence of disability and adoptive family building in twentieth-century America. The history you will read in the forthcoming pages is the outcome of my decade-long inquiry into this topic.

Even though the Hansen case involved transnational adoption, the story raised questions for me as a historian about the conceptual, contextual, practical, institutional, evaluative, and discursive issues relating to the entanglement of disability and adoption.[6] These dilemmas are historically tenacious; they have reverberated in the adoption of children labeled disabled for decades in America and are still very much alive today. Although only a very small percentage of adoptions have historically ended in what social workers called "failed placement," for much of the twentieth century the specter of "adoption failure" deeply concerned adoption professionals, implicitly and explicitly. These social workers understood that adoption was a high-stakes endeavor. It entailed a legal act that takes a child "of another into his own family and gives [the child] the rights, privileges and duties of his own child."[7] Part of adoption professionals' calculus surrounding adoptive family building had to do with deciding which children and which adoptive parent applicants were fit to form a cohesive family unit that would last. From the early years of agency adoption in America, social workers were cautious about the long-term viability of adoption for children labeled disabled because they questioned whether adoptive families with such children could grow, flourish, and remain stable.

Much of their worry derived from two overarching assumptions that persist in the current moment: that both child and parents needed to be able-bodied and healthy for a family to fully thrive, and that the future for a disabled child was likely bleak and intractable.[8] The strength of these assumptions for adoption professionals—but also for prospective and adoptive parents—has fluctuated throughout the twentieth century. Frequently, these assumptions were wholeheartedly embraced; sometimes they were challenged. Nevertheless, much like in the more recent Hansen case, health and disability have played a central role in determining which children could gain entrance to a permanent adoptive family.

This book brings that role into sharp focus by analyzing the complex historical dynamics of disability, adoption, and family. It shows that the story of adoptive placement is, both in discourse and in practice, inextricably connected to and shaped by issues of disability. It concentrates on how adoption professionals and prospective adoptive parents explicitly weighed the implications of disability and difference for building and sustaining families in the United States during the twentieth century. It examines how and why adoption professionals created practices and policies shaped for the children they thought would be desirable and suitable for adoption. To be sure, their views drew from era-specific notions of desirability and broad, but changing, notions of family, childhood, and parenthood. For their part, prospective parents' preferences for certain children throughout the twentieth century derived from notions about love, belonging, and potentiality within a shifting American cultural, medical, and economic terrain. For the American public, the child figured as the object of parents' and society's desire; thus, Americans bestowed "the child" with societal and personal meaning, aspirations, projections, and expectations.

Disability was deeply ensconced within these broader societal notions. As a category that is "at once both biologically grounded and socially parsed," the presence and treatment of disability and the disabled child shaped social hierarchies regarding child eligibility.[9] Like race, disability was imbricated in decisions about a child's value and in the ranking of a child's fitness for adoption. As we will see, potential adopters, social workers, and medical practitioners "inscribed" evaluative judgments about a child when they determined who was an adoptable or unadoptable child; signifying stratified worth, the label of disability induced certain time-bound decisions about the boundaries of inclusion and exclusion in agency adoption and their consequent pathways.[10]

Disability constituted a social formation in adoption as much as a corporeal one; much like racial formation, there was nothing essential or
fixed about the treatment of disability and of children labeled disabled.
Instead, it was strongly tied to both cultural representation and social organization, and its implications for permanent placement shifted in history.[11] Perhaps most importantly, society's changing views of disability
translated into tangible adoptive practices and had significant material
implications for children labeled disabled. These changing views determined whether a disabled child would be placed in an adoptive family at
all. In essence, they affected disabled children's ability to access permanent family life throughout their lives.

Such access to the social institution of family is an understudied yet
fundamental issue for disabled children, and it remains salient today. Familial fitness, I propose, is *the* first access point to the "benefits and status
of the properly human."[12] The story of disability and adoption uncovers
how disability operates as a fundamental category in the making of the
American family. It reveals that concerns about and actions related to disability invariably shape the contours of American familial belonging and
worth and arouse deep feelings of reticence and love. This book explores
the complex dynamics of disability's place in adoption history as a way to
help us rethink what constitutes the American family itself.

To tell this story, I am indebted to the rich scholarship in adoption
studies, a field that provides new ways to think about kinship in its separation of family from biological affiliation.[13] Adoption studies scholars have
looked at how race, class, age, gender, and sexuality have intersected in
multiple ways to transform the fabric of adoptive families and the contours
of the adoption experience.[14] But whereas researchers have acknowledged that these categories shape and structure American adoption practice, disability's similar role has been overlooked until very recently.[15]

I fill this gap here by bringing to light the history of disabled children's
placement in adoptive families from the Progressive Era to the Adoption
and Safe Families Act of 1997. I ask whether adoption professionals and
parents considered children labeled disabled worthy of an adoptive family
and I inquire about the changing reasons and historical contours behind
the inclusion or exclusion of certain children.

I argue that adoption practice gradually moved from widely excluding
children that social workers labeled disabled in the early twentieth century to *partially* including them at its close. I trace this trajectory on two
registers: the changing definition and scope of adoptability (eligibility of

a child for adoptive placement) throughout the century; and the key conceptual role that the concept of risk played in determining that dynamic.

The trajectory from excluding children labeled disabled from adoption to partially including them followed a long and uneven path; it was ridden with fissures, exceptions, contradictions, and much variability. Before World War II, adoption agencies and prospective adoptive parents generally assumed that children labeled disabled were unfit for adoption. But during the postwar period and beyond, this assumption slowly underwent a major change. Adoption professionals determined that disabled children's fitness rested on two major considerations: first, whether agencies and adopters regarded these children as desirable candidates for placement, and second, whether the growing number of programs and policies to facilitate placement were effective. Various other forces shaped this story of familial fitness, including fluctuations in the demographics and policies of adoption, changes in the idea of an "authentic" American family, the role of custodial institutions, financial constraints and medical insurance, institutionalization and deinstitutionalization, disability stigma and rights, broad disability and child welfare policies, and wide-ranging changes in foster and adoption care. Despite all its complexity, the story of the adoption of children labeled disabled during the twentieth century offers readers a chance to think broadly about the place of disability in American family formation; that is, how the presence of disability is accommodated or not in areas of family building, how that treatment changes over time, and ultimately what the answers to these questions reveal about Americans' treatment of disabled people and disability in society.

Belonging and the Disabled Child in Adoption Practice

Underpinning adoption professionals' cautious discussions about how disabled children might be incorporated into and belong in an adoptive family are implicit cultural ideas about the adopted child as akin to the "stranger"; neither a biological child nor a child that physically resembles her adopters. Georg Simmel's idea of the stranger is instructive here. He describes a stranger as a person who does not organically belong in the group (here, the adoptive family) but comes to it and stays. As such, the stranger embodies the simultaneous positions of both nearness and remoteness, of familiarity and of distance.[16]

The stranger in Simmel's discussion is conceptualized as a nonrelation, but in adoption she becomes a legal relative with all the inheritance rights of biological children. Worries in adoption about bringing a nonbiological child—able-bodied or not—into one's family reflected the historically uncomfortable question of belonging *in* a family despite not being *of* it. Social workers' and adopters' anxieties about adoption derived from a fundamental assumption in American kinship formation that biological ties are "real" and "authentic" and are fundamentally based in corporeality. Nonbiological familial ties are somehow inferior or inherently unstable.[17] They worried about the potential for failed integration and continuity and about continued marginality. The historically inferior status of adoption influenced social workers and prospective adoptive parents to conform to a normative notion of family, and within that idea a normative notion of corporeality in the family.

Adoption stigma itself conjures up the role of the stranger. According to anthropologist Jessaca Leinaweaver, adoption incorporates the "little stranger" and personifies the uneasy status of a non–blood relative by constructing practices that "kin." Analyzing the dynamics of international adoption, Leinaweaver notes that racial and ethnic differences have often complicated this form of family building.[18] Adoption historians Ellen Herman and E. Wayne Carp describe a similar phenomenon in American adoption, arguing that adoption is fundamentally about difference, stigma, and kinship that is visible.[19] As Herman states, the "struggle to make adoptive kinship look and feel as real as the 'real thing' has been a virtual obsession in law, language, and literary representation as well as in the social practices that make families up."[20] Key to that historical quest for authenticity has been a standard of able-bodiedness as well as physical and cognitive resemblance.

As a result, disability compounded adoption's sense of strangeness, even during moments when the latter became more common.[21] This observation is consistent with the work of other scholars who have shown that disability quintessentially and inescapably embodies the foreign; that the history of foreignness is inseparable from the history of disability.[22] A distinguishing feature of the story of disability in domestic American adoption is that social workers saw the child with a disability as doubly the stranger, not only because of natal differences but also because of corporeal ones.[23] They viewed disabled children as departing from "a standard script of human form, function, behavior, or perception." They therefore did not treat them as automatically eligible candidates for adoptive placement.[24]

Like children of color, disabled children—an adoption category that also included children of color—were the focus of social workers' constant contentious debates about whether and where they belonged in families. Their presence in the adoption story tested the scope of American pluralism and the dimensions of the acceptable American family.[25]

Social workers throughout the twentieth century understood what anthropologists Rapp and Ginsburg have so clearly noted for recent times: that the inclusion of disabled children in families "rearranges presumed narratives of 'normal' family life" and "changes the horizons of the family and the horizons of the future of one's child."[26] At different points in history, social workers hesitated to provoke a rearrangement; at others, they actively worked to challenge what "normal" family life meant or could be. Similarly, while some adopters rejected disabled children so as to avoid changing the "normal" family life they expected, others insisted upon accepting and placing disabled children into their families, thus making the child stranger into one of their own.

The Adoption Triad: Risk, Adoption, and Disability

Adoption studies scholars often refer to the child, biological parents, and adoptive parents as the adoption triad. For the purposes of this history, I suggest an additional triad: risk, adoption, and disability. Adoption's status as an alternative form of family, combined with the historical notion of disability as inferiority, makes this triad an especially potent heuristic framework.[27] It is at the analytic juncture of these three components that we can see how the meaning of each of these terms varies across time and what the practical implications of their entanglement are.[28] At the intersection of disability, adoption, and risk, we see how adoption professionals and prospective adoptive parents variously constructed, reproduced, and sustained this link across different time periods. Considering these three categories together also reveals how social workers saw the viability of the adoptive parent-child relationship as dependent upon the presence or absence of disability.

Unquestionably, evolving notions of risk structured the historical trajectory of twentieth-century adoption and disability. To be sure, the discourse of risk suggested that adoptive kinship was inherently fragile.[29] Adoption discussions about child eligibility were routinely couched in the language of risk, particularly the risk of disability.[30] Certainly there were

many other risks in adoption, such as the chance of a birth mother changing her mind about relinquishment, risks associated with the act of legal
relinquishment or with transracial placement, or risks related to placement and the demographic characteristics of a child, like her age or sibling status. Each risk has its own history, but social workers considered all
the children who were defined by marginality as among those for whom
it was difficult to find families. Disability intersected with many of these
stated risks, especially those correlated with a child's age and race.

Adoption professionals, doctors, and psychologists all framed disability as a major risk of (and to) adoption, for it epitomized the inherent
uncertainty of the adoption endeavor. Discourses of disability as risk
were culturally significant ways to negotiate, as sociologist Deborah Lupton observed, the "dialectic between private fears and public dangers."[31]
Throughout this book, I refer to this risk as *disability risk*. Disability
risk played a central role in expressing the anxieties and hesitancies surrounding adoption and in translating them into practice. Notions of risk
and disability, and the classifications to which they were applied, indeed
arose, functioned, and were reconstituted within adoption practice; like
other concepts and categories, they worked within a "cultural matrix of
institutional practices."[32] Social workers' discussions about risk in adoption wrestled with the problems of control, of fate, of autonomy, of undesirable outcomes, and of belonging.[33] They also pointed to questions
of culpability and of social workers' desires to manage and control the
future.

The way adoption professionals conceptualized risk was linked to medicine's embrace of normality and ability. In medicine, the risk of disability
connoted (and still does) damage, undesirability, and inferiority.[34] Social
work integrated and utilized these medical meanings as part of its own con-
tinuous attempts to legitimate itself as scientific and as a profession based
upon the model of medical practice.[35] But ultimately the idea of disability
as risk mobilized the weighty goals of family building within an enterprise
where social workers wanted to avoid, predict, and protect against what
they saw as the potential for any misfortune, particularly one involving an
adoption's demise.[36]

These concerns about a placement's "success" or "failure" were tied
up, again, with the adoptive family's authenticity and legitimacy in American life. As Herman observed: "Because adoption is a purely social relationship created by law, lacking the biogenetic premise that underlies
American kinship ideology, it has been consistently viewed as more risky

(because less real) than either kinship cemented by nature alone (which even law cannot eradicate) or kinship defined at once by nature *and* law."[37]

As the notion, perception, and treatment of risk changed, so did the particular disabilities that adoption workers referred to and were worried about. A shifting profile of acceptable or excludable impairments related to advancements in medical technology; new treatments made some medical risks modifiable or correctable. This changing list of impairments was also related to the kind of child that adoption professionals and prospective parents considered acceptable for a white middle-class family to raise in America at given moments in time.

At various historical junctures during the twentieth century, adoption professionals saw risk as either possessed *by* the child or a threat *to* the child; that is, from being something a child embodied to something that affected the child but was located within society.[38] But with either directionality, social workers assumed that the risk of disability potentially hampered adoptive parents' ability to form and sustain a functioning family. Social workers understandably tried hard to avoid adoption dissolution because of its adverse effects upon the child, the adoptive parents, and the agency. They wanted parents to avoid such risks for the sake of building a stable family.[39] Disability risk compounded any unease that prospective adoptive parents had about integrating the "little stranger" into their family, much less one with an unfamiliar or opaque medical history.[40]

Social workers invoked risk in numerous ways. The discourse of risk, for example, justified adoption workers' decisions relating to the differential eligibility of children. Before World War II, adoption experts tolerated very little risk. They promoted what I describe as risk avoidance and minimization. By associating what adoption professionals termed the "pathological background" of a child's birth parents with a child's disability status, social workers believed that the child possessed those risks and was inevitably defined by them.[41] Once the age of risk avoidance receded, social workers used a language of risk to denote one's lack of control in determining the health of one's biological progeny. Thus, in the postwar era, experts espoused a concept that I call *risk equivalence*. Social workers argued that in order to adopt, adoptive parents would have to accept the same risks of having a disabled child as biological parents did. As doctors, geneticists, psychiatrists, and psychologists became increasingly engaged in adoption after World War II, they weighed in on which children with pathological backgrounds or with known impairments would be the greatest risks for adoptive placement.

Their appraisals of acceptable and unacceptable risks reveal the key role experts had in making knowledge claims around disability risk.[42]

After 1960, however, adoption professionals advocated a stance of risk acceptance: parent applicants would have to accept disability in a child before adopting her, while adoption workers would have to simultaneously reevaluate and reconfigure their own perceptions about disability. Risk acceptance continued until the latter part of the twentieth century. At that point, adoption professionals used the notion of risk to identify conditions that posed a threat *to* children, thus relocating risk outside of the body and marking society as culpable in the making of disability and social vulnerability.[43] This shift marked a major transformation in the way adoption professionals conceptualized and utilized risk in adoption. Social conditions like discrimination and foster drift (moving from foster home to foster home) made it difficult for some children to be chosen by parent applicants for adoption. Medical and child welfare professionals worried that long-term foster care could, in turn, lead to disability and thus create a never-ending cycle of impermanence for the child.[44]

Disabled Children and the Demographics of Adoption

The historical trajectory from exclusion to partial inclusion was shaped not only by ideological and conceptual factors, but also by practical ones. Its cadence followed the changing demographics in adoption and numerous sociopolitical, economic, and reproductive trends in the United States.[45] The balance between the number of children legally available for adoption and the number of eligible prospective adoptive parents significantly influenced decisions about whom to include or exclude from adoption. Generally speaking, when there were fewer parents than children, the inclusionary criteria were restrictive, but when the reverse was true, criteria were more liberal.

Developments in the mid-nineteenth century set the stage for this book's twentieth-century phenomena. Amid the widespread use of almshouses and orphanages to manage urban poverty and state dependency, child welfare reformers posited the family as a better alternative to childcare institutions since they believed the family could more readily produce upstanding citizens. In fact, America's first legal statutes about adoption came in response to an increase in farmers' demands to legalize the integration of such children into their families.[46] These state laws laid out fundamental principles surrounding the formation of the "substitute families" that structured adoption for decades to come, including protecting the child's welfare and positing the necessity of fit and suitable adoptive parents. Loring Brace's well-known "orphan trains" (New York Children's Aid Society), for instance, sent urban children to western states to provide a home environment for them, take them out of city life, and supply farm labor.

Child welfare reformers' emphasis on the home continued during the Progressive Era. Adoption reform efforts began in response to what they saw as the dangers of institutionalized life and so they increasingly advocated "placing out" children in paid foster homes. Reformers criticized Brace's imprudent placement practices, as many children he placed still had living biological parents. They strongly espoused standardizing adoption practices to uphold child-centered precepts. Their efforts profoundly changed adoption practices.

Adoption also became a popular topic of discussion in the public sphere during the Progressive Era.[47] Still, it was decidedly not the family building option of choice. A bias for biological kinship rendered adoption as "flimsy and inauthentic—not just different . . . but deficient."[48] In fact, adoption was still quite uncommon during this time; when it did occur it mostly transpired privately and through independent brokers. During a time when social workers were professionalizing and there was a patchwork of adoption practices, leaders in the field tried to dispel public prejudices against adoption in order to convince prospective adopters that raising a nonrelated child in their home was not abnormal.[49] Yet societal views that adopted children had inherited mental defects because of "bad heredity" only compounded Americans' broad rejection of adoption and made prospective adoptive parents hesitant to go through with it. As a result, there were more children available for adoption than adoptive parent applicants during the Progressive Era.

In these early years of child welfare reform, the topic of children's health and welfare gained public and governmental attention. Such national focus on children led to the establishment of two major organizations: the US Children's Bureau, the main government agency that undertook child welfare reforms and provided the public with information about adoption, and the Child Welfare League of America (CWLA), the nonprofit umbrella organization for private and public adoption agencies in the United States. These organizations worked to reduce mother and child government dependency, preserve birth families, and, when necessary, facilitate adoptions. Emerging professional adoption agencies used principles that included obtaining biological parental consent for relinquishment, investigating the adoptive parents' homes before placement, and curtailing third-party adoption brokers as a way to safeguard prudent adoptions.[50] The CWLA licensed adoption agencies and became the main governing body of adoption practice. As adoptions increased, the CWLA set adoption standards for child eligibility and casework and established other adoption policies to systematize adoption practice in America.

As social workers professionalized, adoption became increasingly regulated, and eugenics weakened, adoptive family-making gained greater societal acceptance. For its part, the federal government infused money into child welfare programs as a way to address the Great Depression's devastating effects upon children and families. This move helped expand adoption programs and create state welfare departments.[51] By 1937 there were approximately 16,000 adoptions annually. The number increased to 55,000 in 1945 as more childless couples sought adoption to form their families.[52]

World War II marked a key turning point, with numerous changes to adoption's demographics and practices. Social work ideas transformed from resisting adoption to accepting it, parents' profiles and motivations shifted, and the stigma of adoption slightly subsided, although it never disappeared. During the war and postwar periods, out-of-wedlock births also grew substantially. Yet social workers viewed unmarried women as unfit, neurotic mothers.[53] The baby boom, economic prosperity, and upward mobility caused marriage rates to increase and interest in adoption to rise, which prompted social workers to reconsider their strict conception of adoptability. For their part, infertile couples sought adoption to address society's pronatalist sentiment.[54] Changes to child eligibility criteria tried to accommodate and respond to the rising number of prospective adoptive parents and their growing preference for infants. In response to these trends, the CWLA broadened the category of adoptable children to include those whose biological families had pathological histories, including criminality, alcoholism, and physical, mental, or cognitive disability. These children did not have diagnosed impairments, but social workers nonetheless considered them disabled. They worried that impairments would emerge that could threaten the integrity of an adoptive placement. But their strong belief in the influence of the home environment and in the "best interest of the child" (centered on the importance of a stable, permanent family home for a child's well-being) counteracted fears and worries about children with pathological histories. In the end, social workers argued that as long as parents could accept them, children with pathological family histories could be placed.[55]

These changes took place during an era when the cultural notion of family in America expanded and adoption as a form of family building grew substantially. In 1955, adoptions numbered 93,000, but by 1965, they had increased to 142,000.[56] Five years later, adoptions reached a total of 173,000, half of which were nonrelative adoptions.[57]

During the postwar period, adoption agencies became overwhelmed, resulting in adopters becoming dissatisfied because of long wait times and what parents saw as overly complicated rules and procedures. By this time, demand for children by prospective white adoptive parents far exceeded the actual number of white healthy infants available for adoption. There were several reasons for this state of affairs, including that fewer biological parents abandoned their children or relinquished them from temporary care, and that social services improved for families. Pro-natal societal pressures, however, led to increased parent applicant demand.[58]

The imbalance between available children and prospective adoptive parents led adoption professionals to expand the definition of adoptability and to make even more serious efforts to place children labeled hard-to-place—that is, minority children, older children, siblings, and children with diagnosed impairments. Social workers' attempts to place this category of children in greater numbers, in turn, shaped the practice of expanding, adjusting, and recruiting a particular parent profile. At midcentury, the number of transracial adoptions rose and agencies eventually began to consider single and divorced parents as eligible adopters, especially for hard-to-place children. New mechanisms in the form of adoption exchanges matched parents and child across state lines while specialized agencies for children labeled hard-to-place facilitated disabled children's permanent placement (adoption) in families.

By the mid-1970s, a downward trend in the number of nonrelative adoptions had occurred; this type of adoptive placement dropped to about 50,000.[59] There were numerous reasons for this decline. As Americans experienced the sexual revolution, abortion became legal, and single motherhood became more widely accepted in the 1970s, birth mothers relinquished their children for adoption much less often than before.

Other adoption practices changed as well. Adoptees fought to have access to identifying information in their records, often citing psychological trauma resulting from not knowing about their biological roots due to closed adoption records. Birth mothers could now choose to disclose their identities with adoptive parents and develop a relationship with the adoptive family.[60] For their part, the National Association of Black Voters tried to stave off transracial adoption and promote same-race placement in the 1970s. Shortly thereafter, Native American leaders argued that child removal was extremely detrimental to their communities—it produced cultural dislocation and poor outcomes for Native American adopted children. Native leaders wanted to maintain tribal jurisdiction over adoptions involving Native American children and for the federal government to address disparities in social services.[61] These objections led to the 1978 Indian Child Welfare Act and to adoption policies that promised to first attempt intraracial placement before transracial ones. As a result, transracial adoption fell from its peak of 2,574 adoptions in 1971 to 1,569 in 1972; by 1975, only 831 such placements occurred.[62]

At the same time as transracial adoption became contentious, many prospective white adoptive parents started to turn to international adoption in greater numbers, particularly from Asia. Intercountry adoptions rose significantly during the 1970s and 1980s, leaving domestic adoptions numbering 118,000 by the end of the 1980s.[63] Scholars attribute this shift to adopters seeking what many would have considered was a more palatable transracial choice (since, they argue, these children were not African American) and to an established rescue ideology in adoption. The shift could also be attributed in part to the discouragement of domestic transracial adoptions. But it is also possible that parent applicants sought what they thought were healthy, available children abroad as compared to the status of American foster children, as described below.[64]

Cultural shifts in reproduction, mothering, and·child-rearing, and new child welfare policies that promoted out-of-home placement, signaled changes in who made up the category of adoptable children. As international adoption increased and domestic adoptions fell, the effects of domestic social welfare policy changes, alongside child welfare's heightened concerns over child neglect and abuse, led to a rise in children's placement in foster care. Urban poverty and growing illicit drug use compounded these trends.[65] Thereafter, adopted children increasingly came from the foster care system, especially during the 1970s and 1980s. While waiting to be reunified with their biological families or placed for adoption, these children often moved through several foster homes because of social and structural barriers and failing institutional systems. These children's long-term limbo status led child welfare workers to deem these minors at risk for behavioral, emotional, intellectual, and physical disabilities. Thus, adoption professionals turned their full attention to tackling the foster care crisis. The federal government also responded by enacting the 1980 Adoption Assistance and Child Welfare Act, which included four provisions: (1) promoting preplacement services to assist with preserving biological families; (2) supporting reunifying birth families when possible; (3) mandating periodic review of long-term foster care cases; and (4) incentivizing states to develop subsidy programs to enable the adoptions of "special needs" children in foster care who could not be reunited with their biological families. By this time, the term "special needs" replaced "hard to place" as a way to emphasize placement needs, rather than a characteristic of the child herself.

From 1980 to 1997, laws, policies, and innovative mechanisms to facilitate special needs adoptions decreased the foster care population, but not nearly enough. Several trends explain why the foster care crisis continued. First, economic retrenchment, conservative measures that were harmful to the poor, the crack and HIV/AIDS epidemics, and mass incarceration broke apart biological families and refueled the foster care crisis. Second, an ongoing downward trend in adoption occurred during the 1980s, when traditionally "desirable" (white and healthy) infants became increasingly hard to find. Third, physicians and social workers diagnosed many foster children as disabled because of behavioral issues related to long-term foster care, HIV diagnosis, and exposure to drugs. Fourth, reproductive technologies offered opportunities to build a biological family to Americans who might otherwise adopt. Fifth, stories emerged of adoptive families dissolving because of their adopted child's behavioral or medical problems. Lawsuits against agencies for "wrongful adoption" because parents were not told the truth about a child's health background also rose. These developments caused adoption professionals to fortify their disclosure practices and to create specific pre- and postplacement services to help adopting parents address the medical, financial, and service needs of their disabled child so that families would remain intact.

By the late 1990s, with the number of children in foster care reaching 500,000, the federal government was compelled to respond to long-term and multiple foster placements. It did so by enacting the Adoption and Safe Families Act (ASFA). This law restricted the amount of time that a child could stay in foster care before the state terminated her biological parents' custody rights. It also sought to prevent children from returning to unsafe biological homes and gave funds to states to promote adoptions. In so doing, the government replaced its previous preference to preserve

and reunify biological families with a strong commitment to placing children in adoptive homes. ASFA drastically changed the landscape of foster
care and adoption, with implications for the status of disability and disabled children in contemporary child welfare debates.[66] Adoption professionals recognized that children labeled disabled were inherently adoptable and endeavored to operationalize this belief, but there were never
enough prospective parents to adopt disabled children in their families,
thus making access to a permanent family for these children incomplete.

Outline of the Book

A physician observed in 1937 that "the problems of adoption practice are
so interwoven that they do not readily lend themselves to formally organized discussion."[67] This could not be truer than when analyzing adoption
practice and disability. Like all historians, my task was to unravel and
make sense and meaning of these entanglements.

To do so, I divided the book into three parts, each of which corresponds
to major shifts in adoption policy, practice, and attitudes about the adoptability of disabled children. This three-part structure follows a story of reluctance, exposure, receptiveness, and then retrenchment in social work
practices relating to adoption and disability. Part 1, "Expecting Normality:
1918–1955," spans the decades during which adoption professionals strove
to create "normal" families—thereby excluding disabled children from
agency adoption. In the early part of the twentieth century, the period of
reluctance, eugenic views about deficiency and defect translated into professionals' and parents' hesitation about including disability and difference
in adoptive families. After this initial phase, they expanded the scope of
adoptive placement to specifically include children with pathological family
backgrounds. Worries about the dual historical dependencies of disability
and childhood further exacerbated professional and parental hesitancies
around such differences and informed adoption principles and practices.

In chapter 1, "Exclusionary Practices in the Age of Eugenics and Child
Welfare," I argue that adoption professionals' concerns about the interface of disability and adoption permeated adoption discussions and practice. Central to their concerns was the assumption that disability posed
a threat to the integrity of adoption family formation, an idea that was
based on common stereotypes of people with disabilities as damaged,
unproductive, and dependent. Between the Progressive Era and World

War II, worries about "feeblemindedness, illegitimacy, and social inferiority" only exacerbated the links between disability and adoption and
the hesitancy surrounding the placement of children labeled disabled.[68]
Adoption professionals therefore implemented casework investigation,
physical and mental testing, and infant observation as mechanisms to measure the risk of disability in order to minimize it and create a normal and
healthy adoptive family. They imagined the latter to be stable, nurturing,
and closely resembling the biological family.

But discerning which children to place to create the "perfect" family
was not so simple, not least because the borders of the normal and abnormal lacked clear definition. Nevertheless, excluding disabled children was
the norm. As eugenics waned towards the end of this period, experts and
social workers began to question the prospect and value of sustaining perfectionism in adoption family formation. Chapter 2, "Risk Equivalence
and the Postwar Family," considers how and why agencies reexamined the
criteria of adoptability and began to employ a discourse of risk equivalence, the social work idea that prospective adoptive parents should take
the *same risks of disability* in their potential child as biological parents.
Adoption leaders' calls for risk equivalence resulted from several changes
to adoption practice, like placing a child in an adoptive home before six
months of age. Broader societal developments, like earlier marriages, rising birth rates, and changing ideas about sexuality, motherhood, family
planning, and child spacing, influenced adoption amid its theoretical and
practical reforms. These societal trends called into question the very conditions of family belonging which, in turn, led adoption leaders and agencies to rethink whether "children with pathological family backgrounds"
should be excluded from adoptive family building. The adoption profession's reappraisal of child eligibility marked a key transitional moment in
disabled children's adoption.

Opening up adoption to "children with pathological family backgrounds"
led to the transformations discussed in part 2, "Working toward Inclusion: 1955–1980." In these years, the scope of adoptability expanded even
more. Adoption professionals' discussions about disability and adoption
shifted from focusing on children with supposed problematic family histories to concentrating on whether children with diagnosed impairments
could be eligible for adoption. Social workers increasingly criticized the
practice of excluding "handicapped" children from placement.

Chapter 3, "Love, Acceptance, and the Narrative of Overcoming," argues that adoption professionals reconfigured their ideas about risk to

achieve a more inclusive child eligibility goal. Instead of conceptualizing the risk of disability as located in a child's "bad heritage," adoption
professionals now anchored risk in social prejudice and barriers to placement, including those related to adoption agency practice. They invited
families to accept handicapped children by arguing that love and acceptance would overcome fears about a child's future development, her belonging in a family, and potential medical costs. I contend that adoption
professionals deployed the same "overcoming" narrative toward parent
applicants that health and education professionals traditionally applied
to disabled people themselves. A distinguishing feature of the adoption
overcoming narrative was that it required *prospective adoptive parents*
to consciously choose a child with a disability and then actively work to
achieve a cohesive family unit. Adoption workers did not presuppose, as
in the biological case, that belonging within the family automatically existed. Rather, they believed that it *had to be created* through love and acceptance, particularly as performed by mothers.

Chapter 4, "From Overcoming to Programmatic Solutions," examines
the institutional and programmatic efforts that helped bring the idea of
overcoming to fruition. As adoption professionals intensified their critique of agencies' exclusionary practices at midcentury, they took tangible, often painstaking steps to include disabled children in adoptive families. They established specialized adoption agencies, a national adoption
exchange, and a national adoption center, and devised outreach efforts
to find families. This chapter examines the ways that social work efforts
to place handicapped children intersected with those designed for other
marginalized children (minority, older, and sibling). During this time,
adoption professionals simultaneously reconfigured their idea of risk to
associate it with social barriers. They gradually began to view children
labeled disabled not as risky per se, or even as "hard to place," but rather
as having "special needs" for permanent placement.

In addition to programs targeting special needs children, the Child
Welfare League of America specifically established an adoption project for the permanent placement of children with developmental disabilities. These children tended to wait the longest in foster care for families.
Through this project, adoption professionals established training programs
intended to help social workers destigmatize disability and learn new,
suitable casework skills to facilitate these children's placement. States
began to offer subsidies to enable families to afford medical and other
care needs. By the end of this period, the federal government passed

legislation providing financial assistance to families. The law restructured incentives so that states would place special needs children in adoptive homes. These initiatives underscored professionals' emerging belief that children labeled disabled deserved families. They were now entitled to loving, stable homes. Because they largely relied upon individualized practices, however, inclusionary programs were somewhat tenuous and particularly susceptible to shifting political and cultural conditions. They failed to keep certain structural, institutional, and cultural barriers at bay in the face of a deepening foster care crisis.

Attention to children with special needs and their adoption significantly developed in the period covered by part 3, "Continued Obstacles: 1980–1997." Agencies, parents, physicians, and policymakers intensified efforts to place disabled children in adoptive families and to characterize them as unequivocally adoptable. On the level of rhetoric, at least, these children finally belonged. The practical reality, however, suggested a different story.

Chapter 5, "Institutional and Structural Barriers to the Adoption of Children with Disabilities" explores the reasons why, despite adoption workers' heightened commitment, parents remained reticent about adopting children labeled disabled and why these children's permanent placement turned out to be more complicated than social workers had originally anticipated. Even though mechanisms existed to successfully facilitate placement, and the number of special needs adoptions increased during these years, stubborn institutional and structural barriers thwarted agency efforts, resulting in an insufficient number of parents to fulfill children's overwhelming need for adoptive families.

Four contributing factors produced this situation. First, the sheer number of children in foster care with physical, intellectual, and emotional disabilities made it difficult for social workers to keep up with the children's placement needs. Second, agency practices sometimes undermined the late-twentieth-century belief that "all children are adoptable," turning it into a prejudicial vision of separate services that worked against full inclusion of children labeled disabled in the American adoptive family. Third, though interested parent applicants existed, there were simply never enough of them to fulfill the critical need. Fourth, numerous structural, bureaucratic, and budgetary obstacles frustrated successful outcomes. Obstacles included a lack of adequate services, expensive medical costs, the uneven provision of subsidies across states, continued agency prejudice, and an overall lack of adequate funding. These challenges put adoptive families under great strain and ultimately reflected the government's lack of commitment to take care of America's marginal children. These contextual factors helped limit parents' ability to imagine disabled children as belonging in their families. They therefore frustrated the children's full inclusion in adoptive family building during this time.

Chapter 6, "The Limits of Inclusion," analyzes select trends during 1980–1997 that formed the social and cultural backdrop in which adopter reticence to children labeled disabled persisted. These trends include: the idea of foster children as damaged, the emergence of the "crack baby" issue and the upswell of infants with HIV/AIDS, the rise of reproductive technologies, and the question of treatment withdrawal for disabled infants. Adoption professionals intensified their focus on disruption and wrongful adoption cases, which emerged in greater numbers during this time, partly as a consequence of these other social trends. Cultural messages of damage, risk, limited futures, and perfection and imperfection help explain why there was always a dearth of parents willing to adopt these children. As a result, children labeled disabled continued to have limited, uneven access to permanent families. By the end of the twentieth century, I contend, disabled children's inclusion in adoption was still only partial, thus sustaining a persistent need for placement in adoptive families well into the next century.

The imperative to understand and address the complexities of disability in foster care and adoption persists. The epilogue considers how the same themes that surfaced throughout the twentieth century are now reoccurring but under new conditions. I argue that as a result of shifts in Americans' conceptual and functional understanding of family, in the notion of risk, in adoption recruitment strategies, in financial programs, and in critiques of disability stigma, disabled children's inclusion in adoption has expanded significantly, but it is still incomplete. Today, all children are considered inherently adoptable, no matter what their disability status. This final, definitional change in the borders of adoptability ostensibly removes ideological and definitional barriers. Yet to materialize this position, it must be matched with stronger community supports, more extensive social services for adopted children labeled disabled, and financial assistance for adoptive families with these children. Moreover, the social meaning of disability itself must be markedly transformed to facilitate even more placements. The epilogue lays out what matters for increased access: a decrease in stigma and changed attitudes, more personal stories, community, advocacy, foster and adoption practices, coordination of child welfare and disability services, and research. Whether in the past or present, these intersecting areas play key roles in determining whether (and which) disabled children have the opportunity to be nurtured in a permanent family.

The epilogue lays out the multiple forces that shaped, and continue to shape, practices to place disabled children. These forces impact parental willingness to accept those children into their family. It reflects the book's underlying policy premise: that understanding past structures and forces that enabled or impeded the integration of children labeled disabled in families can inform serious efforts to map accessible programmatic and societal structures in the future. With such understanding, researchers, activists, parents, and practitioners in child welfare and disability can demand more supportive pathways to attain and sustain a spectrum of diversity in familial fitness, one that can thereafter produce new forms of situated knowledge about family relations.[69]

A Final Note

Readers will notice that the voices of children labeled disabled are rather silent in this manuscript. Such absence tends to pervade histories of adoption and childhood, not only histories of disabled adopted children. This relative absence is fundamentally a methodological issue. Individual case records are very difficult to access if one is not a birth parent, an adopted child, or an adoptive parent; even for these members of the adoption triad, access can be arduous.[70] Inasmuch as I am committed to privileging the voices of people with disabilities in historical writing, such voices were difficult to find for the twentieth century, perhaps because the children are often too young to write or because social workers and parents thought of them as too vulnerable to quote them in archival documents.

Indeed, scholars of childhood have acknowledged that adult desires, beliefs, and investments about the future are often the constructs that cohere in the figure of the child and descriptions of childhood experiences. We know much more about children as "objects of health-and-welfare interventions" than we do about their own interpretations of their lives.[71] This, as Alison Kafer has observed, is also true for disabled children, and perhaps even more so given that disability often culturally signifies "what ends one's future" rather than a quality that enables critical insights about one's past, present, or future and about the American family writ large.[72]

Memoirs written by adoptees emerge in greater numbers in the twenty-first century, and works by adoptees with disabilities are still largely uncommon.[73]

As such, this history is based largely upon the writings of experts, social workers, and adoption organizations with quotes from adoptive parents drawn from studies examining them, and stories and descriptions of birth mothers (not usually fathers) embedded within, and filtered through, social workers' writings. Using these archival and published sources, I employ what disability studies scholar Aly Patsavas has astutely termed a *disability analytic*; that is, a form of scholarly analysis that utilizes a critical disability studies lens that always considers the multiple interests of, and impacts on, disabled people. Scholars' use of a disability analytic is motivated by the goal to pursue social justice by and for the disability community.

Furthermore, this book explores the macro-dynamics of the adoption of disabled children. Given that this is the first social history of disability in American adoption, I do not derive my material from one adoption agency's archives to then illuminate general questions. Rather, I chose to examine generalized policies, structures, and transformations pertinent to this story to lay the foundation for further study. With a broad perspective in mind, I use the terms *social workers*, *adoption professionals*, *child welfare workers*, *prospective parents*, and so forth to reflect points of general consensus. Readers should understand, however, that there were always diverse positions among and between these historical actors, which a more localized project could uncover. Further research could certainly delve deeper into a variety of disparate perspectives, the contributing factors of social workers' racial and embodied identities, and the fragmentary, state-based nature of American adoption. Scholars could investigate state, city, or agency histories—hopefully and particularly special needs adoption agencies—to give further texture to this subject. With access to internal agency records in a particular city, scholars could more extensively trace and analyze the numbers and status of children whose identities crossed racial, age, sex, sibling, and changing disability classifications with more granularity.[74] Hopefully, my work will inspire these microhistories.

Because this book is a broad look at adoption, disability and family, it is primarily focused on the child. Though the suitability and eligibility of prospective adoptive parents, including those with disabilities, is an important factor in adoption, that angle deserves a separate study. Similarly, birth parents and their motivations, thoughts about disability, and reasons for relinquishment feature less prominently in this book. When birth parents' presumed disability or their status and decisions affect children's eligibility, I discuss them. But my primary concern here is to chart the adoption debates, policy decisions, and contextual factors that surround the fitness of the *child* for permanent placement. I hope that this book will open numerous new avenues for a wide range of inquiries on this very rich and complex subject. In the meantime, I trust that through this history, the far-reaching relationships between the child, disability, family, society, access, and equity become clear.

PART I

Expecting Normality: 1918–1955

CHAPTER ONE

Exclusionary Practices in the Age of Eugenics and Child Welfare

Writing in 1922, Honoré Willsie, a women's magazine editor and adoptive mother, recalled that suggesting to her spouse to adopt "conjured up a horrid picture of discomfort, of responsibility, and of risk."[1] Those considering adoption and those working in adoption saw the venture as full of hazards and risks. Florence Clothier, a key commentator on adoption and a psychiatrist at the New England Home for Little Wanderers, warned in 1942: "There is risk in adopting a child and there is risk in being adopted . . . we can struggle ceaselessly to minimize them [risks]."[2] Clothier conceded that although agency adoption would "remain a hazardous relationship," it was much less dangerous for children than the usual alternative of living in an orphanage.[3] Clothier's words typify the social work attempt to minimize and avoid risk in adoption, from the early decades of the twentieth century through World War II.

According to Clothier, social workers and parents based their feelings about adoption's danger on the recognition that there was a grave responsibility in placing a defenseless child with unrelated parents for life.[4] As much as permanence in a family was social workers' goal for children without permanent homes, it was also fraught with serious reasons for hesitation. The motivated act of placement in adoption—in contrast to the inability to choose to have a biological child—increased public and professional fears about it.

Adoption professionals who discussed risk certainly included social and legal factors, but by far they focused most on the risk of disability. There is not one moment, or one piece of evidence, when it is clear that professional social workers "discovered" the question of disability and adoption. However, collective concerns about the interface of disability and adoption—both conceptually and materially—permeate the practices of American agency adoption from the Progressive Era until the end of World War II.[5] Adoption workers believed it had a strong potential—if not outright inevitability—to jeopardize the integrity of family formation.

This judgment was based on numerous assumptions about disability and about families. Adoption professionals believed that even the placement of children with suspicious heredity would likely fail because adoptive parents would judge a child as damaged. These practitioners concluded that taking in a child with a problematic heredity or body was an obvious and avoidable risk of adoption.[6] Some practitioners believed that placing a child considered handicapped "by mental defect or bodily disability" was *unjust* to the adoptive family and the child because adoptive parents might return children who they felt "did not fit in."[7] They worried that parents would be constantly dissatisfied with a disabled child, which would result in the adoption falling apart.[8]

Practitioners' worries that including a disabled child would lead to a problematic or even unraveled placement were not altogether unfounded. Given that prevailing expert and public attitudes supported institutionalizing children with "mental defects," and that communal supports for adoptive families with disabled children were poorly lacking, adoption workers rationalized that it did not make sense to place a disabled child in an adoptive home when parents would likely remove her to a custodial setting.[9]

Adoption workers implemented casework investigation, physical and mental testing, and infant observation to achieve lasting adoptions and obviate ones they suspected would not last. Strategies in adoption to create certain families and to discourage others were conceptually and practically two sides of the same coin; they closely resemble eugenic ideologies around biological reproduction and highlight how eugenics itself was a flexible ideology and a set of practices that was adaptable to numerous social formations. Indeed, by employing eugenic tenets and goals about family-making in the 1920s and 1930s and integrating them into their investigation, testing, and observation practices, many adoption professionals effectively treated adoption as an alternative form of reproduction that closely aligned with eugenic goals relating to biological reproduction.[10] They delineated which children were suitable for adoption as a way to achieve their primary task: to find the "right home for the right child" and to create adoptive families that were likely to be stable

SUGGESTIONS FOR SUMMARY OF INFORMATION
AS TO
FAMILY HISTORY

(In addition to that called for on record blank.)

NOTE—This is not a blank form to be filled out but a suggestive outline of information to be sought for.

Brothers and sisters

1. Addresses absolutely necessary as well as name of people with whom living.

Relatives

1. Interview if possible. Brief summary of type of family.
2. Good or bad characteristics, in order to know what value to give statements.
3. Relatives' story of family situation, its causes and solution.

Additional information about family

1. Home life of parents before marriage, including:
   a. General type of home
   b. School life
   c. Physical condition
   d. Defects
   e. Mental capacity
   f. Occupation

2. Parents in home
   a. Characteristics
      (1) Truthfulness
      (2) Honesty
      (3) Morality
      (4) Temperance
      (5) Industriousness
      (6) Gambling
      (7) General weakness of character
      (8) Attitude toward family.

3. History of present crisis in family.

Additional information about child:

1. Physical and mental history as completely as possible.

2. Personal Characteristics.
   a. Truthfulness
   b. Honesty
   c. Morality
   d. Industriousness
   e. Affection for parents, brothers and sisters
   f. Obedience
   g. Unselfishness
   h. Application to work
   i. Fondness for reading
   j. Ability to do manual work
   k. Past opportunities for recreation
   l. Leader or plodder
   m. Attitude toward children
   n. Attitude toward adults

Mention all forces that have been important in making child what he is.

FIGURE I. Suggestions for Summary of Information as to Family History. From Bureau of Children, Commonwealth of Pennsylvania Department of Welfare, "The Significance of Children's Records," Bulletin No. 32 (February 1928). CWLA Collection, Box 56 Folder: Admin Recording 1928, Social Welfare History Archives.

and enduring.[11] But discerning which children to place to create a normal family and which to avoid was not straightforward, especially because the standards for adoption, including on child eligibility, were only vaguely outlined as late as 1938.[12] Furthermore, many factors—like the definitional parameters of what constituted normal and abnormal; child welfare notions about proper American childhood; larger societal, medical, and economic developments; and prospective parents' views—all themselves in flux, shaped the contours of child eligibility.

Fundamentally, adoption professionals strove to guarantee a healthy, nondisabled, suitable child for prospective adoptive parents as a way to mirror what they imagined was a "normal" biological family.[13] Their model for such a family was rooted in what child welfare reformers imagined an ideal biological family to be. A complex set of variables and a larger narrative involving the regulation of adoption, the professionalization of social work, and the making of twentieth-century childhood structure this entanglement, but the zeitgeist of both eugenics and child welfare ideology about normality played particularly key roles in formulating child eligibility. Indeed, these two conceptual frameworks and their practical implementation jointly prevented the disabled child from being adopted in agency practice during this time.[14]

Eugenics is generally defined as the modern science of selective breeding for the betterment of society. But within different historical periods, there were "competing and evolving varieties of eugenics," thus pointing to eugenics as a flexible ideology and as a set of practices with multiple permutations.[15] As historian Paul Lombardo has argued, eugenics "borrowed meaning from the social and political agendas of the people who found practical uses for it no less than from those who first offered it as an idea."[16] Whatever their leaning, users of eugenic ideas shared the propensity to biologize social problems along the axes of race, gender, class, and disability and to prioritize concerns about reproduction and the family.[17] Influenced by scientific racism, eugenicists believed that essential biological differences existed between white Protestant American-born middle- and upper-class citizens and people of other races and classes. They eschewed investments to improve the living conditions of the poor and of people with disabilities because they believed in a deterministic view of heredity; as such, they saw any investment to ensure improved conditions as a waste of time, effort, and money. Eugenicists argued that policies promoting the propagation of superior groups and the hindrance of inferior groups would help rid the country of its stubborn social problems.[18]

Eugenic understandings of disability (which included a variety of impairments but also alleged questionable heredity) as undesirable, risky, different, and defective, with a strong emphasis upon normality, played prominent roles in underpinning, fortifying, and cementing exclusionary agency practices.[19] Using eugenic notions about difference, defectiveness, and especially (ab)normality, adoption professionals during this period employed a discourse of "disability risk" to discuss children's desirability and to build adoptive families. These practitioners conceptualized disability risk as embodied and individualized, yet also group-affiliated; risk was intrinsic to the child yet collectively attached to the marginalized group of children with disabilities. Disability risk as an embodied peril essentially replicated operative ideas about disability itself, as a (medicalized) problem located in the individual that resulted in suffering, incapacity, and inferiority.

Child welfare and adoption professionals of the time seemed to think of disability risk as static, objective, and self-evident. To them, disability predicted an undesirable future.[20] On this they concurred: disabled children had limited or even "tragic futures" that would burden, overwhelm, and cause adoptive parents to reject them. They saw this outcome as desirable for neither the child nor the parent. Putting aside whether such negative imputations about disability were just or accurate, adoption professionals applied these standard ideas to the practical issue of adoptability, the term they used to denote child eligibility for adoptive placement. They feared that the presence of disability would inevitably pose a significant risk to adoptive parents' ability to build and sustain their family. What most professionals failed to weigh—or perhaps saw as outside their purview—was that the *unadoptable* label severely constrained the trajectory of a child's life, producing the very "tragic future" it predicted. The label determined where the child resided, what opportunities she had, the scope of her social relations, and even whether she survived.

To understand how and why disabled children were excluded from agency adoption, we need to first examine modern adoption in the Progressive Era, during which time the landscape of adoption grew from a patchwork of haphazard practices to a field in which professional social workers began to standardize agency work. From the Progressive Era and through World War II—and much like their counterparts in other social work spheres—adoption professionals continued to refine the field's principles and tools, to systematize adoption practices.[21] Within that set of efforts, they articulated inclusionary and exclusionary child eligibility criteria in which the discourse of disability risk played a key part, and which ultimately negatively affected disabled children. Throughout this process, ideas from eugenics and child welfare about the normal child, the defective child, and the normal family pervaded the logics of a developing normative adoption practice.

Child Welfare Reform and Adoption

One of the transformative nodes that introduced the subject of adoption eligibility occurred even before the Progressive Era, with the 1851 Massachusetts adoption law. The law stressed the welfare of the child as a primary adoption concern and posited the importance of evaluating adopters' qualifications. It instituted judicial supervision of adoption, directing judges to ensure that adoptions were "fit and proper." It did not mandate or delineate the processes by which the state should place a child in a new family, however.[22] In the absence of such legal direction, unsupervised private adoption agencies emerged. They were primarily run by philanthropic, sometimes religious, amateur women volunteers. Newly trained professionalizing social workers at the turn of the century scrutinized these agencies and were loath to accept them. Their criticisms reflected a larger paradigm shift in social work that moved from a practice based on individual moral judgments to one based on organized practice wisdom.[23]

Professionalizing social workers were working within an era marked by reform on a number of societal issues that responded to industrialization and urbanization, including poverty, harsh working conditions, public health, and child welfare. Reformers were also extremely distressed about public dependency among poor children.[24] Towards the end of the nineteenth century, orphanages and almshouses served most dependent children whose parents could not care for them. The conditions in these institutions were terrible. Progressive Era reformers harshly criticized the moral failures of these institutions, yet they also held the newfound belief that the family could rehabilitate dependent children. These two dynamics led to the home-finding movement, where charity organizations preferred to "place-out" "normal needy and homeless" children in foster homes, boarding care, and adoption instead of in child-caring institutions.[25] Even though Progressive Era reformers tried to offer alternatives to orphanages, dependent children's institutionalization between 1900 and 1930 nearly doubled; in 1928, for instance, approximately 250,000 children were being cared for outside of their biological homes.[26]

During this time, a "dependent child" denoted one under seventeen years of age who received economic and social assistance from outside of the family. Child welfare workers commonly considered these children "victim[s] of various calamities, social deficiencies, or parental failures."[27] The dependent child category included children deserted by their parents, needy or neglected children (children born to poor, immoral, criminal, diseased, or feebleminded parents), abandoned babies, orphans, delinquents, and defectives. On the other hand, Progressive Era reformers also had concerns about the "defective child"; one who had a serious disease, was epileptic, mentally ill, or cognitively disabled, or was "physically crippled or deformed."[28] They recommended segregated institutions as the best residential option for these children. Institutionalization would also relieve the burden reformers believed these children posed to their families and to society.[29]

Such views were repeated in the public sphere. Americans perceived people with disabilities as unproductive citizens, and reformers cast disability as a social problem that caused and was caused by poverty. They both worried about the extent to which people with disabilities were, or could become, dependent upon public funds. But reformers enacted policies and programs that, ironically, ended up aggravating the problem.[30] Given that the orphanage served as the most prevalent child-caring residential location for all dependent children, recommending another form of institutional living for defective children was not unusual, especially since these institutions additionally served nondependent disabled children.

Still, reformers understood the detrimental effects of institutional life and so they repudiated this option, but only for normal dependent children. They advocated for the social rights of the child and proposed public health interventions to address the structural and environmental drivers that led to such placement.[31] The 1909 White House Conference on Children and Youth, for instance, focused on the biological family as a central social institution, and child welfare professionals urged their colleagues to stop using poverty as a reason to remove children from their birth families. Along these lines, the US Children's Bureau, established in 1912, fought to reduce poverty and supported efforts to preserve biological families.[32] A national agenda supporting child welfare reforms continued with a second White House Conference in 1919. A year dedicated to improving the state of children's health and well-being culminated in the 1919 conference report, which set health and welfare standards for the

American child to experience "normal family life."[33] The report failed, however, to extend this commitment to disabled children, particularly those considered "mentally defective."

Amid a child dependency problem that persisted into the interwar period, child welfare reformers turned their attention to the growing problem of out-of-wedlock births. These births had always occurred, but increased numbers derived from a cultural shift in the 1920s that relaxed norms around sexuality and decoupled reproduction from sexuality. The number of white unmarried women who wanted to relinquish their out-of-wedlock children for adoption also steadily grew. As a response to this trend, a network of maternity homes where unmarried white women could give birth proliferated across the country during the 1920s.[34] Generally speaking, these homes were segregated by race; although some Black women sought the protection of maternity homes, social workers presumed that there was little stigma about illegitimacy among Black communities that would warrant mother-child separation.[35] The Depression only deepened this pattern of racial segregation, as economic woes made it difficult for unwed mothers and even intact families to care for their children. Because orphanages and agency adoption were closed to Black communities, Black children in need were regularly cared for in boarding homes.[36]

· "Illegitimacy," the term used at the time, revealed Americans' attitudes about what professionals and the public considered legitimate, normal family life. To eugenicists, psychiatrists, and social workers alike, promiscuity and illegitimacy threatened the institutions of marriage and family and stimulated fears about changing norms of gender, class, race, and disability. Amid rising divorce rates, decreasing birth rates, and increasing out-of-wedlock births in the 1920s, their sights fell upon the unmarried mother as the cause and result of these trends. Eugenicists and psychiatrists advocated for sterilization, but professional social workers promoted rehabilitative programs for the unmarried mother instead.[37] Social workers took a rehabilitative approach because they believed their main task to be preserving the biological family whenever possible; they saw adoption as a last resort.[38]

Preserving the biological family was such a priority that child welfare reformers asserted in the 1919 White House conference report, *Standards of Child Welfare*, that social workers should not separate a child from an unmarried mother who possessed even "a passable degree of intelligence."[39] Upholding a belief in the power of maternal instinct, reformers contended that a mother had a duty to care for her child and that the child had a right to receive that care. They also saw motherhood as a pathway to strengthen a woman's character.[40] In 1929, adoption professionals went even further, stressing that the social and character development of a child relied on her residing in her biological home. If she had to leave her biological home, she would suffer from a "profound emotional and social disturbance which can never be altogether compensated."[41] Preserving the biological family was therefore fundamentally about protecting normality and preventing disability.

Conserving the biological mother-child bond also stemmed from child welfare officials' assertions that keeping mother and child together was the most effective way to secure the child's "normal" growth and future and counter the alarming high rates of infant mortality for children born out of wedlock during this time (two to three times higher than those born to married couples rate; the mortality rate was high among all infants at 85.8 per 1,000 live births in 1920, with disparities among classes, races, and regions).[42] Child welfare reformers believed that these high rates were caused, in part, by the stigma of unmarried motherhood, which led some women to avoid prenatal care, and by separating mother and child in early infancy. Social workers also worried that separation required the baby to stop breastfeeding. Several states had already passed laws in the 1910s that forbade mother-child separation before six months of age because reformers saw breastfeeding as preventing and decreasing infant mortality.[43]

Once effective infant formula became available by the 1920s, however, the tie between the rate of infant mortality and family preservation to secure the child's normal growth loosened, and social workers' resistance to separation began to unravel.[44] Though most social workers still did not tout adoption as the best solution for illegitimacy or unwanted births, others like Alberta Guibord and Ida Parker saw adoption as a way to reconstitute the social validity of the child and mother. In this view, a minority one for the most of this period, adoption served as a normalizing agent that made the transgression of out-of-wedlock birth invisible for both mother and child.[45]

By 1938, a study on adoption in New York City by the Child Welfare League of America (CWLA) found that most doctors objected to agency efforts to keep mother and baby together during the nursing period, believing that this delay would make it harder for the two to separate later.[46] With more prospective adoptive homes than available children, social

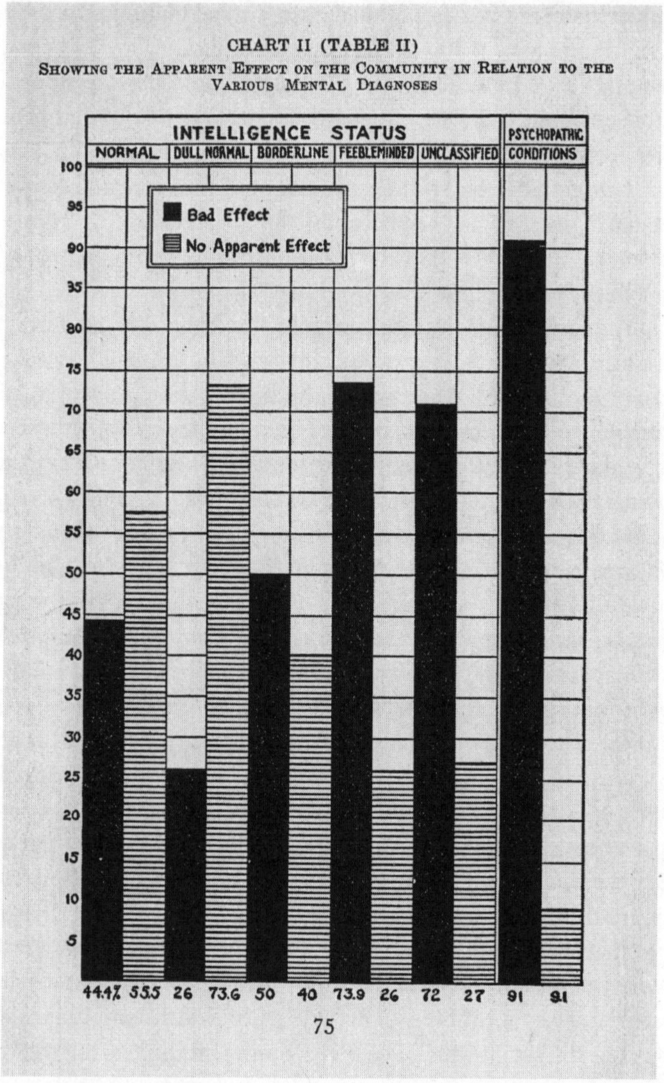

CHART II (TABLE II)

SHOWING THE APPARENT EFFECT ON THE COMMUNITY IN RELATION TO THE VARIOUS MENTAL DIAGNOSES

INTELLIGENCE STATUS — NORMAL | DULL NORMAL | BORDERLINE | FEEBLEMINDED | UNCLASSIFIED — PSYCHOPATHIC CONDITIONS

■ Bad Effect
▤ No Apparent Effect

44.4% 55.5 26 73.6 50 40 73.9 26 72 27 91 9.1

75

FIGURE 2. Effect on Community in Relation to Various Mental Diagnoses. Alberta Guibord and Ida Parker, "What Becomes of the Unmarried Mother? A Study of 82 Cases" (1922), 75. CWLA Collection, Box 44, Folder 44-6, 23, Social Welfare History Archives.

workers recommended that an unmarried mother should wait until after the baby was born to make a decision about relinquishment.[47] In 1944, Henrietta Gordon of the CWLA asserted that every child needed to feel she belonged to her own family and that blood ties formed the basis for family stability. But, she added, children also needed to be loved by parents who would nurture them.[48] Gordon stated that if biological family stability did not exist, then adoption could take its place.

Just because professional social workers ideally wanted to keep mother and child together during most of this period did not mean they always did so. Americans' acceptance of eugenics and psychometric testing influenced social workers' decisions to separate birth mother and child when circumstances warranted it, leading them to make exceptions to the family preservation mandate.[49] Certainly, social workers did not believe in forcing an unmarried mother to keep her child if the mother insisted upon giving her up for adoption. But when weighing concerns about defectiveness against separating mother and child, the consensus was that "if normal, they [the child] haven't a chance at home; they will repeat the mistakes and sins of their parents."[50] Social workers justified this decision by deeming biological parents who were criminals, had contagious diseases, were labeled immoral, or had intellectual or mental disabilities as "unfit to bear or rear children."[51]

Safeguarding the Normal Family

Adoption professionals' concerns about the effects of a child's defective heredity on the adoptive enterprise competed with forces that worked against their bias toward family preservation. First and foremost, adoption agencies wanted to offer prospective adoptive parents a "normal" child in part as a counterweight to the stories of unregulated placements that involved disabled children. Professional social workers denounced unregulated adoptions—arranged by maternity homes, legal aid societies, hospitals, family welfare agencies, court probation departments, agencies staffed by untrained private citizens or doctors or lawyers, and other commercial entities—on several grounds. Social workers argued that they contributed to infant mortality, kept the child from her biological family, undermined the work of competent adoption agencies, and "foisted feebleminded children onto unsuspecting adoptive parents."[52] Such accusations underlined their position as professionals with the training and skills necessary to create a "sound" adoption, especially as the field developed standardized adoption practices. Yet even by the late 1930s, amid a continual decline in the birth rate, high rates of childlessness, and increased demand for nonrelative adoption, prospective parents and unmarried mothers did not regularly use professional adoption agencies in half to two-thirds of all adoption cases. Speed and secrecy were two factors that caused these actors to turn to unregulated intermediaries.[53] Professionalized social workers wanted to resist these patterns to safeguard the normal family.

Within this landscape, disabled children became flash points in professional and public discussions about child eligibility. Magazine articles, for instance, warned of unscrupulous commercial brokers who placed children without scrutiny and left adoptive parents to experience what authors described as calamitous circumstances. Much of the disaster cited in the press was about disability risk and the use of reputable agencies to minimize it. An article from *Collier's* in 1939, for instance, featured a case in which physicians at the Babies' Hospital at the Medical Center in New York City observed a child who had been adopted from a commercial maternity home and was diagnosed ten months later with "hypoplasia of the brain and [she] may never develop normally."[54] Learning this, the baby's adoptive parents asked to annul the adoption, as state laws like those in Minnesota, Kentucky, Iowa, Wisconsin, Alabama, Louisiana, and New Mexico allowed in such cases.[55] The Minnesota Children's Code (1917), for example, stated:

> If within five years after his adoption a child develops feeblemindedness, epilepsy, insanity or venereal infection as a result of the conditions existing prior to the adoption and of which the adopting parents had no knowledge or notice, a petition setting forth such facts shall be filed in court which entered the decree of adoption, and if such facts are proved, the court may *annul the adoption and commit the child to the guardianship of the state board of control.*[56]

Responding to these laws, adoption professionals like Clothier and Parker and child development experts like Arnold Gesell called for a probationary period of one year before legally finalizing an adoption to ensure that the child was not disabled and to evaluate whether parents and child were compatible. The probationary period, they contended, could help prevent adoptive parents from dissolving an adoption.[57]

Collier's cited another case that involved a syphilitic birth mother who gave birth to a "monstrosity," but the adoptive parents had no recourse because the adoption was arranged by a doctor who circumvented any court proceedings.[58] Authors of articles like these implored prospective parents to adopt from a reputable agency; one that "deals fairly with the real parents, [and] safeguards the child's interests by making sure there's no syphilis, insanity, or chronic alcoholism in the baby's inheritance."[59] The message was clear: it was better for the child to be excluded from adoption than to have the adoption eventually annulled.

Adoption leaders made consistent calls to establish and maintain "safeguards" in adoption to regain control over what they saw as the dangerous, sentimental, and delegitimizing behavior of unregulated brokers who, they contended, created "abnormal" family units. They recommended that parents shift toward reputable agencies who produced "normal" families. They argued for casting aside feelings of sentimentality and embracing scientific methods to build thriving families.[60] Leaders insisted that nonrelative, professional agency adoption instilled a "measure of security" for parents and child and minimized what they considered the deleterious outcomes of pure chance and emotionalism.[61] Eleanor Gallagher, who wrote the first popular manual for prospective adoptive parents advised applicants to go to a reputable adoption nursery to secure a baby who is "physically sound and mentally normal" in order to prevent tragedy.[62] When her book was reviewed in the *CWLA Bulletin*, the reviewer wrote: "Of course, the giving of a defective child for adoption is to be avoided by the use of every safeguard that the present state of science suggests."[63]

The CWLA also instituted practices to minimize disability risks, including legal regulation of who could place children in state supervision; a probationary period before finalized adoption; thorough casework about the biological parents; the physical fitness of the adopters, their background, and the state of their home; and the "suitability of the child for adoption."[64] Such safeguards could prevent cases like that of a couple in Wisconsin who suffered a "pitifully unfair outcome of a warm human impulse." The couple adopted a baby from a private agency who failed to secure any information about their child's background. The baby turned out to be a "congenital idiot. He has never sat up, walked, or talked." The statute of limitations to annul the adoption on these grounds passed and so the couple had to "bear the burden and expense of an ignorant but innocent mistake."[65]

To avoid more cases like these, in 1938 the CWLA asserted official minimum safeguards in adoption for the child, the adoptive family, and the state to ensure the building of a "normal" family. Embracing a new notion of childhood and of a child's rights, the safeguards stated that the child had the right to be wanted not for her labor (as in the first decades of the century) but to complete a family that would accord her an education, love, and security. The CWLA safeguards also declared that adoptive parents could expect anonymity from the birth mother and had the right to a child who had the physical, mental, and intellectual background and condition to meet their expectations.[66]

Building the Normal Family

Within this reformist context, adoption leaders applied eugenic suppositions to articulate standards for adoption work that were consistent with the overall child welfare agenda of the time.[67] To address the capricious nature of private adoptive placement, professionally trained social workers sought to produce a systematic, scientific form of adoption, one that would estimate an idealized conception of the biological family to authenticate the adoptive family as a socially legitimate unit. They aspired to have scientific adoption "conquer chance and vanquish uncertainty," a risk-averse approach that paralleled—and extended—Progressive Era thinking about controlling nature to craft a healthy society.[68]

Adoption professionals' objective to solidify adoption standards that drew from eugenics, however, was not a straightforward venture; eugenics' evolutionary explanatory framework sometimes collided with child welfare's ideas about the causal factors of society's ills and its maternalist notions about an innocent childhood, domestic privacy, and the basic rights of the child. At the same time, these two frameworks converged when it came to enforcing an ideology of normality, and it is here that adoption professionals seemed to have sidestepped any tensions.[69]

Normality derived from the modern concept of "normal," which became a fundamental notion in almost every societal sphere as it offered an "objective" way to understand human bodies and behavior. While the "normal" denoted an average, its meaning also came to strongly imply a moral quality and became closely intertwined with a linear notion of progress. Its meaning was also one intimately entangled with its opposite: abnormality.[70] Eugenicists defined defectives—the insane, epileptic, feeble-minded, blind, deaf, alcoholic, diseased, deformed, orphans, and criminals, to name a few—as consistently falling short *compared to normal* persons; those who could never become useful members of society.[71]

In adoption, the conceptual relationship between the normal and the abnormal child translated into drastically different fates. Whereas the normal child gained access to family because of and through her diagnosed normality, adoption professionals believed the disabled child did not belong due to her alleged defectiveness. Adoption leaders effectively inscribed compulsory normality, whatever its historically contingent incarnation, into its practice standards.[72] Early standards of professional adoption clearly articulated that child candidates for adoption had to be "normal"; birth parents had to be unredeemable to warrant separating mother and child; and prospective adoptive parents had to be financially stable, nondefective, and willing to educate their child.[73] In many ways, determining eligibility functioned like medical prognosis: if physicians diagnosed a child as clearly eligible for adoption, by implication she was assumed free of disability, which attested to the extent to which compulsory normality was embedded in agency adoption.[74]

The opposite was also true. As E. Wayne Carp has noted, "professional social workers strongly ruled out the possibility of adoption for what they called 'defective' children; it simply was not an option."[75] The executive secretary of New York's Catholic Home Bureau also unequivocally stated in 1919: "No child should be placed out who is suffering from any physical or mental defect."[76] For her part, Clothier detailed "worrisome" impairments that necessitated exclusion, including "gross handicaps," Friedreich's ataxia, Huntington's chorea, hemophilia, congenital syphilis, congenital blindness and deafness, and degenerative diseases of the nervous system. These excludable impairments were a mix of specifically identifiable risks (e.g., syphilis, ataxia, hemophilia) and vague categories (e.g., emotional problems, feeblemindedness, criminality).

The mixture of specific and vague risks demonstrated disability's utility as a simultaneously fixed and flexible category, a quality that enabled social workers to apply an expansive understanding to their work while still demarcating the parameters of the normal.[77] Unlike other adoption leaders, however, Clothier made exceptions to the ineligibility of children who might have had congenital disabilities like deafness, blindness, or heart defect, but only when adopters wanted to care for a "crippled child to satisfy an inner need of their own."[78]

Adoption professionals who focused on excluding disabled children and upholding normal childhood mirrored the eugenic impulse to see only certain bodies as fit to biologically reproduce or, in the case of adoption, to be part of a family. Instead of being concerned with reproducing *humans*, they applied eugenic thinking to reproduce particular kinds of heteronormative, nondisabled *families*. Within the context of reproducing what they saw as normal families, social workers used the eugenic mechanisms of investigation and restriction to build and promote socially desirable, adoptive families and to impede other adoptive families they considered unacceptable from being formed.[79] Agencies tried their best to provide prospective parents with a child that could "have been born to them" so that she was "in truth one of them and not a stranger among them."[80] This mission took on particular significance during the Great Depression. Amid the Depression's destabilizing effects, the normal, intact family became even more important as a way to counterbalance and stabilize otherwise uncharted territory. As such, the normal family gained even more credence among the American public as an essential ingredient of society.[81]

A Normal Match?

In an age of keeping adoption secret and trying to "pass" adoptive parents and children as a biological family, social workers believed that conspicuous differences between parents and child could jeopardize adoptive family belonging and cause a failed placement.[82] They used principles of matching, which involved pairing adoptive parent applicants with a child along the lines of religious, ethnic, and racial traits, and physical characteristics like eye color, body type, and hair color to create what they imagined were normal (biological) families. Matching adopters to children unequivocally sought to minimize difference in the process, including the difference of disability, and to make the adoptee less of a stranger. Since prospective parents had to be generally healthy to adopt, children with potential or known medical or mental issues could automatically complicate matching measures, because their adoption would mean integrating dissimilar physical or mental profiles.[83] Adoption workers therefore set out to create families devoid of disability, particularly for nonrelative adoption, because they believed the latter was more fraught and in need of supervision.

Matching inherently promoted upward mobility for a child for whom the agency thought "placement was deserved."[84] Thinking of themselves as social engineers, social workers could "raise [a child's] life to its highest value" by building what they saw as the best, middle-class adoptive families.[85] Indeed, professionals agreed that adoption should not give families an opportunity to "rise above their genetic station."[86] To their thinking, this was predicated on only placing a child who they deemed suitable for a particular family. Fitness, suitability, and normality translated into being within the range of parent applicants' class expectations.

Social workers also matched prospective adoptive parents with a child based on her purported intellectual capacity for the same reasons. Intellectual matching correlated a child's supposed mental capacity with parent applicants' economic and professional status. Agency workers sought to avoid under- or overplacement, meaning placing a child with a high mental capacity in a home with parents of low mental capacity or vice-versa, respectively. Otherwise, a child would feel inferior and overwhelmed (overplacing) or extremely frustrated (underplacing) because the family would fail to encourage the child to live up to their potential. Either scenario of mismatch, workers believed, could lead to unfulfilled expectations, child maladjustment, and unhappiness for all parties.[87]

Matching also enabled prospective adoptive parents to voice their own preferences for a child's physical appearance or demeanor. Many times, their preferences had to do with not only physical or cognitive characteristics but also future ones. Educated parents, for instance, often asked agencies and consulting psychologists if they could expect educational achievements from their child.[88] Through matching, adoption workers thus tried to fulfill prospective parents' expectations by making even the potentials of home and child compatible.[89] Agencies also looked into the emotional dynamics of the parent applicants and tried to fit those qualities with what they thought was the child's personality.

The project in adoption to ensure normality applied not only to adoption applicants but especially to children. Since eligibility for adoptive applicants meant they had passed the agency's screening as nondefective, agencies felt that such parents were entitled to "non-defective children."[90] Social workers tried to carve out what they believed the "normal" and "abnormal" child to be. They consistently differentiated between these two labels, using them to determine adoptability. In this framework, the normal child might have a range of qualities and personalities, but being healthy, behaviorally age appropriate, and of average intelligence were necessary for this label. By contrast, social workers configured the abnormal child as unhealthy, and cognitively or behaviorally below age appropriate expectations. Labeled unfit, they deemed these abnormal children unsuitable for adoption.[91]

Normality, Flexibility, and Perfection

In their work to build normal families and contemplate child eligibility, adoption workers drew from psychological notions of child development and public anxieties about being morally, physically, and cognitively fit and about having normal children. To articulate the scope of the "normal" child and to pursue professional legitimacy, agency workers kept pace with the shifting theoretical and practical currents of psychology and psychiatry, particularly in the 1920s, when experts studied this question. They also based their ideas upon psychologist G. Stanley Hall's fluid notion of child development as a series of developmental stages, a pioneering idea that he proposed in the Progressive Era but that significantly influenced child welfare policy during the interwar period.[92] Thus, notions of what the body and mind of a child *should* be remained powerful forces within the American cultural and professional imagination.

These emphases reflected larger currents in the United States, where Americans feared threats that could destabilize their homes and families, like child delinquency.[93] In the 1920s, for example, behavioral psychologists recommended that child rearing should be based on rigid, standardized routines to prepare children to function in an adult world.[94] Against the backdrop of the Depression, however, support for strict child training subsided. Child psychologists reconfigured the family as a refuge from the country's social and economic dislocation. They called for a less regimented, more nurturing, flexible approach. This perspective quickly gained favor among the child development expert community. By this time, support for psychoanalysis and the mental hygiene movement had also increased among experts and social workers, leading to theories of parental and child adjustment, where "normality" meant the ability to adjust to and cope with one's environment.[95] With the advent of World War II, and in continued opposition to behaviorism, physicians and psychologists promoted the use of more relaxed, democratic child-rearing styles that they posited as a form of maternal patriotism.[96]

Following these trends, social workers treated the notion of normality variably. Some treated it as fixed, while others increasingly saw normality in a family as a more flexible concept, dependent upon the child's personality, the adoptive family's priorities, and their general home environment. Jesse Taft, the director of the Child Study Department of the Children's Bureau and Children's Aid Society, for instance, challenged the "cast iron" idea of normality for the dependent child, acknowledging the mistake that she felt social workers made when they spoke of the normal dependent child as one who was unproblematic when it came to placement. She argued, "No child is so normal as to be proof against the upsetting effects" of adoption. Adoption fundamentally involved a disruption from, and loss of, a child's birth mother, which Taft believed naturally stirred disquiet even in a "normal" child.[97] That was why, she contended, finding a suitable home was essential. Social workers, she warned, should not assume normality for children eligible for adoption, with "normality conceived of as something not requiring analysis and able to adapt itself to any home."[98] Rather, she explained, social workers should always investigate the child's background and perform a mental test, rather than assume that everything would be fine because the child seemed ordinary. They should realize that normality was dependent upon a child's feelings of security, stability, and belonging. Taft cited a case showing that a normal child could suddenly become a problem child, acting out in ways that would otherwise have made the child ineligible due to suspicions of mental or emotional disability. If adequate casework had been done, the social worker would not have suspected disability as the cause of the trouble but would rather have looked to the dynamics in an unsuitable home.[99]

Although Taft's ideas about normality were less rigid than most, agency workers' ideas about normality and the normal child were generally located within a certain range; they were always within the "prevailing ideology of the family" of the time.[100] Social workers did not distinguish between the normal and striving for the ideal; according to adoption historian Brian Paul Gill, their moralism prevented them from explaining why a "'normal' child or parent meant the *best* child or parent."[101] This "cult of normality," as Gill explains, impeded them from building atypical families, like those with children with disabilities or those with children of mixed race. Workers simply assumed that "the unusual family was a *bad* family."[102]

Feeblemindedness and the Elasticity of the Normal Child

Numerous child welfare and adoption leaders, along with child development specialists, cited "feeblemindedness" as a distinctly grave threat for the adoption endeavor.[103] These leaders' construction of feeblemindedness as a key danger of and to adoption, however, was based on an anxiety about how the normal child in adoption practice could be variously interpreted; that is, they feared that there was an inherent elasticity to what and who agencies could determine as normal and how that understanding could shape various agencies' child eligibility criteria.

The diagnostic category of feeblemindedness probably added to this sense of instability regarding the category of normality. It embodied a variety of alleged deficiencies and conferred a diagnosis imbued with a certain morality and "social inadequacy."[104] It could connote either a person with low intelligence or behaviors that signaled degeneracy, like alcoholism or criminality. In any configuration, the feebleminded person lacked a level of self-control, including sexual, and was deficient in common sense and initiative.[105] Feeblemindedness was also a particularly gendered category, one that referred to young women who supposedly had loose morals and heightened sex drives and who were pregnant out of wedlock. Experts believed that feebleminded women had a "differential fecundity" and therefore argued that their reproduction should be controlled.[106]

Feeblemindedness referenced all forms of mental deficiency, but eugenicists then further delineated degrees of feeblemindedness: *idiot*, *imbecile*, and *moron*. They defined idiots as those functioning below the level of an average three-year-old and who required institutional care. They diagnosed imbeciles as having a mental age between an average three- and seven-yearold, requiring custodial care, and deemed morally deficient by psychologists and psychiatrists. Finally, they set the mental age of morons as between eight to twelve, a level that likely necessitated the child's transfer to an institution but also meant that the child could also be trained to do certain tasks.[107] Once these definitions were developed, mental health experts articulated more granular classification schemes by further demarcating idiot, imbecile, and moron as high-, medium-, and low-grade. They divided borderline cases (those people who tested between the feebleminded and normal scores) into the subcategories of dull, backward, or unstable.

This specificity created a firm metric for diagnosis with the IQ test and a higher level of testers' and social workers' confidence in IQ tests' prognostic capability. But such assurances also obscured the "elasticity with which experts applied their methods."[108] Those classed as morons were particularly worrisome to eugenicists because their status was liminal and slippery. They were difficult to detect, could pass as normal, had no "few or no obvious stigmata of degeneration," and therefore could procreate without anyone stopping them.[109]

In their ability to pass as normal, morons embodied the elastic nature of the concept of the normal child. Despite challenges to eugenic claims about the menace of the feebleminded that arose in the 1920s and strengthened in the 1930s, the figure of the moron persisted as a threat in the American cultural imagination *precisely* because the construction of the moron rested at the cusp of normality. Indeed, if people *thought* morons were normal, then could they be? What were the boundaries of this supposedly axiomatic diagnosis? Given the conceptual ambiguity of the moron, the invisibility of any impairment, the level of disability risk it personified and created for the adoption endeavor, and the unpredictability of the moron's future, most adoption experts agreed that this class of mental defectives should not be placed in adoptive families.[110]

Although they were undoubtedly concerned about children with noticeable impairments, professional social workers were very worried about placing children who, with no evident bodily differences, possessed a family history of deviancy or disability. Clothier, for instance, believed that a child who bore "seeds of known familial or hereditary disease" should not be offered for adoption. She recommended that agencies very carefully assess children whose biological family history included psychosis, feeblemindedness, emotional problems, criminality, addiction, or epilepsy, even if the child herself did not exhibit any impairment.[111] Gallagher agreed with Clothier, arguing that she would be the last person to advocate placing a child whose family history "shows a strain of insanity or definite feeblemindedness." In Gallagher's view, the social worker had to know every aspect of that history before she made a final judgment.[112]

Some psychiatrists in the 1920s started to counter this type of hereditary determinism, however. They argued that as long as the children of feebleminded parents were brought up well, any disability risk posed by inheritance could be mitigated.[113]

Most adoption professionals, however, believed that there was a strong link between illegitimacy and feeblemindedness. They employed a gendered understanding of this link, relying upon the idea of an unmarried woman as sexually promiscuous but also upon the idea that a feebleminded man was unattractive. In this way, they cast the correlation between sex drive and men as inconsequential.[114]

In this context, a child's normality was not just a function of her own body or mind but contingent upon her biological mother's marital status. As Ruth Workum, executive director of the Ohio Humane Society in Cincinnati, attested in 1924, the "handicap of illegitimacy" for children began in the period of gestation.[115] Workum posited that many unmarried mothers were "victims of mental diseases and venereal conditions, [and] their children should not be given in adoption unless the clinical and medical findings show that the agency is not giving out a piece of 'damaged goods.' "[116] Although not all unmarried mothers were considered feeble-minded or of lower intelligence, many who took mental exams received such a diagnosis. Adoption agencies explained that they gave mental exams to unmarried mothers as a "diagnostic aid in helping to understand the girl for the purpose of making a satisfactory program for her future," but they also administered them to find "defects" in the mother and make predictions about her child's future.[117] Often, when psychiatrists found "mental defect" in an administered mental exam, mother and child were separated and the woman was put into custodial care. Still, there were exceptions where agencies arranged foster care for the child or relatives took care of them both to prevent separating them.[118]

The tie between female feeblemindedness and illegitimacy—steeped in eugenic anxieties about immorality, degeneracy, female delinquency, sexual precociousness, and social change—clearly formed the basis of American society's stigma on adoption as a suspect way of forming a family. From the Progressive Era until World War II, the American public not only openly reproached unmarried mothers but largely condemned their offspring, deeming them abnormal and defective.[119] To be sure, Americans' deep suspicions of the adoption enterprise and of adopted children stemmed from a cacophony of questionable adoption practices. But because Americans considered illegitimacy a disgrace, the stigma affixed itself to the affected child. As a result, as Carp explains, adopted children carried a double stigma: "They were assumed to be illegitimate and thus mentally deficient by inheriting the genetic trait of feeblemindedness, and they were adopted, thus lacking the all-important blood link to their adoptive parents."[120]

Experts' fears about adoption thus influenced a majority of childless, married partners in the mid-1920s because they thought that factors of bad heredity "may crop out" of a child later.[121] Applicants who recognized that adoption involved certain risks searched for a child with good inheritance while others were hesitant about adopting a dependent child at all. They were often surprised to find out, as Ida Parker, associate director of the Research Bureau on Social Case Work, observed in 1927, that "normal families of good stock seldom give away their children."[122]

Measuring Risk to Control Abnormality

Controlling disability risk was part and parcel of discerning child eligibility for adoption. Physician evaluation at the time a child-placing agency received a child, IQ tests, and infant observation (up to two years) could provide evidence of normal or abnormal child development. These tests measured the physical and cognitive status of the child, measured the level of disability risk for adoptive placement, and shaped the agency's view of her future prospects. Agencies' reliance on these assessments reflects Deborah Lupton's observation about the synergy between a discourse of risk and the strategy of diagnostic testing, and a dependence upon expert, scientific knowledge to discern risk.[123] Given that adoption professionals were themselves trying to legitimize their field and authorize themselves as serious and scientific, it is not surprising that employing these tests gave credence to their endeavor. Though they did not resolve all the issues inherent in child adoption, such clinical safeguards could, according to a leading child development expert, "steadily improve its methods and make them both more scientific and humane."[124]

Physicians and psychologists who contracted with an adoption agency to perform an initial medical exam of the child looked at all parts of the child's body: teeth, lungs, heart, nose, ears, eyes, skin, feet, and digestion.[125] They performed a Wasserman test, tuberculin test, and urinalysis.[126] According to Clothier, a good pediatrician had to:

> identify any gross abnormalities of structure or congenital disease processes. Certainly no baby should be placed for adoption who has not been examined by a competent physician. . . . Thoroughgoing physical and laboratory examinations, combined with an adequate medical family history (usually absent from social records), should rule out from blind adoption placement of a group of grossly handicapped children. This group includes children suffering from hereditary degenerative disease of the nervous system, Friedreich's ataxia, congenital blindness and deafness, Huntington's chorea, congenital syphilis and hemophilia.[127]

For its part, the CWLA believed that testing, evaluation, and observation "should be routine for all children considered for adoption."[128] A thorough child study that could enable agencies to sufficiently evaluate adoptability had to include casework, a medical exam, and observation. Casework had to look at a child's heredity and the likelihood of impairment (particularly epilepsy, syphilis, feeblemindedness, or insanity). It also had to include an assessment of the child's life in the biological home and, when possible, her preferences and personality. The medical exam needed to thoroughly evaluate not only the child's physical condition but also her "mentality" in order to gauge her relative mental age and aptitude. Finally, the child study involved physician observation for a lengthy period to confirm normality or abnormality, to correct any minor defects to restore normality, and to make sure that no new impairments arose.

Along these lines, some state adoption laws required investigatory practices into the child, the birth parents, the adopters, and their home. Clothier extolled the 1936 law in Massachusetts, for instance, for mandating such thorough study. She sadly acknowledged, however, that by the late 1930s only twenty-two states required that the department of welfare or a court-appointed person or agency investigate the clients in the adoption triad (birth mother, child, and adoptive parents). Twenty-three states had no provisions at all, and only nineteen mandated a probationary period in the adoptive home (technically foster home) before the adoption could be finalized.[129] Despite attempts to standardize and regulate American adoption, then, practices ultimately depended as much upon state law as on local agency practice and CWLA recommendations.

Measuring Risk through Casework

Comprehensive casework involved an inquiry into the legal status of the child, a study of the "child's family history, environment, and personality, and in a general way its physical, mental, and moral condition."[130] Adoption leaders recommended that casework for adoption go as far back as possible and extend beyond the nuclear family, "for this helps us to evaluate the strength of genetic forces expressed in physical make-up, interests, abilities, intelligence, etc."[131] Pursuing extensive information about the child's birth family provided details to adoptive applicants about a child that, if placed for adoption, could be later communicated to the child once she had grown. It was also a way to assure the adoptive couple that the child was normal and that her natural endowment would meet the prospective parents' expectations. Furthermore, it helped practitioners screen out those children they regarded as abnormal.

Performing casework also addressed cultural fears about unknown or suspicious heredity that practitioners assumed would make adoptive parents hesitate to raise an adopted child in the first place.[132] The first comprehensive guide to adoption for social workers, by van Senden Theis, recommended in 1921 that agencies exclude children with unknown or problematic heredity because of the common belief that all sorts of "bad heredity" could be passed onto one's progeny. This history could include having a birth mother who had mental illness or "mental retardation," or a record of alcoholism or criminality. Even though these children did not have diagnosed impairments, professionals labeled them as having "pathological family backgrounds."[133] Clothier also believed that certain conditions in a family history posed a risk too high for adoptive placement, including unexplained conditions like manic-depressive psychosis or schizophrenia, feeblemindedness, alcohol or drug addiction, emotional inability, criminality, and epilepsy.[134] Speaking to this range of typical impairments and exclusions, the well-regarded journalist Dorothy Thompson published an article titled "Fit for Adoption" in the *Ladies' Home Journal* in May 1939 in which she strongly condemned the strict eligibility criteria of adoption agencies. She noted that the definition of "'fit subject for adoption' is, among many social agencies far, far stricter" than even German eugenic directives.[135]

The similar exclusionary treatment of children with bad heredity and those with impairments speaks to the fluidity of disability as a social construct and reflects the belief that both groups of children presumably possessed disability risk. Indeed, the category of children with pathological family backgrounds in adoption moves us beyond the common understanding of disability as a medicalized deficit to a historically contingent "social location complexly embodied."[136] In other words, a person did not have to have an impairment to be disabled. Rather, it is through the stigmatizing attribution of disability and the "spoiled identity" such attribution conferred—compounded by the subsequent process of exclusion—that the social location of disability was formed in adoption during this time.[137]

Casework might have been a way to avoid adoptive parents "getting stuck" with a problematic "abnormal" child or a child with a pathological family background but it also legitimized adoption by explicitly distinguishing it from charity and by aligning itself with scientific fields.[138] The Study Group on Adoptions of the Cleveland Conference on Illegitimacy, for instance, agreed that upstanding adoption agencies should not sacrifice scientific casework in favor of "hasty" sentimental placement decisions to avoid "failures and sad results." Like the CWLA, the group recommended that agencies perform a thorough physical exam on the child, a Wasserman test (for syphilis), an intelligence study, and a social investigation of the child's biological parents. It also strongly suggested that the agencies select respectable foster parents deemed physically, mentally, and financially suitable—that is, similar to the child.[139]

Casework could never be entirely scientific or conclusive, however.[140] Physicians and adoption professionals alike admitted that it was often difficult to attain a full accounting of a child's family history, typically because the record of putative fathers for children born out of wedlock was either nonexistent or hard to come by. In fact, inadequate genetic information was the rule rather than the exception, a reality that heightened social workers' anxieties about children with pathological family histories and increased their worries that they might place a disabled child in an adoptive home by mistake. As adoptive applicants increasingly pressured agencies for infants, agencies often had to choose between waiting to see what a physician observed about a child's mental and physical status or taking a chance and placing an infant in a home. One geneticist, for instance, noted that in the face of an incomplete record he would never adopt a child whose family background indicated "nervous disorders" like Huntington's chorea, spinal ataxia, paralysis agitans (Parkinson's disease), and amaurotic juvenile idiocy (Sandhoff disease). Similarly, he would not adopt a child with any unexplained psychosis in their family background. If he were ever to adopt, he would only use a reputable agency that made sure to gather a child's records and would avoid children with "bad" family histories and definitely those without any records at all.[141]

For his part, Hyman Lippman, director of the Amherst H. Wilder Child Guidance Clinic in St. Paul, sent out a questionnaire in 1937 to thirty mental hygiene experts to determine how they dealt with child adoption and adoptability (see appendix 1).[142] Lippman's results clearly depended upon the expert's eugenic leanings and his notions of the hereditary transmission of certain traits; for Lippman, the degree of risk for feeblemindedness depended upon how many sides of the family were affected.[143] Some of Lippman's respondents acknowledged that the decision to adopt a child with feeblemindedness in her family history should be left up to the parents rather than the social worker, thereby challenging the social workers' full control over determining eligibility.

Lippman not only asked about feeblemindedness but also asked experts to discern whether serious delinquency, incest, transvestism, homosexuality, or other "bizarre behavior" in the immediate biological family background could also rule out a child. Answers to these questions were mixed. While some experts who believed that criminality was not inherited would deem a child with that history adoptable, others could not recommend a child with a history of family delinquency if it was judged "fundamental" to the family's character.[144] Respondents replied even more harshly to instances of incest, stating that they would look out for "serious character pathology" if the child resulted from an incestuous union. But other experts offered more complicated answers, noting that it depended on which family members engaged in incest.[145] In an incestuous relationship, both "sides" of the family were the same and therefore mental health experts raised concerns about a child having a twofold risk of exaggerated negative characteristics, especially for psychosis and feeblemindedness.[146] Experts also disqualified children with family histories of conditions considered particularly problematic, like hereditary degenerative diseases of the nervous system, congenital blindness and deafness, Huntington's chorea, and epilepsy.

No matter the particular impairments, adoption workers listened to experts' overwhelming opinion that children with disabilities should be excluded. Yet they also encountered competing priorities that they tried to fulfill. Casework took a long time for agencies to do, creating long waiting periods for adoptive parent applicants to attain a child. Though applicants appreciated how careful reputable agencies were, the wait frustrated many. This practical reality prompted some physicians, applicants, and even the press to contend in the late 1930s that agencies should be a bit less cautious, so as to make adoptive placements "with more dispatch."[147] The casework process also frustrated biological mothers. Unmarried mothers complained, for instance, that the adoption agency asked too many intrusive questions about themselves and their relatives. The time casework took also made it difficult for biological mothers to settle on adoption plans, because they often had to wait "a year or two to find out whether the baby is going to be a blonde or a brunette."[148]

Lengthy casework, first mandated with the Minnesota Children's Code of 1917, also extended to prospective adoptive parents, including visitations by a social worker to the prospective home to assess suitability.[149] Measures of the home's suitability changed from emphasizing parent applicants' education, class, and religious qualities in the first part of the twentieth century to highlighting the potential emotional stability in the home in the interwar period. Furthermore, psychology's focus on the individual, starting in the 1920s, shaped agencies' queries into the emotional makeup of the applicants, the couple's relationship, and their motivations for adoption.[150] Evidence of disability would exclude adoptive parent applicants just like it did for a child. Adoption professionals regarded potential foster parents with disabilities as unable to "insure the child of proper physical care, wise training and a reasonable degree of economic security," and as such they were ineligible to build a family of their own.[151]

Measuring Risk through Cognitive Assessment

Psychologists hired to test a child for adoption used IQ tests to assess a child's cognitive capacity in adoption. Like their counterparts in other areas of applied psychology, psychologists' repeated reliance upon this instrument ended up naturalizing the notion of intelligence and enforcing normality to make life-changing decisions based upon it. Although IQ tests could be used to verify that a child was normal, agencies also used them to avoid having children pass as normal in cases when they were not. In a context where feeblemindedness, particularly the moron, posed a threat for the adoption endeavor, practitioners saw IQ tests as a particularly powerful tool.

Experts believed in the ability of IQ tests to determine a child's developmental potential and future, and to manage prospective parents' expectations. They were particularly necessary to "forestall serious errors of selection in over-sanguine foster parents who may have their hearts set on putting their child through high school or through college."[152] Arnold Gesell noted that it was a mistake to believe a good home could determine the "caliber" of the child, even though he acknowledged that heredity and environment interacted.[153] According to Gesell, IQ and developmental tests, aided by infant observation, had the power to "confirm normality when it is obvious or taken for granted" or to discover "subnormality" when it is less obvious because of the "general ambiguousness of infancy." The tests could even uncover "normal or even superior endowment" in cases when social workers did not suspect it because of a child's poor family background.[154] In other words, IQ tests could confirm biases but also counter them. He believed that clinical tests offered adoption workers some solid scientific guidance for placement decisions, even though he also recognized that no one could entirely predict a child's future.

A 1928 mental exam administered by the Bureau of Child Welfare in Connecticut, for instance, required the social worker to answer questions about and record the child's intelligence and educational outlook: Was the child superior or inferior? Normal or dull normal? Feebleminded (high-, middle-, or low-grade)? Could the child complete grammar school, high school, or college? Or was she more likely to undertake vocational training?[155] Fifteen years later, that same state legally required all agencies to perform preadoption medical and psychological screening.[156] For its part, the Children's Aid Society, the pioneer in efforts to intensify the role of the psychologist in adoption in the 1940s, had the psychologist see the infant at one month of age, and thereafter monthly if there were developmental issues. If no issues were detected, the psychological service would continue every two or three months until retesting was deemed no longer needed.

To assess a child's intelligence quotient, adoption agencies used the Binet-Simon test, the Kuhlmann-Binet test, or the Stanford-Binet test. The intelligence quotient measured as mental age divided by chronological age multiplied by one hundred, enabled adoption workers, psychologists, pediatricians, and schoolteachers to discern what they deemed was a child's innate intelligence so they could either exclude her or place her in a matched "suitable" home with adoptive parents who had a similar intellectual profile.[157] The Stanford-Binet test, for example, determined mental age using its scale by dividing large numbers of normal (white) children into age groups "in such a way as *to bring it about* that the *average* child of eight years will earn by the scale [of the test] a 'mental age' of eight years."[158] Despite such determinism, the tests purportedly provided "evidence" of (ab)normal child development and measured the extent of disability risk for adoptive placement.

Testing was a tool to manage disability risks that many experts expected from the progeny of poor, unmarried mothers; it was a mechanism to make legible those problematic embodiments. Such practices enabled Mrs. Willsie, an adoptive parent applicant, to reassure her husband that agencies worked to minimize disability risk. She wrote that agencies using scientific forms of adoption had "reduced the gambling element to about fifty-fifty with the own-child hazard. You ordinarily know far less about the eugenic history of your husband's family than you do about the ancestry of the child you have adopted under proper conditions!"[159] Similarly, Agnes K. Hanna of the Children's Bureau warned listeners in two radio talks in 1935 not to adopt a child unless "careful tests" could assure "his mental abilities." Hanna claimed that IQ tests, even for children under one year of age, could ensure against such disability.[160]

Adoption professionals took this responsibility very seriously. Within the context of unregulated adoption brokers, IQ tests allowed agencies to detect an invisible disability like intellectual disability *prior* to placing a child in a permanent home. In an article published in the *Journal of the American Medical Association*, R. L. Jenkins of the Institute for Juvenile Research in Chicago tried to acquaint physicians with "good adoption practice" and implore them to cooperate with child-placing agencies.[161] He believed that to ascertain fitness and adoptability, a child needed two IQ examination sessions, one before and the other one year after placement. If a child was younger than four years of age, Jenkins suggested that the child take two tests at each examination session.[162] Jenkins recommended "reasonably cautious" parameters for eligibility, with an acceptable IQ as a main factor. His eligibility requirements depended not only upon intelligence but also upon age, likely because of psychologists' beliefs that the older the child, the more stable, representative, and predictive her IQ would be. When intelligence was stable, social workers could better assess fit for a certain adoptive home.

Thus, for Jenkins, eligibility scores should decrease with age. For children at age one year and beyond, for example, a child could be eligible for adoption if she received a score denoting "superior intelligence." For children aged eighteen months or older, a test score of 110 or above qualified the child for adoption. While an IQ score of 100 or above was "adequate for adoption" for children two years old and older, at three years of age and older a child could qualify with a score of 90 or above. With children four years and older, "indication of intelligence falling at or above the middle of the grouping 'dull and backward' (intelligence 85 or above)" made a child adoptable.[163] Finally, for children ages five or older, a child had to be above "borderline defective" for Jenkins to consider her eligible for adoption.[164]

According to the physician, children with IQs of 70–80 were considered suitable for adoption only when certain circumstances were "favorable to the adjustment of such children."[165] Jenkins's one caveat to this schedule was that where there was an attachment already formed between the foster parents and the child, the child could be adopted against expert advice in cases where the child might not test sufficiently. Though uncommon, there were cases where foster parents contested social worker's concerns about "less than perfect" children. In 1934, for instance, eager to finalize the adoption of a girl named Catherine whose mental tests proved ambiguous, the foster father stated, "Even if she is a moron we want to keep her."[166]

Catherine's foster father was an exception. Agencies who used IQ testing sold their service as safe for prospective parents; they claimed they were providing a guaranteed fit child to secure the adoptive family's integrity and sustainability.[167] Women's magazines like the *Woman* reinforced claims of agencies' absolute reliability. In a mid-1940s article, for example, the author claimed that no child placed through an adoption agency could be feebleminded.[168] Of course, this promise's power rested on available cultural images of disabled children during this time as burdensome and pitiful, perpetually suffering by virtue of their disabilities. The American public considered families with disabled children victims, with disability posing an intractable barrier to their own normality.[169]

As shifts in understanding intelligence and feeblemindedness occurred, psychologists and geneticists began to question the limits of the IQ test. Studies of IQ, adopted children, and adoption outcomes increasingly showed that the home environment played a more significant role in child development and intelligence than previously acknowledged. With these discoveries, adoption professionals changed their position to duly consider the adoptive home they were building over discrete, assumedly objective and predictive demographic profiles.[170] "All of these studies are reassuring to families who are interested in adopting children," stated Frances Lockridge and Sophie van Senden Theis of the New York State Charities Aid Association. "They seem to prove the fundamental soundness of human nature and its capacity to blossom when given the right soil in which to grow."[171]

By 1940, psychologists recognized that although the IQ test was the only tool they had to estimate a child's intelligence, knowledge of the mental capacity of a very young child could in fact be unattainable. Adoption leaders therefore began to warn parents that they should not try to rely on definitive developmental predictions because each child matured at her own pace. "Beware the danger of accepting IQ tests as in the least final," warned a manual for adopters. "Do not be discouraged if your child is reported slightly under the average rating, or smugly content if he is reported normal, or too proud if he is reported superior."[172]

Reexamining the IQ test was closely related to a scientific paradigm shift: strict hereditarianism in psychology had given way to the idea that heredity influenced, but did not necessarily determine, behavior.[173] Consistent with this trend, Thompson tried to reduce public fears about hereditary transmission by writing, "The heredity of these children is no better or worse in the sum of its chromosomes than the heredity of the rest of us."[174] With such rethinking, coupled with a continued lack of definitive scientific knowledge about the hereditary etiology of certain conditions, some adoption professionals suggested softening exclusionary standards so that, although children with problematic birth family histories should still give social workers pause, they should not necessarily be considered "absolute contraindications to adoption."[175] Others took the middle ground, arguing that normal children could be shaped by positive environmental factors but genetics wholly determined the (static) futures of "defective" children.[176] Fundamentally, however, this transformation offered the implicit message that things could change; disability is fluid, able-bodiedness provisional, and adoption eligibility changeable. This outlook grew louder and more frequent in the postwar era.

Measuring Risk through Physical Observation

Prolonged medical observation was another part of the child study. A long observation period was justified not only in terms of allowing the birth mother to definitively make up her mind about relinquishment but also of thoroughly evaluating the child's health. But it often delayed adoptive placement, from four months to two years.[177] Most agencies kept a new-born for six months to a year to have physicians and psychiatrists observe and perform additional tests to assess a child's disability risk; that is, any (ab)normal or inadequate development. Doctors engaged in adoption ef-forts gave the children vaccinations and performed routine examinations each month for those under one year. They looked for signs of apathy or a lack of vision or hearing acuity to assess if the child was mentally normal.[178]

Despite parental pressures to shorten the time of observation, prolonged medical detection provided agencies with the assurance they needed to en-sure a healthy child to parent applicants. Gesell remarked, for instance, that "the improving standards of child placement work throughout the country are placing more and more demands upon psychological and developmen-tal predictions."[179] Gesell noted that prediction was important for adoption but that there were also difficulties inherent in the task, especially when adoptive parents sought very specific qualities in their potential child, like college educability. He conceded in 1928 that "the intelligent foster parent is entitled to at least reasonable assurance as to the health and develop-mental potentialities of the infant," but then asked, "Can we supply this assurance? We can at least reduce the risk."[180]

Long observation also gave agencies the necessary medical information they needed to redirect a disabled child to an institution or other setting since to most, "a child with noticeable defects would never be offered for adoption."[181] One piece in the *Minnesota Children's Home Finder* (1947) captured the consequences of these views and the trajectory such deci-sions commonly produced during this period. It stated: "These are the children with deformed hands or feet, hair lips, allergies, heart defects, or whose hereditary backgrounds make them 'unsuitable' for adoption."[182] Because the children have disabilities, the piece went on, they are "con-demned to go through childhood" with the additional challenge of "be-ing shunted from one boarding home to another," often ending up in an institution and "denied the right to a home and parents of their own."[183]

Although agencies contracted with physicians to perform these evalu-ations, doctors did not always wholeheartedly agree with the extent of the agencies' assessments. One 1938 CWLA study on adoption in New York

Form Ca—(1937 revision)   **CHILD'S MEDICAL RECORD**   Number_____
Face Sheet

Name _____   Sex ____   Date of Birth _____   Nationality or Race of: { Father_____ Mother_____ }

Family History:

Mention any physical or mental defects (especially insanity, feeblemindedness, epilepsy, tuberculosis, rheumatism, chorea, heart disease, syphilis, gonorrhea, alcoholism) in the family or relatives or in others who have lived or are living in contact with the child

	Living	If dead, cause of death
Father		
Mother		
No. of Children		

Child's Developmental History and Habits: Birth: Term_____Wt._____Condition_____Delivery_____

Infant Feeding: Breast_____Weaned at_____Formula (State what, if patient is an infant and still taking)_____

Began Orange Juice at_____Cod Liver Oil at_____Cereal at_____Vegetables at_____Plain milk at_____

Development: First tooth at_____mos. Sat alone at_____mos. Walked alone at_____mos. Talked at_____mos.

Growth regular?_____Loss of Weight at any time?_____

Habits: Sleep adequate?_____Regular?_____Meals adequate?_____Regular?_____

Bowel movement regular?_____Constipated?_____Urination normal?_____Enuresis?_____nocturnal?_____diurnal?_____

Nervous habits: Nail biting?_____Tic?_____Masturbation?_____Other?_____

Behavior: Any special problem?_____

Health:

Diseases:	Years of Age																Exposed (date)	By Whom Exposed
	1	2	3	4	5	6	7	8	9	10	11	12	13	14	15	16		
Chickenpox																		
Diphtheria																		
Discharging Ears																		
Frequent Colds																		
German Measles																		
Influenza																		
Measles																		
Mumps																		
Pneumonia																		
Rheumatism																		
Scarlet Fever																		
Smallpox																		
Tonsillitis																		
Whooping Cough																		

Accidents, Injuries, Operations or Illnesses other than above	Nature	Age	Result	Nature	Age	Result
Circumcision						
Tonsillectomy						

Tests and Inoculations:	Date	Result	Date	Result	Tests and Inoculations:	Date	Result	Date	Result
Audiometer Test					Toxoid (diphtheria)				
B M R Examination					Tuberculin Test				
Blood Smear					Typhoid Fever Vaccine				
Blood Wassermann					Vaccination (smallpox)				
Dick Test					Vaginal Smear				
Scarlet Fever Vaccine					Vision Tests				
Schick Test					Whooping Cough Vaccine				
Stool Examination					X-ray of Chest				

Subsequent Tests with Dates:_____

Mental Tests:	Date of Exam.	School Grade At Time of Exam.	Name of Test (Specify whether Group or Individual)	Chronological Age	Test Result	Name and Title of Examiner (Psychologist or Teacher?)

Issued by Child Welfare League of America   Printed in U. S. A.   (Over)

FIGURE 3. Child's Medical Record—Face Sheet. Form C: 1937 revision. CWLA Collection, Box 39, Folder 39-3, Publications 1927–1954, Social Welfare History Archives.

City, for instance, found that many of the doctors they interviewed did not understand the rationale of a lengthy observation period; they claimed that the process delayed placement and prevented adoptive families from receiving small infants. They believed that a physical exam and family history should suffice to determine adoptability. Yet the CWLA stood firm in their recommendation. The organization explained that these physicians just did not understand the importance of following children to detect abnormalities; the CWLA believed that physicians who were educated about the advantages of this approach would change their minds.[184] Still, with shifts in the perceived value of IQ testing and the parental pressure to shorten observation, some adoption professionals in the 1940s proposed placing children earlier to facilitate bonding with adoptive parents more quickly, lessen the time applicants had to wait, and relieve foster parents from the state's purview.[185]

Restoring Normality

Some adoption professionals understood that their work was constrained by the pool of children available to them. On the one hand, this heightened "eugenic anxieties about the quality of available children," but on the other, these practitioners had to relax their idea of the ideal child with what they faced in reality in order to avoid being intolerant of *all* "imperfections."[186]

Adoption and child welfare professionals, like child reformer W. H. Slingerland, suggested that children who had a correctable or curable minor illness could, in theory, be eligible for adoption. Physically "defective" children, according to Slingerland, could be divided into two groups: the diseased (those with acquired or constitutional serious ailments; e.g., anemia, malnutrition, tuberculosis, syphilis), and the physical defectives (those who had deformities or sensory or mobility impairments; e.g., club feet, blindness, deafness, scoliosis, loss or weakness of limb).[187] Slingerland recognized the invisible/visible divide among defectives, acknowledging that some "diseased" children could look "normal in body, and many are healthy although bodily abnormal."[188] Where treatment was available, he believed that diseased children could recover and "become normal." But those who were "crippled, deformed" or diseased and incurable should be sent to institutions.[189] Similarly, he argued that "mental defectives" possessed a spectrum of capacity. He contended that efforts should be expended for a "merely backward" person to restore her to normality, but a "constitutionally backward" person should be placed in an institution.

Still another set of children suffered from neglect or abandonment and often exhibited "minor imperfections" like decayed teeth, low height and weight, rickets, or adenoids and were not considered defective; they too could, and should, according to Slingerland, regain normality through speedy treatment. Such imperfections were not altogether uncommon. School exam findings in 1918 during the national Children's Year campaign, for example, showed that 50 to 67 percent of the general American child population exhibited an array of uncorrected physical ailments.[190] By 1940, 10,000 school age children required eyeglasses and 1 percent had strabismus, which required treatment.[191] Given these high rates, the school hygiene movement and school medical exams tried to address these illnesses and restore health and normality to children so that they could learn. Similarly, adoption experts wanted to observe adoptive candidates for a period of six months to a year so that doctors could perform any necessary minor medical fixes that would restore the child to what they considered was a state of normality. Once a child was "fixed," the life of a normal family could proceed; that is, a safe, secure place where the child was accepted and loved and could grow.[192]

Restoring children's state of health to normality gave adoptive opportunities to children whom applicant parents might otherwise initially reject. Here, the imperative to restore normality resembles what Anne Waldschmidt describes as "flexible normalism," where the conceptual boundary that separates the normal and abnormal can be redrawn to become less rigid.[193] Waldschmidt warns, however, that flexible normalism can invite a backlash where there is resistance and insistence to return to narrow and fixed ideas of the normal; to regain, as Davis contends, the "hegemony of normalcy."[194] With adoption professionals' insistence that children *had to become* normal to be adopted, they highlighted this goal's centrality in forming adoptive families. In essence, restoring normality ended up reifying the normal, lifting the idea of normality to a compulsory status.[195]

Restoring normality was not limited to agency adoption; it also existed for unregulated placements. An adult adoptee whose adoptive mother had engaged an independent adoption broker, for instance, cited the pressure on brokers to balance adoptive applicants' demands for normality with the availability of children. She told of a young couple who made an appeal for a baby girl who had blue eyes and curly hair. Understanding the impatience of the couple, the independent broker offered Rosalie, a "sound, healthy, and intelligent, but still definitely underweight, scrawny, hairless, and toothless" child; she was, admittedly, "as far as the poles from one's dream of one's own baby." The couple took one look at Rosalie and, in shock, left quickly, saying that Rosalie "wouldn't do." They wanted to wait instead for a baby who fulfilled their personal requirements. With time, Rosalie fattened up and developed a fun personality, so the broker invited the couple back. She promised them she had the perfect baby and showed them Rosalie again, all dressed up and rosy. Rosalie was now the "perfect picture of beautiful, healthy, happy babyhood." The couple immediately embraced her, without knowing that this was the same baby they had rejected before.[196]

Even when they acknowledged that not all children would be perfect from the start, some professionals who wrote about the issue agreed that agencies had to confirm that children were in superb condition before being permanently placed in adoptive homes. If they weren't, as one adoption expert explained, exceptions could be made, but agencies would have to tell adopting parents about the condition and the parents should promise that they would do everything necessary to "remove the condition."[197] The CWLA advised that a physician reexamine the child at the end of the probationary period (before finalization) to make sure that all defects had been corrected and normality had been achieved.

Other adoption practitioners believed that rendering a child normal before proclaiming her eligible made her desirable for a family and thus able to function within it. The superintendent of the Children's Home Society of Minnesota wrote in 1920 that because mental states could be caused by "malnutrition, over-wrought nervous system, or even eye strain, adenoids and a dozen other things," child-placing societies had to be extra careful to require physical and mental examinations of all children to determine eligibility. They had to put these children in "*100 percent condition* before sending them into family homes for adoption."[198] Normality was the key that opened the door to a permanent family.

Correctable impairments could justify exceptions to exclusion, but there were other reasons as well. For example, if an agency found that there weren't enough public funds to support a child with a pathological family history in foster or institutional care, they could consider her for permanent placement because it was the only solution.[199] Or, according to Gesell, if applicants insisted on adopting a child diagnosed as "mentally defective or hereditarily handicapped," then agencies could let them adopt that child as long as they were clear-eyed about the "risks" that disability posed to adoption's success and as long as they forbade their child from marrying or procreating so that defective traits would not be transmitted. As with correctable impairments, the agency in this case would have to disclose all medical information.

In 1932, the CWLA made Gesell's condition into policy, thereby sanctioning the issue of parental risk-taking rather than just focusing on the presence of disability risk inherent to the child.[200] Most agencies remained cautious about this exception, however. For their part, parent applicants had a variety of responses to accepting children with problematic heredities who had nowhere else to go. While some only cared about a child's personality, others wanted to know information about family history but were open to seeing how a child developed during the probationary period. One woman's agency, according to van Senden Theis, warned her about a child's problematic heredity. Although she took a more relaxed attitude about the child's label of disability than other parents, she espoused a religious notion of disability as punishment. It was within the purview of God to cure. She said: "Oh, well, I'll have him baptized and then I guess he'll be alright." By contrast, another applicant reviewed every detail of the entire family history, including mother, grandparents, aunts, and uncles to discern if this was a risk she would take.

Though not the norm, these responses reflect a set of competing epistemologies of disability that coexisted within the period's much broader medicalized views. Within this range of responses, adoptive applicants who decided to "take the risk of trying" a child with a pathological family history still hoped, perhaps unsurprisingly, that a child's normality would remain.[201] Despite this spectrum of prospective parents' views, and despite some movement toward flexibility, most adoption professionals took the position that normality *had* to be restored; they agreed that children who had conditions that could never be restored to normality embodied too much disability risk to achieve a successful placement. Their assumptions that the adoptions of children labeled disabled would end in "failure" also tended to persist throughout this period. Adoption workers largely assumed that those needs had to remain within normative parameters of American family life.[202]

Given the cultural power of the innocent child and of childhood as a projection of parents' ambitions or insecurities—what Henry Jenkins calls the "semiotically adhesive child"—the assumption that disabled children were inadequate to fulfill the goal of mutual satisfaction between adoptive parents and child may not have been altogether wrong.[203] At a 1941 New York State conference, Lucie K. Browning, supervisor of the foster home care department of the New York Children's Aid Society, noted that among twenty-four children who were considered problem children in her work, the inability of the adopting parents to accept the child "fully and wholly for himself" was one of the main reasons that placements did not work out. The adopted child in these cases was "destructively entangled" with parental anxieties about tainted heredity; that is, with parents assessing any peculiarity coming from a child's family background in deterministic ways. Although Lee and Evelyn Brooks disagreed with Browning's eugenic views, by the late 1930s both the Brookses and Browning warned parents to keep their fears in check; *their* perfect child might "be a misfit in most homes!"[204] This attitude shift marked a move away from a child as risky to consideration of the parents' and social workers' culpability in formulating and upholding normality, risk, and success in ways that blocked children with disabilities from growing up in adoptive families.[205]

Unfastening Links with Changing Adoption Patterns

Exclusionary agency policies for children labeled disabled remained prevalent for a third of the century. Standards of adoptability did not go entirely unchallenged, however. Later in this period, some social workers in New York criticized agencies for using inflexible criteria. They complained that some agencies would only accept desirable babies for superior homes and challenged an agency's right to be so selective about their inclusionary and exclusionary standards.[206] But the balance around selectivity was also not entirely up to agencies. Even if social workers had agreed to place disabled children more regularly, the children's chances of being adopted were slim. Within a cultural context where babies functioned as investments in the family and the nation, many prospective adoptive parents cared about a baby's appearance so much that they even rejected children with what social workers considered minor imperfections.[207] Instead, prospective parents imagined the ideal adoption as "happy-go-lucky and care-free, the family was a unit and did everything and went everywhere together."[208] Still, this image of a cultivable all-American family also faced the limits of reality because adoption workers fundamentally recognized that (normal) children needed families. Agencies, therefore, tried to manage the delicate balance between adopters' demands and children's needs so that they could deliver what they considered an optimal outcome for both.

Cracks in the project to create ideal families began to surface by 1938. Experts acknowledged that there were limits to agency attempts to manufacture an adoption's success. Despite agencies' efforts to formulate ideal families and to respond to the pressures and fears of adopters and the community, Ora Pendleton, executive secretary of the Children's Bureau of Philadelphia, warned that "responsible adoption agencies cannot create children for parents wanting them, any more than it can create exactly the parents it might desire for a child. The limit for the agency is set by the fact that it must work with real, human people, not with ideally created puppets."[209] Six years later, Constance Rathbun of the Boston Children's Aid Society went even further, arguing that adoptive parent applicants who sought perfection were likely to be obsessive and unrealistic. In contrast to social workers' earlier attempts to appease adopters because of a particular vision of adoption's main purpose, Rathbun warned social workers to be suspicious, rather than welcoming, of these types of applicants.[210] Here Rathbun and Pendleton implicitly argued that the normal did not mean the ideal. The promise of perfection and normality was starting to fray.

In part, this trend followed the erosion of eugenics' stature as this period progressed. Adoption professionals, for instance, begin to question the original hereditarian and racist underpinnings of feeblemindedness. Geneticists and psychiatrists alike began to acknowledge that the categories of feeblemindedness were arbitrary and had no scientific basis; intelligence was not a fixed entity but rather ran along a spectrum of mental development. They came to understand that feeblemindedness was a concept with both internal heterogeneity and inherent instability. As disability philosopher Licia Carlson has observed, the concept of feeblemindedness encompassed a vast array of causes, severity, and links to different types of moral character and therefore lacked clarity about its locus of impairment.[211]

With these shifts, adoption professionals reexamined their ideas about feeblemindedness, widening their outlook to consider environmental influences on the etiology of social pathology and family relations. Americans' views also transformed. They now demarcated between "good" sterilized feebleminded persons who could engage in normal life in communities, and "bad" individuals who needed to remain in institutions.[212] By recognizing the influence of environmental factors, experts within and outside of adoption reconsidered how families functioned and endured.

The decrease in suspicions about illegitimacy shifted adoption trends as broader socioeconomic conditions transformed. Patterns changed such that by World War II many birth mothers relinquished their children at much earlier ages, and adoptive parents' preferences shifted.[213] The war itself caused other changes in the social and economic fabric of the country, including a foster care crisis, a housing shortage, a rise in the number of mothers with young children, a more mobile population, and generally more pressures upon families.[214] Women widely secured jobs in the war economy, giving unmarried women more financial stability to keep their children if they wanted. But the lack of guaranteed childcare support complicated this choice.[215] From 1943 to 1944, the United States also saw its first large increase in out-of-wedlock births, about seventy thousand children born annually, partly because many Americans postponed marriage in the midst of war. The class profile of birth mothers who decided to keep or relinquish a child also changed: more white middle-class women became pregnant and sought permanent adoptive placement to counter the cultural shame of out-of-wedlock births, like working-class women had done before. Married women who had had extramarital affairs while their husbands were serving in the war also had children out of wedlock. Some of these women sought adoption to save their marriages.

The patterns of adopters also transformed. With the diminished social stigma of adoption and the greater acceptability of this form of family, more families sought children to adopt, which changed the balance between infants available and parent applicants.[216] A larger percentage of adopters were increasingly older as well (thirty-five years old on average), and so they felt a stronger urgency to bring a child into their homes to pursue the normative life course of white middle-class citizens. Whereas before the war adoptive parents were open to adopting older children because their health and survival could be measured and because they feared caring for an infant, in the aftermath of the Great Depression and during World War II, adopters clearly favored infants. The low birth rate during the Depression and new economic growth with wartime drove this shift.[217]

Influenced by these demographic changes, developing psychoanalytic ideas, and shifts in the hereditarian/environmental debate about IQ, social workers in these later years came to reinterpret the causes of illegitimacy, recasting it as a function of women's supposed neuroses and immaturity rather than inherent defectiveness or sexual delinquency.[218] Furthermore, social workers now recognized that not all children with unknown or poor backgrounds turned out badly. As a result, instead of privileging family preservation, they actively encouraged these women to give up their children for adoption, address their neurotic behaviors, and move on to lead a normal life.[219]

The Consequences for Normality

In the first decades of the twentieth century, adoption professionals configured disability as a major risk to adoption and as a threat to the integrity of
the adoptive family. They envisioned the child as embodying risk rather than
seeing risk as emerging out of agencies' or parents' biases against imperfection. These beliefs justified their decision to deem disabled children undesirable for adoptive homes. They assumed that the adoptive family was already
vulnerable to unknown pressures, risks, and eventualities—it was complex
enough to build a normal adoptive family, let alone to place different kinds
of children who would challenge the notion that members of families looked
alike; that is, those who possessed similar levels of intelligence and exhibited
congruent forms of behavior. For some, the way to rectify this risk was to
restore the child to normality through surgical or medical means. But for
others, there was no way to resolve disability risk outside of exclusionary
practices and/or removing the "defective delinquent" to an institution.[220]

By engaging with these discourses and practices, social workers routinely determined that disabled children were not desirable for adoption,
a decision that ultimately affected these children's access to adoptive families for many years to come. In the end, adoption in the age of eugenics
and child welfare was a family-making project of "normativity and exclusion" that consequently produced "hierarchies about [the] worth and
worthiness" of children.[221] Circularly, restricting disabled children's access
into the candidacy pool also helped establish what counted as fitness for
belonging in an adoptive family.[222] Exclusion left only able-bodied children in the pool of eligible candidates, thus establishing normality as the
rule in adoption practice. Essentially, fitness and exclusion reinforced one
another to make disabled children unsuitable for adoption.

Although the concepts of normality, abnormality, difference, and defectiveness persisted throughout this period to shape adoption practices,
they were not altogether static ideas. In fact, over this period, their fluidity
became more evident. (Ab)normality was, in fact, dependent upon expert
opinions, shifts in the demographics of adoption, understanding of the
nature of intelligence, and a recognition of the limits of adoptive practice.
Furthermore, there were consequences to expecting and upholding normality in adoption. Professional adoption agencies' and prospective parents' expectations of normality drove the rationale for exclusion, which in
turn significantly affected the contours of these children's futures.

As became increasingly evident, expecting normality was not something that could be sustained for the long term, either for agencies or for parents. Both started to realize that they could not guarantee a perfect child. As more adoptive parents wanted children to adopt, they had to let go of unbending expectations for a certain type of child so that agencies could fulfill the sheer need.

As we will see in the next chapter, amid challenges to the IQ test and to a strict hereditarian understanding of intelligence, agencies slowly began to acknowledge that difference in adoptive families did not necessarily lead to dissatisfaction or a broken placement. Without relinquishing their comparison to the biological family, adoption professionals instead argued that prospective adoptive parents had to take the same risks of disability that biological parents did when embracing a child as their own.

CHAPTER TWO

Risk Equivalence and the Postwar Family

In 1947, Belle Wolkomir, supervisor of the intake department of the Jewish Child Care Association of New York (JCCA), published what became an extremely influential article in the field of adoption. The piece, titled "The Unadoptable Baby Achieves Adoption," challenged the idea that some children should be excluded from adoption.[1] Wolkomir asked: what happens to those babies rejected by adoption agencies because of hereditary and developmental risks? How can *they* best be served? Can they ever be adopted? She called for adoption professionals to adjust their policies for children with "pathological heredity," to rethink their anxieties about hereditary transmission, and to consider these children eligible for adoption. She reassured adoption professionals that placing these children in adoptive homes could be successful.

In a radical move for the time, Wolkomir argued that adoptability (child eligibility) was not a static, narrow, or natural concept but rather a malleable state. She proposed that adoptability depended upon the home environment and the adaptability of adoptive parents. It also depended upon the social worker's assessment of the child, which was usually done after birth but before adoptive placement. As we learned in chapter 1, such casework involved having the agency investigate the birth parents, study and evaluate the child, assess the adoptive parents, and observe the new family for a year until the adoption was legally finalized.[2]

At least, this was how the process worked for "adoptable" children. Children with pathological heredity had their fate decided by their birth parents' history (another synonymous term social workers used was *pathological family backgrounds*). Which conditions included within the category

of children with pathological heredity varied, but could include birth families with syphilis, gonorrhea, tuberculosis, epilepsy, drug addiction, alcoholism, psychosis, feeblemindedness, emotional instability, and "dull normal mentality."[3] Wolkomir noted that many of these babies became black
or gray market babies, meaning they were adopted through baby selling
or independent means, or were placed in boarding care, rather than entering the formal adoption system.

Wolkomir based her ideas about adoptability upon a limited, experimental adoption program carried out by the JCCA. From 1938 through
1947, the JCCA placed over one hundred "unwanted children whose heredity showed considerable pathology" in foster homes. The study found
that they made stellar social and physical developmental progress.[4] A
problematic hereditary profile did not make these children unadoptable,
their environment did. Once social workers found homes that could be
adapted to their needs, the children became adoptable.[5]

Wolkomir's move to reconceptualize child eligibility impacted not only
adoption policy but also how adoption professionals formulated risk in
the decade to come. Yet even Wolkomir thought some children posed
risks "too great" for *immediate* adoption. Reasons to delay placement in
her view could include a possible physical disability, a birth mother with
a history of syphilis, or the vague precept that a child had "heredity or
development [that] made it inadvisable to consider an immediate adoptive placement."[6] Postponing the determination process gave agencies the
time to further evaluate the child.

Although Wolkomir acknowledged that the JCCA program involved
risks, she noted that the risk of abnormal child development was one that
"every parent faces."[7] She implied that a child did not always embody a
birth parent's impairment and that impairments did not always appear at
birth. In essence, she reconceptualized risk from a notion that only affected prospective adoptive parents to one where biological parents could
be impacted too. In this way, she upended the idea of health status as a
predictable fixed entity.[8]

After the war, adoption professionals joined Wolkomir to embrace what
I call *risk equivalence*, the social work idea that adoptive parents needed
to take the same risks of disability in their potential child as biological
parents. Risk equivalence capitalized on the central adoption principle
of estimating an ideal (and idealized) biological family. By using risk
equivalence to widen parent applicants' notion of a desirable child, adoption workers continued to make the biological family a main referent in

discussions about risk, disability, and adoptability. Even if adopters and the child did not physically or intellectually resemble one another, prospective adoptive parents could mimic biological parents' orientation to the risk of disability.[9] For their part, agencies used risk equivalence as a rhetorical tool when they asked applicant families to adjust their expectations and consider new sets of children who were increasingly made available for placement after the war.

Risk Equivalence and Expanded Adoptability

Before agencies embraced a discourse of risk equivalence, they first redefined the purpose of adoption and broadened the definition of adoptability. At the first CWLA workshop on adoption (May 19–21, 1948), eighty attendees of member agencies from twenty-one states and Canada posited adoption's purpose as finding a home for *every* child who could benefit from "normal family life."[10] Most significantly, the attendees reconceptualized child eligibility and successful placement to include any child *"as long as a family could be found that could accept her with her capabilities and background"* (my italics).[11] They believed, in theory at least, that adopters had the right to any information necessary to raise a particular child.[12] Reflecting broad currents in psychology that challenged strict hereditarianism and the etiology of mental retardation, and with some evidentiary success in these children's placement, most attendees believed that children should not be penalized for their hereditary profile; they should, rather, be afforded the chance to develop in the best possible environment for them. Further, they acknowledged the need for experts to figure out how to weigh any "pathological" factors in a child's background against observations about the child's development and the "ability of the prospective adoptive families to assume the risk involved in accepting such a child."[13]

Accordingly, the CWLA officially redefined adoptability to include "any child who needs a family and who can develop in it, and for whom a family can be found that can accept the child with its physical or mental capacities."[14] This represented a dramatic change from its previous definition of a "normal healthy baby without parental ties, legally available for adoption, who has had a stable family background."[15] The CWLA's reappraisal of family belonging marks a key transitional moment in disabled children's access to adoption.

Despite these changes, the "as long as" clause in the new definition of eligibility, perhaps unintentionally, still allowed social workers to exclude children they labeled disabled. This clause harnessed postwar notions of family love—where parents now believed that a child should be a source of pleasure to her parents—and thus made eligibility contingent upon normative notions of which children could benefit from family life and which could attain parental acceptance.[16] Social workers like Lucie Browning, supervisor of the department of foster home care of the Children's Aid Society in Buffalo, believed, for instance, that a child had to *give* pleasure to her parents while the parents had to satisfy her needs. This dynamic captured the varied expert efforts in the postwar period to articulate the importance of mother-child interactions and roles. These efforts differed somewhat from attachment theorists' conceptions, where a mother primarily gives and a child receives.[17] Instead, Browning conferred agency to the child; she constructed family love and living as a give and take, a mutual, consistently gratifying interaction between parent and child.[18] Not a passive precondition, then, the CWLA's new eligibility definition required that a child be able to *fulfill her role* to "benefit from family life."

Since social workers ultimately determined adoptability, the phrases "benefit from family life" and "who can develop in it [a family]" depended upon their biases, and their assessments of these terms could potentially leave out a wide range of children. For example, they could easily interpret the need to "benefit from family life" through the lens of long-standing cultural ideas of people with disabilities as incapable of contributing to or benefiting from family life. Since they saw these children as predominantly the *recipients* of family joy, rather than also its givers, social workers could often exclude these children from the outset.[19]

Adoption agencies, moreover, continued to distinguish between adoptability and placeability. Helen Hallinan, supervisor of the adoption department of the New York Catholic Home Bureau for Dependent Children, acknowledged in 1951 that:

> Our knowledge that a handicapped child can constructively use family life does not help this child if we are unable to find a family with sufficient love and longing for a child to make them want to build their future around him.[20]

Adoption psychiatrist Viola Bernard concurred, noting that a child's adoptability was lessened by "the degree and kind of physical, mental and emotional pathology he may present, as well as the amount and nature of pathology in his family background, and sometimes by the composition of his racial heredity." The child's placeability, however, was dependent upon many extrinsic factors, like "the desires, capacities and fears of adoptive parents and the home-finding zeal and skill of the agency."[21]

The transition from excluding children with pathological heredity to including them was slow. Many social workers at the beginning of this period continued to debate the new definition of adoptability's parameters and emphasized the importance of healthy children in families. They remained reluctant to place children with pathological family backgrounds because they believed these children were "handicapped" by "unhealthy backgrounds." They often denied them placement because they did not consider the children a "safe" risk for adoption.[22] Others were a bit more open. At the CWLA workshop on adoption (1948), for instance, attendees agreed in theory that a child's family background should not deter her from being placed. They concurred that the key in adoption was to find parents who would accept the child's risks. Yet nationally, a 1947 CWLA questionnaire showed that forty-two agencies (out of sixty-seven) felt that the biological parent(s) could not be "obviously retarded." These agencies maintained that birth parents needed to be in good physical, intellectual, and emotional health for the child to be considered adoptable. Thirty-two agencies out of the sixty-seven reported that they eliminated children whose parents had mental illness. Nineteen agencies reported that they had no criteria, but where doubt about a child's biological family existed, agencies embraced a longer probationary period before the adoption was legalized.[23] Only twelve of the sixty-seven agencies that responded stated that poor health or "defects of the child" should *not* exclude her from adoption.[24] More agencies agreed to include these children in the 1960s, but in the late 1940s and into the 1950s, the majority considered children with uncorrectable medical issues or congenital disease unadoptable.[25] By contrast, agencies fully considered children with no "hereditary hazards" and no complications at birth, and who were "physically normal at birth" for adoption. Some agencies even directly placed these children from the maternity home to an adoptive home after only two weeks.

Ideas of risk equivalence factored into social worker decisions about adoptability and placement. As Browning noted as early as 1944: "They [children] are offered . . . to adoptive parents if the doctor, psychologist, case worker and supervisor feel confident that these babies will present *no more* and perhaps *less risk* to the adoptive parents than they would be facing in the procreation of a child of their own [my italics]."[26] When a social worker felt that a child had more disability risk than an imagined biological child, she could exclude her. Irma Simonton Black, who performed research in child development at the Bureau of Education Experiments of New York City, gave an environmental rationale in 1947 for equating risks between biological and adoptive parents.[27] According to Black, risk equivalence was based on new scientific knowledge that showed that personality traits were not necessarily inherited but emerged from a child's life experience. A child's relationship with her parents, whether biological or adoptive, was as important as heredity. Thus, having a biological child was "as great a gamble" as adopting one. The caveat for Black was that the child had to be "healthy" and "normal" for the risk to be on par with a biological family. She assumed the latter to be without disability and assumed that a family could not have disabled members if they were to achieve belonging.

Other practical constraints complicated agencies' desire to implement new adoptability standards. Agencies often argued, for instance, that limited time and money left them only able to place children for whom they could more or less easily find a home; most agencies at this time did not actively seek a home for children who had "some special problem."[28] The provision "as long as a family could be found" allowed social workers to determine that a child for whom it was difficult to find a home, or for whom there was difficulty finding adopters who could accept the child as she was, was unadoptable. Forty-two of the sixty-seven agencies at the CWLA's May 1948 workshop stated, for instance, that when they decided a child was unadoptable, they required the biological parent to work with the agency toward another plan, including taking back the child.

Because the new definition of adoptability was ambiguous, the CWLA sponsored a special workshop in 1949 to flesh out its specifics for children with pathological heredity.[29] Agency representatives at the 1949 workshop made clear judgments about who fit within and outside of the new category of adoptable. They agreed: "all those, *but only those* [my italics], children who can benefit by family should be considered adoptable." Other children needed a more suitable form of permanent placement.[30] The attendees stressed that a disabled child was clearly unadoptable if she had a poor prognosis for life or if she could not "use family life—for example, the feeble-minded child, or the emotionally disturbed child who cannot bear close attachments."[31] These representatives constructed a hierarchy of disability wherein some children's futures were "ends without possibility."[32]

To specify the meaning and impact of adoptability, the CWLA asked the workshop participants to bring an actual case or home study to the meeting so that they could present it to their peers. Attendees could then consider the various issues they had to face when placing children with pathological backgrounds. Henrietta Gordon, for instance, focused on the prospective adoptive parents and *their* abilities, driving home the point that family environment was what ultimately mattered for a successful adoption. She presented the case of Mary, who after a stint in a loving foster home was placed in a supportive adoptive home that accepted her developmental issues. Despite the workshop's intended focus on children with pathological heredity, Gordon described Mary as a child diagnosed as "dull." Mary's case pointed to the few exceptions where children with diagnosed impairments could be adopted; here the agency considered children with "congenital abnormalities" adoptable.[33] Once the agency found a suitable home for Mary, Gordon remarked, the girl functioned "as a normal child" in the family unit. Mary's adoptive parents were suitable in this case because they accepted *her* as a child, rather than focused on her "dull" IQ. Their emphasis on Mary as a whole child enabled the three of them to develop into a "well-integrated" family.[34]

Unfortunately, Gordon's emphasis upon the family environment was largely lost on the workshop group. Attendees reverted to focusing on the individual child, stressing perhaps too literally that adoptability depended upon the *ability of children* who could benefit from family life, not the ability of parents to adapt. By contrast, Gordon introduced the idea that it was parental environment that enabled the child to benefit from family life. Gordon's point, like Wolkomir's, was that the child's ability was not static or predetermined but rather shaped and nurtured.

While certain health conditions in a child's birth family concerned attendees more than others, many attendees were also troubled by the stigma, bias, and prejudice in adoption that disabled children faced.[35] But because prejudice affected agencies' ability to find willing families, so too did it affect a child's ability to "benefit from family life." Perhaps paradoxically, even though attendees focused on impairments and their eligibility ramifications, they also recognized that disability stigma was a constitutive part of a child's unadoptable status. They debated how to get a fair medical prognosis and acknowledged that physicians' and psychiatrists' own biases about disability (optimistic, pessimistic, etc.) influenced their assessment of eligibility and so agreed to consider such input critically.[36] The pervasive prejudice against disability particularly threatened the eligibility of a child with certain conditions in their family background, including an unpredictable syndrome (dwarfism associated with feeblemindedness), a communicable disease (syphilis), a mental breakdown by the birth mother, a controllable hereditary disease (diabetes), and a hereditary and recently controlled disease (epilepsy).[37]

Workshop attendees tended not to acknowledge their own prejudice. Viola Bernard, chief psychiatric consultant of the Louise Wise Adoption Center, presented a case that showed how social worker prejudice impacted children. The case involved Jimmy, placed at age three and seven months after a stint in foster care. Social workers described Jimmy as having a "convergent squint" and an "open bite." Although one social worker noted that the open bite was cute, another felt that it took away from his appearance; each appraised Jimmy's "physical defects" in completely different ways. Bernard argued that even if their bias was implicit, when a social worker had a negative attitude about a child, it could "tip the scales for the clients" and could have clear implications for including disabled children in adoptive families.[38]

The CWLA continued to work out the criteria for adoptability in a series of workshops in the 1950s. Distinguishing various degrees of impairment became a way for social workers to limit the full expansion of adoptability during this time. In 1951, for example, workshop participants distinguished between "handicapped" children ineligible for adoption and those with "minor" impairments who were adoptable. This type of distinction was reminiscent of attempts to restore normality to children with common conditions before the war. Adoption workers' attention to severity here, though, created both a ranking of child eligibility and a more specific delineation of a child's health status. Indeed, that severity/correctability began to factor into adoptability assessments pointed to the beginning of what would a decade later become a fine-tuned risk-coding gradient whose purpose was to determine whether a child could "benefit from family life."[39] Classifying impairments by severity/correctability likely resulted from emerging medical treatments and technologies in the 1940s and '50s, like cardiac surgery that corrected some children's congenital heart problems or advances in audiology that led to treatment services like speech and auditory training. Some of these therapeutics enabled disabled children to survive. Furthermore, better knowledge about certain physical conditions (e.g., heart disease, diabetes, and cancer) could also mitigate an agency's judgment of how risky a child was to the success of her placement. But the inverse was also true: a dearth of medical knowledge about mental conditions and their effects upon a child's development, for instance, led agencies to think the worst about those children. The latter led to "fear and insecurity . . . real and imagined" about certain children.[40]

After much debate about child eligibility, by the mid-1950s it was common practice to place children with pathological family backgrounds. A 1954 survey reported that between 93 to 100 percent of respondent agencies did not automatically rule out adoption for a child with a family background that included neurological defects, "mental defectiveness," incest, epilepsy, heart disease, cancer, diabetes, venereal disease, a history of mental illness, or tuberculosis.[41] Indeed, by 1955 most agencies tended to display more openness and flexibility about their adoptability assessments, considering the child's total needs rather than concentrating on one aspect of her profile.[42]

These deliberations, and the decision to change official CWLA policy in the first place, underline the contingent nature of assessing eligibility. To be sure, shifts in practice sat alongside resistance to change during the 1950s. But compared to the previous decade, the CWLA's new position on adoptability prompted more agencies to loosen the power of the perfect child "guarantee."

The Changing Landscape of Postwar Adoption

Adoption professionals' willingness to enlarge the category of adoptable children and to invoke risk equivalence in the postwar period cannot be understood apart from the larger context of changing adoption demographics. After the war, Americans increasingly accepted adoption as a legitimate alternative form of family. Amid a sense of national prosperity and increased opportunity, domesticity reigned and a baby boom resulted. American society's emphasis on couples that reproduce and raise healthy and normal children filtered into adoption.[43] The pressure to reproduce and to have a family, and to strive for upward mobility, led infertile couples to seek adoption in numbers. By one measure, Americans' appetite for adoption had quadrupled from 1938 to 1948; it continued to grow through the 1950s.[44] Adoptions rose nationally from 50,000 in 1944 to 90,000 in 1953, and to 93,000 in 1958.[45] In 1956 about 90,000 children were eligible for adoption, but an overwhelming 800,000 couples applied to adopt.[46]

Social workers also saw adoption as the best solution to the problem of white out-of-wedlock pregnancy, which became a primary reason mothers relinquished their children for adoption during this time.[47] The picture for African American birth mothers, however, was different. Historian Regina Kunzel argues that whereas social workers constructed white out-of-wedlock pregnancy as a symptom of individual pathology, they understood Black out-of-wedlock pregnancy as a symptom of cultural pathology.[48] At the same time, however, social workers acknowledged the growing need to place minority children in Black homes.[49] This need resulted from African American migration during World War II from the south to northern and western cities and from the Children's Bureau's decision in 1948 to begin including the category of race in their adoption reporting, which brought the issue to the fore. The reporting exposed the deep racial disparities in adoption services and the serious needs for Black children's permanent placement.[50] Child welfare agencies consequently had to provide services to these children, even though casework remained unequal.[51]

Placement needs of white children depended upon age. Before World War II, some couples preferred not to adopt newborns because of high rates of infant mortality and any "defective" heredity that could show up later with a baby's development. But, according to Carp and Leon-Guerrero, due to "the low Depression birth rate, wartime prosperity, and baby boom pronatalism that put a premium on family and home life," prospective parents shifted from giving instrumental reasons for adoption (work) to sentimental reasons (companionship, love of children, altruism). This made parent applicants strongly desire healthy infants and eschew other types of children, including older ones. As Florence Brown, executive director of the Free Synagogue Child Adoption Committee of New York, remarked in 1951, "We have few applicants who are willing to accept an older child or one with a handicap" [meaning here a child with pathological heredity].[52] A few prospective adoptive parents desired a young infant so strongly that they preferred to accept a younger infant who might later develop an impairment rather than wait to secure more physical and cognitive testing.[53]

In all, even with out-of-wedlock relinquishments, the number of parent applicants outpaced the number of available white healthy infants.[54] Agencies and child welfare specialists had to change their own practices, including the definition of adoptability, in the face of these pressures.

Changing adoption demographics forced agencies to reconsider the adoptability of several different groups of children previously excluded from agency adoption to potentially meet the rise in applicants' interest in adoption. To reflect the relative "neglected" status of these children

(including those with pathological heredity), adoption professionals created a new category called the "hard-to-place" child. Social workers used
the descriptor "hard-to-place" to describe minority (African American,
Native American, and mixed-race) children, older children (over two years
of age and mostly boys), siblings, and "handicapped" children. The latter included children with pathological heredity and those with diagnosed
impairments, even though agencies still commonly excluded the latter
during this time.[55]

Agencies labeled all of these children hard-to-place because applicants
desired them the least. As one attendee at the 1955 National Adoption
Conference admitted: "hard-to-place" implied that the social worker saw
the child as a "problem." She and her colleagues tended to "place the
burden on the children rather than our own lack of skills in finding homes
for this group of children."[56] Because agencies gradually affirmed these
children's eligibility for adoption but generally faltered in placing them,
hard-to-place children had an overwhelming need for permanent homes
in the late 1940s and 1950s.

In their position on the hierarchy of desirability, hard-to-place children
held a subordinate position to able-bodied whiteness, to the ideal child
who was easy to place, who had no background or evidence of imputed
pathology.[57] The further away a child was from the default position of
able-bodied whiteness—which social workers coded as having no risk for
placement—the more risky social workers believed that that child was to
family intactness. Intercategorical identity markers of hard-to-place children certainly complicated the chances of placement, but evidentiary constraints make it difficult to grasp specifics. As an umbrella category, however, hard to place collapsed the often diverse positions of these children
and the various reasons they were hard to place. The term obfuscated the
conceptual and programmatic differences between and among the child
groups for the larger purpose of placement.

Such elision had consequences. As historian Karen Balcom has pointed
out, "the conflation of physical and mental disability with minority racial
status in *hard to place* [italics in original] left the impression that nonwhite racial status was a pathology that needed to be/could be overcome
through the intervention of social workers."[58] This conflation echoes
what disability historian Douglas Baynton so adeptly describes as society's imputation of disability to minority groups in order to discriminate
against them. Yet descriptions like Balcom's also tacitly distance race
from disability/pathology as a way to rehabilitate nonwhite children's social

legitimacy. This kind of move ends up implicitly locating disability as the rightful bottom level in a hierarchy of marginalization.[59]

When social workers did not conflate subcategories (minority, siblings, handicapped, older), it seems they chose only one subcategory to describe the child, even if the child inhabited many subcategories at once. For instance, when social workers classified hard-to-place children for adoption exchanges, which were mechanisms to facilitate placement for these children across state boundaries, as explained in chapter 4, they described healthy children of color as "minority" and disabled children of all races as "handicapped."[60] In later periods, social workers acknowledged that a child who crossed subcategories (e.g., children of color with disabilities) were the hardest to place. But in this period, social workers rarely explicitly referenced children who traversed subcategories; they either referred to one subcategory or to the whole category of hard to place.[61]

Still, adoption professionals often ideologically and programmatically treated hard-to-place children similarly. For one thing, they imagined and managed mixed-race and "handicapped" children in parallel ways. Couples' and social workers' anxieties that mixed-race children may develop "Negroid" features, for example, mirrored their fears that children with pathological heredity would manifest diagnosed impairments at a future date. In both cases, couples and social workers assumed that the potential allegedly undesirable characteristics could surface and cause a threat to family integrity and to the adoption itself. These racial-ableist logics and fears led agencies in this period to enlist experts like anthropologists, physicians, and geneticists to examine mixed-race children and children with more pronounced pathological heredity to discern the unknown and often unknowable.[62]

Beyond the new demographic picture of adoption, nonagency adoption (independent adoption) influenced CWLA and agency arguments about risk equivalence, normality, and placing children with pathological family backgrounds. Independent adoption competed with agency adoption by diverting both birth mothers and applicants away from agencies to independent brokers, which in turn forced agencies to consider marginalized and riskier children. Professional adoption agencies partnered with state welfare departments and licensed private agencies to place children. Some private agencies only engaged in adoption work, while others included adoption as part of a larger set of child welfare programs, including caring for neglected, dependent, or delinquent children. In contrast, physicians, lawyers, clergymen, nurses, midwives, and birth parents typically facilitated independent adoptions, also called the gray market. Until 1955, independent brokers managed about 75 percent of all adoptions in the US.[63]

Independent adoption posed such a threat to agency adoption that states and the CWLA studied existing adoption practices, strengthened adoption laws, and changed policies to better protect the adoption triad (biological mothers, the child, and the adoptive parents).[64] In addition, the CWLA was deeply concerned about black market adoption practices (baby selling). To protect the adoption triad, the CWLA recommended that agencies counsel birth mothers to confirm their decision to relinquish and investigate the motivations of adoptive parents. It also advised agencies to determine children's adoptability by administering medical and developmental examinations. As a result, social workers essentially saw themselves as "risk-managers" who could shield families from avoidable disability risk, even as they paradoxically and simultaneously promoted the principle of risk equivalence.[65] This inconsistency reflects just how in flux adoption practice was during this period.

Prospective parents were attracted to independent adoption because of quick placement times. Birth mothers preferred it because it was less intrusive and offered rapid closure. In contrast, agency adoption often required birth mothers to wait months for a final agency decision about her child's adoptability because of the battery of tests it gave to certify a child's health and development. In the interim, a birth mother had to cover the expenses of her child's care and experience the uncertainty of whether the agency would accept her child. This burden worsened if an agency deemed the child unadoptable.[66] Maud Morlock of the Children's Bureau reframed the four- to six-month wait as a positive step, arguing that it not only helped assess normality in the child but also allowed birth mothers to make arrangements to keep their child if they decided to do so. It also enabled experts to "make provision for defective children"; that is, make arrangements to admit the child to a custodial institution.[67]

In 1950, *Woman's Home Companion* published a scathing critique of adoption agency practice that reflected these concerns. The article, "Why You Can't Adopt a Baby," pointed out that long placement times for prospective adoptive parents and strict but inconsistent applicant eligibility practices were major reasons why parent applicants turned to independent adoption. Quoting a New York City Committee on Adoption Report, the author noted, "Less than one family in ten applying for a child receives

one. But at the same time fewer than half of the children offered to agencies for adoption are placed."[68] Even after the New York City Department
of Welfare referred 730 children, excluding "mental defectives, those with
marked physical defects," and "problem children," to a licensed private
agency, the agency still returned 276 as unsuitable.[69] Adoption professionals responded to the critique, arguing that nonagency adoption increased
the risks of an inappropriate and potentially dissolved placement. They
contended that, if they were to compete with independent adoption brokers, agency adoption needed to widen its scope of child eligibility and
accept all unmarried mothers.

Much of the debate about the competition between independent and
agency adoption rested explicitly on concerns about disability. Adoptive
parents who turned to independent adoption often wanted a child at a
very early age (often right after birth) to avoid having the birth mother
change her mind. In their haste to complete the adoption, one adoption
official noted, prospective parents did not attain sufficient knowledge
about the child's "mental endowment" or emotional stability, often leading to a placement that was "more of a gamble" than it needed to be.[70]
According to the adoption official, a lack of information was unfair to
both the prospective parents and the child because needs could go unmet
or the adoption could fray.

To steer adoptive applicants away from independent or black market
brokers, licensed adoption agencies portrayed their ability to evaluate babies for their normality as a distinct advantage. One source, for instance,
warned that independent adoption multiplied the number of risks, including the inadvertent possibility that an independent broker could place a
"mentally deficient" child: "This danger is particularly acute in the case of
independent placements with non-relatives, often made when the child is
less than a month old, because feeblemindedness can rarely be detected
under the age of three months." Adoption leaders believed that regulations needed to "protect the adoptive parents from assuming responsibility for a child whose mental and physical condition is questionable and
from interference by the natural parents after the child has been satisfac-
torily established in his new home."[71] By trying to demonstrate that agencies exposed applicants to less disability risk than independent brokers,
however, adoption professionals inadvertently undermined their claims
of risk equivalence.

Two physicians, Joseph Baldwin and Catherine Amatruda, conducted
a study to make a case for agency placement over independent adoption.

Baldwin and Amatruda compared the two types of placements, finding that in independent adoption some of the "good" babies ended up in "poor" (unsuitable) homes and some of the "poor" babies ended up in "good" homes (which social workers called under- and overplacement). By comparison, agencies that made an "honest effort" to "screen out the babies who are poor risks" and came from unsuitable homes (birth parents who had rocky marriages, psychiatric health problems, alcoholism, prostitution, domestic violence, drug addiction, or prison records) had a 75 percent success rate in matching the "goods" together.[72]

The media followed professional agencies' lead. It featured stories about the dangers of failing to use an accredited adoption agency, with disability highlighted as one of the main dangers. In December 1944, for instance, *Woman's Home Companion* illustrated the risks and "tragedies" of independent adoption by featuring children who turned out to have various impairments.[73] One case involved a family who adopted twin boys before they were born. One died shortly after birth due to hydrocephalus and the other was diagnosed with the same condition. The author wrote that parents now bore the costs of institutional care of the surviving twin, "who may live for eight or ten years with an enormous grotesque head," even though they were not actually going to be raising him. "If they had waited for a few months, put up with the red tape involved in supervised adoptions, the family would have the assurance that the child they adopted was free from disease."[74] A letter to the editor of the *Cleveland Press* advocated the same sentiment. A couple wrote that they did not mind getting a child that was slightly older since they felt it was better to know that they were adopting an intelligent and healthy child, rather than risk getting one that was "abnormal."[75]

Even the Kefauver Senate oversight hearings, held specifically to address the dangers of independent adoption, covered how disability was entangled with deceptive adoption practices. For instance, Mrs. Epps, a boarding mother for wards of Richmond County Juvenile Court in Augusta, Georgia, testified that she stopped being a foster mother because she heard that many of the children were being sold. All of the four children placed with local people from her boardinghouse between 1940 and 1951 were "afflicted" with some sort of impairment. According to Epps, the children would not have been "presentable" to most couples, but one couple wanted a baby so badly that they would "take anything they could get."[76] Another witness, the judge of the Augusta juvenile court, agreed that most prospective adoptive parents found disabled children undesirable. When asked what types of children prospective parents most wanted in Richmond County, the judge responded that couples desired infants and children who were physically "very normal." When asked if he had any difficulty placing children with serious "defects," the judge responded that he did. But then the judge relayed the story of a woman who adopted a girl with a cast in her eye. The judge asked the woman why she wanted to adopt the child and she responded, "She is a little ugly duckling and I do not think anybody would have her." After her adoption, the girl had surgeries to correct her eyes.[77]

The point of the Kefauver hearings was to show how unfair, unscrupulous, and problematic these adoptions supposedly were, but testimonies like these inadvertently provided some evidence that a minority of prospective parents knowingly adopted children with diagnosed impairments through independent brokers. At the same time, all of the stories, whether in the hearings, in the media, or among experts, suggested that protecting parents against disability was a valid and forceful argument against independent adoption.

Early Placement, Futurity, and the Nature of Risk

The move of adoption professionals toward "early placement," defined as the practice of placing infants by six months of age, influenced their calls for risk equivalence because the short time span precluded a number of tests that psychologists now argued simply could not be conducted in any meaningful way before the age of six months. Thus, early placement made it hard for agencies to promise prospective adoptive parents a perfect child and more difficult for applicants to demand one.[78]

Adoption professionals' calls for early placement emerged not only in response to parent demand for infants, but also because of practical realities at the end of the Second World War.[79] As social workers became more open to adoption rather than keeping birth mother and child together, unmarried women who wanted to relinquish their children felt freer to do so at stages earlier than before. A shortage of foster homes "which must be freed for the use of incoming infants" also forced social workers to place healthy infants in adoptive homes at earlier ages. They would place such children only if their family and health profile seemed satisfactory, but adopting parents had to be comfortable with having limited knowledge about the child because of the shortened observation period.[80]

Nevertheless, adoption leaders posited that placing children early conferred developmental and emotional benefits. This idea rested on the results of several sets of ideas emerging from psychological research. First, studies showed that keeping children in orphanages had negative effects on children. Second, adoption leaders supported the theories of maternal deprivation and maternal attachment espoused by John Bowlby, author of the famous report *Maternal Care and Mental Health*, among others. These theories suggested that children needed quick but permanent family substitutions when "normal and natural ties" were broken.[81] Most psychologists contended that early placement closely mimicked the conditions of biological parenthood, thereby allowing for immediate maternal-child attachment.[82]

Adoption leaders thus determined that placing a child in early infancy with loving adoptive parents provided the best chances for an adoptive child to develop like biological offspring.[83] Weltha M. Kelley of the Catholic Home Bureau of New York wrote, for instance, that early placement ensured that the "totality of the infant's dependence," the "charm of his helplessness," created a deep, mutual love between mother and child.[84] Others reiterated this point, arguing that through caring for an infant, couples would feel that they "could not have produced a finer baby."[85] In an age where medical advice widely encouraged mothers to bottle-feed their infants, Lucie Browning, supervisor of the department of foster home care of the Child's Aid Society in Buffalo, contended that early placement was important because giving a bottle to a baby early would stave off any feelings of libidinal loss so that damage to the infant's mental life could be avoided.[86]

Adoption professionals' concern about any psychological harm resulting from broken attachments conflicted with their anxieties about the potential for an adoptive child to become disabled. The earlier the placement, the harder it would be for agencies to recognize disability, especially for invisible disabilities like deafness, blindness, and mental retardation. For this reason, Kelley reassured fellow social workers that early placement did not necessarily clash with estimating a child's potentiality. Agencies could still acquire a lot of information about a baby and her background:

> The choice has not seemed to be between more risk or less risk for the baby. He still is selected on the basis of known and favorable hereditary facts, on evidence of an uneventful pregnancy and birth, and finally on the grounds of his beginning health and early normal development.[87]

Even with early placement, social workers still gathered information about the health status of the child, including a full physical and mental health history of the birth parents, the baby's weight and length at birth, head measurement, the condition of the fontanelles, a Wasserman test, data on feeding habits, chest measurement, a record of any operations and the child's discharge weight and examination. Kelley reassured adoption workers that the Catholic Home Bureau had great success with early placement; for the ninety-seven infants it placed over a three-year period, only one adoption ended because of a suspected diagnosis of microcephaly.[88] Thus, in the late 1940s and early 1950s, adoption professionals increasingly began to believe that for most children "the risks of not placing him [the child] until he is older are immeasurably greater" than placing him early. Adoption leaders argued that if there was a chance to be in a stable family early, the child would have the best opportunity to "develop strengths that will go far to counteract any adverse tendencies in his background."[89]

Casework practices changed to accommodate anxieties about disability and "fit" in an age of early placement. Taking the recommendations from the CWLA workshops, the Children's Aid Society (CAS), for instance, used the prenatal period to attain more precise social histories so that it could more efficiently match parent applicants to a child upon her birth. Histories also included birth family information that reached farther back in time. When social workers could not obtain paternal information, they offset the gap by gathering even more information about the birth mother. Some agencies also allowed prospective adoptive parents to see or meet the prospective child so they could become acquainted with the child's appearance and determine whether or not they wanted to move forward.[90]

Some agencies even started to consider placing newborns directly from the hospital (an approach known as *direct placement*) if they were normal.[91] They promoted direct placement to reduce the number of multiple foster care placements or avoid institutionalizing the child before adoption.[92] Certain conditions had to be met to directly place a child in an adoptive home: the child's full birth history had to be available, her birth parents had to be of at least average intelligence, there could be no pathology in the birth family's history, and there could not be any pathology in the medical exam.[93]

By 1955, agencies also began to accept that tests only measured a child's current development. They did not predict the future. Although agencies could use tests for planning, they could not rely on test results alone.[94]

Psychologists' recognition that the IQ test was unreliable became especially acute in the context of early placement. Given that the test could
not predict future intelligence, and given applicants' desire for infants, the
only option left was for prospective adoptive parents to forgo agencies'
earlier promise against disability. As such, many agency workers believed
that adoptive parents' intelligence, rather than birth parents', might be a
"better index of criteria" for development. This was one of the ways they
began to recognize that the emotional environment in the adoptive home
mattered.[95] This openness to environmental influence on intelligence and
behavior reflected an emerging focus in psychology on the interaction between heredity and environment in the 1950s.

Social workers' inability to use the IQ test to predict a child's intelligence reflected the particular challenge disability posed for the adoption
enterprise. Experts who continued to use infant tests insisted that even
a child's present development had predictive value and, in all likelihood,
couples probably took a child's present development as a way to imagine
her future.[96] "Prediction is inherent in adoption planning," declared Voskine Yanekian of the Child Adoption Service of the State Charities Aid
Association of New York. "We all use it consciously or unconsciously."[97]
Indeed, placing a child into an adoptive home involved seemingly incongruent elements: an assumption of risk, the reduction of uncertainty and
risk, and a benefit analysis of "good" and "bad" risks.[98] When a social
worker engaged in this benefit analysis, she did so to determine a child's
adoptability. The absence, potential, or presence of impairment fundamentally influenced whether a child could be adopted or probably sent to
an institution.

Invisible disability, however, disrupted the benefit analysis process; it
problematized a static notion of futurity and of risk. For instance, Sheldon Reed, director of the Dight Institute for Human Genetics, asked how
one could tell which babies having "mentally retarded mothers" were going to turn out to have cognitive impairment themselves:

> Those with obvious physical stigmata such as are found in Mongoloids, micro-
> cephalics, hydrocephalics and so on, can be screened out at birth. However, the
> mentally retarded without physical defects will probably be indistinguishable
> from the normal until they are one or two years old.[99]

A preliminary report on the 1955 CWLA conference also spoke to the issue of detecting disability at birth or after and its implications for decisions

about adoptability. It stated: "It is known that 95 percent of the children are in good condition initially and that they continue normal to 3 months. Only 5 percent show some defect (not all serious) by 3 months. Should agencies hold up 95 percent because there is a risk for 5 percent?"[100] This questioning eventually led the CWLA to clarify and solidify its adoptability criteria in its 1958 Standards for Adoption Service:

> There are no hereditary factors which should automatically rule out adoption. Qualified consultants should be relied on to decide which hereditary conditions may be considered risks because they may limit life expectancy or adversely affect normal development. Such conditions should be carefully evaluated, recognizing that there are adoptive parents who may be willing to accept children with special needs.[101]

If a physician suspected that an infant had an impairment, agencies required a longer waiting period to do more psychological, neurological, and pediatric testing, to attain medical and social histories, and to observe the child again.[102] Many agencies used foster family homes as temporary care during this waiting period. It took one to eight months to complete the testing and other casework, with an average of six months. Other agencies used institutional care as a form of preadoption care.[103] These, however, were exactly the kinds of temporary arrangements that early placement tried to avoid.

Adoption professionals continued to debate the benefits and hazards of early placement well into the mid-1950s. While most agencies considered a period of between three and twelve months enough to ascertain the child's development, some other agencies still tried to minimize any risk in adoption placement.[104] For those agencies, early placement had significant hazards that included uncertainty about the child's development, possible removal if a child showed abnormal development (even when adoptive parents wanted to keep a child), and a potential mismatch between parent and child.[105] Still other agencies delayed placement in order to address worries about children suspected of having physical or cognitive disabilities, behavioral problems, or pathological family backgrounds.[106] By 1954, most agencies did not outright deny a child with a pathological background, but delayed placement to address uncertainties in a child's developmental or medical status.[107] Other reasons for delay included the inability of the caseworker to find a home, legal issues, psychiatric problems of the birth mother, and agency staff shortages.

However, by the mid-1950s, an increasing number of adoption professionals objected to delayed placement because of fears that this practice would make children even harder to place; they worried that these children would be older or would have suffered from deprivation by the time they were considered adoptable. Many adoption workers agreed, arguing that later placements could disrupt normal development and interrupt early love relationships.[108] John Bowlby, for instance, had serious reservations about psychological testing and delayed placement. He argued not only that psychological testing before eighteen months had no predictive value but also that delayed placement could actually *produce* mental retardation; deferring placement to give social workers time to gather more conclusive evidence of a child's intellectual capacity could ironically make an adoptable child unadoptable in the end.[109] The logic of delayed placement had been flipped; instead of using delayed placement to best evaluate an infant for impairment and possibly exclude her, by the 1950s experts believed that delayed placement could produce the exact undesirable condition agencies tried to avoid.

Adoptive Parent Eligibility and the Best Interests of the Child

Given the number of parent applications to adopt a child, the needs of hard-to-place children, and the new definition of adoptability and its conditional clause "as long as parents can accept them," adoption professionals set out to delineate the desired postwar characteristics of adoptive parents. Through their choice of applicants, they believed, agencies could protect the "best interests of the child," a standard of child welfare that first developed in child custody law in the mid-nineteenth century and then made its way into modern adoption law.[110] One of the key desirable qualities of prospective adoptive parents that these professionals identified was their ability to manage and accept certain reasonable risks.

Adoption professionals changed their assessment of suitable applicants in response to new trends in psychology that challenged earlier notions about heredity and eugenics. Influenced by the work of Rene Spitz, Anna Freud, Margaret Ribble, and John Bowlby, among others, adoption leaders emphasized the importance of the mother-child tie for normal child development.[111] They saw this bonding as unquestionably in the "best interests of the child." This stance, however, led to seemingly conflicting positions. Because social workers wanted to avoid depriving the child of a maternal figure and tried to promote early bonding between the adoptive mother and child, they began to interpret "best interests of the child" to mean separating the biological mother and child, rather than striving to keep them together, as earlier in the century.[112] Adoption as a solution to white out-of-wedlock pregnancy—so the woman could return to her community, life, and prospects—also factored into such separation.

At the same time, psychiatrists, adoption professionals, and psychologists believed that the "trauma" and "wound" resulting from losing a biological mother created a particular psychology for the adopted child. They argued that the child marshaled her ego to compensate for the loss of a birth mother, producing an "unknown void" that would separate the psychologies of adopted children from the nonadopted.[113] Adoption professionals believed that this void made adoptees especially fragile and therefore in need of special care and attention. But they also saw adoption as "preventive therapy" for maternal deprivation.[114] Adoptees' fragility necessitated that adoptive parents fully accept them. A child needed to feel that she completely belonged to the family; she needed to feel that the "kind of person [s]he is, is a good kind to be."[115]

By 1955, the Child Welfare League of America sought to systematize adoption practices nationwide to implement the best-interests principle.[116] By focusing on the best interests of the child and on new dimensions of parenthood, the CWLA endorsed a version of risk equivalence where, according to Mary Fairweather, the supervisor of adoptions at the Children's Services of Cleveland, children do not come with guarantees. By this logic, parents who could not accept the "normal risks of life" would be "poor risks for our children."[117] In an era when psychologists more widely scrutinized maternal fitness and behavior, agencies concluded that they had to select parent applicants who could "take risks" and share that risk with the agency; parents had to be mature enough to "accept the normal risks of life" because "to give complete assurance of normal development, we should have to place adults, not children."[118]

Other adoption leaders echoed Fairweather's sentiments.[119] They maintained that if prospective adoptive parents requested an infant, they would have to accept the "added risks" that the baby could develop a disability in the future. What these applicants gained, leaders like Viola Bernard contended, was the "reduction of risks of another sort"; that is, a purportedly greater sense of connection from the beginning of the child's life.[120] This condition also allowed agencies to weed out more applicants, especially given the disproportionate postwar number of white adoptive parent applicants compared to healthy white children.

Agencies translated the tenets of risk equivalence and best interests of the child into applicant eligibility criteria. A growing number of agencies revised their parent applicant eligibility criteria to incorporate positive parent attitudes, believing successful placement depended upon them.[121] Agencies privileged flexibility and rejected prospective parents who struggled with not definitively knowing a child's intelligence. Social workers at the Free Synagogue Child Adoption Committee, for instance, explained to parent applicants that the same inability to know a child's mental capacity would have also extended to children born to them. To the agency's mind, rigidity on this point exposed applicants' shallowness, which it believed was anathema to parenthood and reflected immaturity.[122] Other agencies saw applicants who approached adoption as though they were "making a purchase" as irresponsible, narcissistic, and unprepared to become parents.[123] For the well-known Menninger Clinic analyst, Dr. Robert P. Knight, for instance, applicants' rigidity about age or physical characteristics such as hair, eyes, or sex signaled that they were, even unconsciously, simply averse to being parents.[124]

An increasing number of agencies joined Knight in contending that applicants who had preconditions for loving a child—what I call *conditional parenthood*—were unable to handle the trials and tribulations of child raising. By contrast, desirable applicants at midcentury were those whose "ideas as they may have about sex, age, social or biological heredity, illegitimacy, potentiality or future life roles for the child" are not motivated by "neurotic needs" or the wishes of the extended family. Ideal parent applicants were not "too preconceived or irrevocable," but were ready to "rear a wide range of children."[125] Ruth Taft, director of the adoption department of Children's Services in Hartford, Connecticut, was one adoption professional who espoused this view. In 1953, she argued that "normal, well-adjusted adults" who want to adopt a child would be "willing to accept risks arising from reasonable unknowns" and could accept the consequences of their decisions. It was rigid adoption workers, according to Taft, who had trouble changing their attitudes about any "risky placements" of previously unadoptable children; in contrast to social workers who were increasingly open to parent applicants' flexibility, they were flummoxed by parent applicants who were willing to take the "normal risks of parenthood."[126] To prove her point, Taft offered the case of a ten-month-old infant whose parents were in mental hospitals. The child had eczema, which experts deterministically believed was caused by a hereditary emotional problem. Physician and psychologist consultants precluded adoptive placement, but social workers found a couple who were "unperturbed" by the baby's problematic family background and felt they could give him "love and acceptance, without fear." And indeed, their love proved therapeutic. Ten months after placement, the infant's eczema had disappeared. She was psychologically "fully normal," and exhibited high average ability.[127]

Agencies wanted prospective parents who had open attitudes, but they also insisted on applicants with a "sound body, normal emotional and intellectual development and freedom from bad inheritance."[128] These factors, many believed, had a "direct bearing on the capacity" of applicants to parent any child.[129] In a 1951 study, Ruth Brenner, a leading adoption worker, noted that a couples' good marriage, realistic ideas about a child's behavior, and an absence of pressure on the child were predictors of a successful placement. Brenner added this extensive list:

> the parents are warm and affectionate; they are admiring, but not without judgment; they are easy and relaxed, for the most part, and enjoy their child; and have no undue anxiety about their parental responsibilities; they are generous with their time for the child; they are mild in their discipline; and they allow a child freedom to experiment and take risks suitable to his age, while setting limits that will contribute to his growth and safety.[130]

Besides these emotional traits, agencies looked for a stable, middle-class income, rather than a minimum income, and required that applicants have medical insurance because problems with insurance access could pose a major barrier to a child's health. For its part, the CWLA reconfigured sound adoptive practice to include communication with the potential parents to give them a better understanding of the variety of children available for adoption. Agencies did outreach to prospective applicants and to the community—including to minority racial and ethnic communities—to attract more families to consider adopting a hard-to-place child.[131] They looked to communities of color in which to place children of color because transracial adoption was not socially acceptable until the 1960s. Such outreach foreshadowed later initiatives like Adopt-a-Child in 1955, which recruited African American and Puerto Rican adopters nationally and highlighted the principle of matching. The program claimed it could find a child "who will blend into your family, grow happily in your home, and may even look a little like you."[132] It also foreshadowed the Indian Adoption Project in 1958, which placed Native American children in non-Native homes.[133]

Although agencies stressed the need for prospective adoptive parents to make decisions for themselves, some also looked upon applicants' motivations with great suspicion. Their mistrustful attitude mirrored Americans' general apprehension about maternal devotion and maternal knowledge at the time. Psychologists, physicians, and social workers warned of mothers who, unhappy in their lot as sole caregiver at home, could be domineering toward their children even if it were under the pretense of complete devotion. Mothers could be the source of mother love that promoted a child's healthy emotional development, but they could also be the cause of a child's emotional problems.[134] These professionals feared that mothers could reject their children, be overprotective, or expect more than the child could achieve.[135]

Disability, especially as it intersected with class and race, factored into these expectations about parent applicants. Adoption experts, for instance, described middle-class white parents and "mentally retarded" children as incongruent. One expert noted that mentally retarded children had much better "adjustmental prognosis" when parental standards were low enough so as to make the disability "inconspicuous." By contrast, a child whose "intellectual handicap places him below the level of the family aspirations" would fare much worse.[136] Social workers had to find the right fit between parent applicants and child so that the family unit could thrive.

Disability, Family Resemblance, and Risk Equivalence in Context

Agency workers went to great lengths to define, create, and elevate the normal family in their selection of prospective adoptive parents and eligible children. For some of them, "adoptive families were modeled on the 'normal,' defect-free biological family: children should resemble their parents, and children with disabilities should not be placed."[137] Disability disrupted the idea of family resemblance and fundamentally challenged the underlying assumptions of intellectual and physical matching that sought to produce "as if begotten" families.[138] The fallacy, of course, was that not all members of biological families look or act alike or have the same level of intellect; as one citizen's critique about adoption's matching practices asked, "Did all your brothers and sisters look alike . . . did your mother get a guarantee of perfection when you were born?"[139]

According to adoption historian Brian Paul Gill, agencies almost never tried to explain why "normal" was considered the best arrangement for a family or a child or why an unusual or atypical family was less than ideal. But social workers' logic about the ideal family seems to have contributed to the relatively slow pace with which they accepted the new CWLA guidelines on adoptability.

In many ways, this makes contextual sense. Social workers were drawing on a broader social devaluation of children labeled disabled. At the time, most Americans considered disability a tragedy. They viewed disabled children as perpetually and completely dependent, and so they considered having a disabled child in one's family a burden. Educator Edward L. Rautman, for instance, claimed in 1949 that omnipresent disappointment could frustrate middle-class parental love and affection to a disabled child, especially one with, or having the potential for, mental retardation. A family's middle-class status itself could be jeopardized.[140] Without affection, how could a child "benefit from family life" in the adoptive family?[141] Other educators worried that mentally retarded children diverted a mother's attention from her husband and other children. Such an adoption could damage the family and break it apart.[142]

While experts, social workers, and parents concentrated on individualized risk and personal decisions, they failed to problematize the societal structures that devalued disability. These views reflected the cold reality that parents found themselves facing limited social assistance for their disabled children in postwar America. Despite a dramatic increase in special education classes, guaranteed public education was not available to *all* children until 1975; only children diagnosed with mild disabilities had access to education prior to that time. Where they existed, special education classes often grouped physically disabled, mentally ill, and "mentally retarded" children with "juvenile delinquents."[143] In practice, excluding disabled children from key social settings meant more responsibility for mothers.

Within this context, many parents institutionalized their disabled children. In the same way that social workers offered a narrative of relinquishment as freedom for birth mothers, physicians counseled parents that institutionalizing their disabled child would allow them to move on with their lives. They could regain their respectability. Physicians often criticized parents who opted to keep their child at home, claiming that they did not accept their child's condition.[144] Given society's push for parents to institutionalize disabled children, the expansion of institutions to house them, and the practice of sterilizing residents who inhabited the institutions (60,000 people from 1927 through 1957), it is no wonder that adoptive applicants would hesitate when contemplating adopting a child labeled disabled.

Disability factored into prospective parents' adoption decisions in other ways. As Mrs. Austin Melford of the National Adoption Society explained in 1951, sometimes families sought to adopt a nondisabled child to compensate, or provide a sibling for, a biological child "with some unfortunate disability, perhaps backward in speech, a little deaf or even mentally retarded; they offer to adopt a child of average development whose companionship will, they hope, be of help to their own handicapped child."[145] Melford remarked that applicants sought adoption to avoid the risk of having another biological child who could be "abnormal." She explained: "Such adopters are accepted [by the agency] only if the abnormal child is permanently looked after elsewhere in an institution; it would be very unfair for a normal child to place him in such [a home] environment."[146] The underlying message was that a normal family's status depended upon its abnormal elements being out of sight. These practical constraints and concerns, and the ethos they reflected, disincentivized many prospective adoptive parents from adopting children with pathological family backgrounds. They also influenced casework decisions about children with mild impairments, even when agencies found them officially adoptable.

At the same time, while many social workers employed a dominant narrative that saw disabled children as the cause of tragedy and disruption in families, a new cultural narrative taking shape in the country may have also influenced their use of risk equivalence. Figures like Pearl Buck, an adoptive mother, a mother to a birth child with intellectual disability, and known for her involvement both in issues of mental deficiency and in adoption, and Dale Evans Rogers, an adoptive parent who also had one biological child with an intellectual disability, started to lift the veil of shame that parents with disabled children had experienced. In their confessional writings, these adoptive parents minimized heredity's role in mental retardation and promoted parents' attitudes of acceptance and transcendence. In the 1950s, national associations of middle-class parents, like the National Association of Parents and Friends of Retarded Children (NARC), argued that rather than fearing these children, Americans should recognize their potential (even as the latter was ill-defined).[147] If middle-class parents and famous people like Pearl Buck, Dale Evans and Roy Rogers, and John Frank could have biological children with intellectual disability, then surely adoptive applicants could end up with a disabled child too. These examples provided the evidence for risk equivalence.

The threat of polio probably also made risk equivalence germane to both adoption professionals and adoptive applicants. Most likely, polio led adoption thinkers to recognize that nonadopted children could be at risk for acquiring a disability. Polio reached epidemic levels in the years following the Second World War. In 1946, reported cases totaled 25,000; by 1952, at the height of the epidemic, that number reached 57,000. In that year alone, 21,000 people developed permanent paralysis and approximately 3,000 died. Incidence rates also rose significantly, from 8 per 100,000 from 1940 through 1944, to 16 per 100,000 for 1945–1949, and 25 per 100,000 for 1950–1954.[148]

The March of Dimes published and disseminated copious information about the disease. Pictures of "poster children" appeared in women's magazines and newspapers. This public health campaign added to national fears about the disease and introduced the inspirational, innocent figure of the child who overcomes her disability into American culture, a figure taken up by adoption professionals in the late 1950s and 1960s.[149] Despite the small probability of any given child becoming physically disabled from polio, Americans experienced great psychological panic; polio threatened, if not tore apart, the fantasy that was the middle-class American family and undermined any attempts by parents (that is, mothers) to protect their children from harm. As historian David Oshinsky explains, there was no way to escape the "damage that polio did, the random way in which it struck, or the gruesome truth that *everyone was at risk*" [my italics].[150] The risk of polio put middle-class adoptive and biological families on the same plane when it came to disability. Even as the threat of polio loomed large, penicillin and other antibiotics, better nutrition, new medical technologies, and public health policies made it more likely that children and adults with disabilities in postwar America survived.[151] The federal government also began to actively fund biomedical research, leading many Americans to believe that a world free from disease and disability was on the horizon.

Risk Equivalence Gives Way to Love and Acceptance

In all, numerous ideological and practical developments came together to make ideas about risk equivalence and expanded adoptability happen and resonate. Even though the mandate of having perfect, healthy babies and being a healthy parent proved exceptionally important during the baby boom, changing adoption demographics, threats to agency adoption by independent brokers, shifts to a child-centered philosophy, challenges to notions of heredity, and new ideas about child development together pushed social workers to gradually consider children with "hereditary handicaps" as potential members of the adoptive family.[152] Although applicants generally first resisted this move, they slowly came to accept that they might have to consider a "hard-to-place" child if they wished to adopt in a timely manner.

By the end of this period, leading adoption professionals increasingly spoke of the necessity for adoptive parents to accept some "reasonable" amount of risk. Helen Marsh, chief psychologist of the Cleveland Guidance Center, for instance, remarked that "well-adjusted adults" could "weigh the risks of reasonable unknowns, arrive at a decision, and find a healthy way to adjust to the results of their decision." She warned that agencies did not have to overprotect their clients and that adoptive parents had a right to autonomy, thus mimicking social workers' presumptions about the autonomy of biological parents.[153] Evelyn Smith of the US Children's Bureau agreed. She remarked in 1951 that even though many physical symptoms were not apparent at birth, prospective adoptive parents should be "willing to assume some risks just as they would in the development of a child born to them. . . . While some of the early placements have turned out badly, in many instances the child has made normal progress and a good adjustment in the adoptive home."[154] Most importantly, risk equivalence resonated for agencies not only because they recognized that predicting impairment was impossible, but also because some adoptive parents did, in fact, take risks.

Adoption professionals' growing acceptance of children with pathological family backgrounds in the postwar era provided the bridge to the wider acceptance of children with diagnosed impairments in the next period, especially those with mild or moderate severity. Indeed, the ideological and material transformations that occurred during this decade set the stage for the next chapter of this story, where adoption professionals touted love and acceptance as having the ability to conquer all parental fears and doubts about the risks adoption workers encouraged them to take.

PART II

Working toward Inclusion: 1955–1980

CHAPTER THREE

Love, Acceptance, and the Narrative of Overcoming

In the fall of 1976, Patricia Kravik, a special consultant for the Community Mental Health and Mental Retardation Services Board in Arlington County, Virginia, wrote a scathing critique of adoption practices (or lack thereof) for developmentally disabled children. "For years, homeless children with special needs stood waiting to hear the affirmation of adoption: 'Yes—you are loved; Yes—you are valuable. . . .' The children were labeled good candidates for therapy, rehabilitation or diagnostic evaluation—but never adoption. What they needed was love."[1]

Kravik's emphasis upon a child's need for love reflected adoption leaders' appeal in the mid to late 1950s for agencies to consider whether children with diagnosed impairments had the potential for adoption. Adoption professionals' new focus on love and acceptance accompanied this rethinking; it signaled a shift in risk discourse wherein professionals relocated risk as situated in social prejudice and barriers to placement as opposed to it residing in an individual disabled child (i.e., a risky child). The individualized framing of risk encapsulated an array of assumptions and concerns: that adopters would find a disabled child difficult to raise, that caring for a disabled child would threaten family dynamics and family cohesiveness, and that these challenges would ultimately endanger placement. By contrast, proponents of the new adoption risk discourse focused on factors outside of the child as they critiqued attitudinal and agency barriers to disabled children's adoption.[2]

Emphasizing this second form of risk discourse in her 1976 editorial in *Adoption Report,* Kravik incisively asked: "What has prevented placement of these children in the past: the child's handicapping condition or

our perception of it, which subsequently determines our attitudes and efforts on behalf of that child?" Adoption workers and parent applicants
had indeed stigmatized disabled children in adoption for decades, with
major consequences for these children's fates. Most adopters and adoption workers, like other Americans, largely viewed these children as a
"burden, a disaster or an object of pity."[3] These attitudes typically signaled
which children social workers considered risky for applicants to adopt.
But as some adoption professionals beginning in the 1960s assessed the
feasibility of disabled children's adoption, they argued that society *made*
a child risky by stigmatizing her.[4] For her part, Kravik implored readers to overcome prejudicial attitudes towards children with disabilities,
to see the child behind the label, and to put the child, rather than the impairment, first. Her call exemplified adoption professionals' growing challenge to disability stigma during this period.

As adoption professionals reconfigured risk, they invited adopters to
accept disabled children into their families. Social workers began to ask
families to overcome their fears about disability's impact upon their adoption: fears about a child's future, her lack of belonging in one's family, or
medical expenses. They proposed that parents replace those fears with
love and acceptance.[5] In essence, social workers deployed an overcoming
narrative with their clients that American health and education professionals traditionally applied to disabled people themselves.

The Overcoming Narrative

What disability studies scholars call the overcoming narrative is a standard trope in cultural representations of people with disabilities that up-
holds the ideals of hope, courage, perseverance, and independence so important in American national mythology. In mid to late twentieth-century
America, this overcoming narrative was a central component of rehabilitation, medical, and special education discourses. By promoting overcoming, professionals in these fields argued that clients could achieve functional independence. They asserted that those who worked hard would,
despite any obstacles, ultimately achieve success and that, conversely,
any disability-related dependency resulted from moral and psychological
failure.[6]

From polio narratives that stressed FDR's "triumph over disease and
disability" to the inspirational stories of children with various disabilities

in telethons, the essential formula of the overcoming narrative for people with disabilities is that to rehabilitate their presumed spoiled identities, they had to overcome their limitations, avoid self-pity by being constantly cheerful, be brave, cope and strive well, and inspire the nondisabled to escape social invalidity.[7] Although a disabled person's overcoming always fell short of the complete validity imparted by medical cure, it conferred "provisional social legitimacy and partial social acceptance."[8]

In the adoption context, social workers primarily addressed the overcoming narrative to parents, and more specifically, to mothers. They utilized this distinct narrative within an environment where adoption professionals saw a stable and permanent family as a precondition to a child's healthy development.[9]

The adoption overcoming narrative involved two basic but interrelated stages. The first stage was the moment of decision, when parents would opt to overcome their fears of the impact of disability upon their family to adopt a disabled child. In the second stage, which centered on praxis, parents would need to continually mobilize love and acceptance to achieve overcoming and a sense of family belonging. To be sure, American society expected parents of nonadopted children with disabilities to push and inspire their children to overcome by exercising love. But the adoption overcoming narrative is distinct from the biological case since social workers not only asked *parent applicants* here to overcome, but they also requested that parents consciously *choose* a child with a disability and then work to *achieve* attachment and family cohesion through love and acceptance.

Furthermore, adoption professionals believed love and acceptance had therapeutic value, not only for children with disabilities but for all marginalized children; this discourse offered a cure for hard-to-place children deprived of family. They thought that bestowing love and acceptance—acts presumably performed by mothers—offered a child protection and facilitated her growth.[10] In this narrative, love functioned as a corrective to applicants' fears about bringing the double stranger (disabled and adopted) into one's family. Specifically, love could mitigate parental fears about the risks involved in raising a child with a disability. A powerful force, love could enable changes to the horizon of family itself.[11] Adoption professionals positioned the act of overcoming as indispensable to evolving adoption conditions since it addressed the problem of prejudice, stigma, and difference and tackled the growing need for these children's placement.[12] Although they applied the mantra of love and acceptance to all children they labeled "hard-to-place" or "special needs"—older, minority and mixed race, siblings, and handicapped, which attests to the entangled and intersecting histories of race, age, and disability—I focus on the overcoming narrative as it applies to adopters of disabled children because practicing love and acceptance for these parents meant, among other things, helping their child overcome her disability. In the case of these children, then, adopters and adoptees engaged in a dual overcoming process.

More expansive notions of adoptability enabled social workers to newly consider certain kinds of children with disabilities, often over others. Researchers sought to identify which parent applicants could overcome their fears and fulfill the promise of love and acceptance. They tried to construct a typology that reflected the attributes of parents who had already adopted children with disabilities as a way to recruit parents with similar profiles. For their part, parents also used the language of love and acceptance to describe their life with a disabled child, even as many challenged the agency obstacles that had stood in their way. Parents seemed to narrate their overcoming stories in more nuanced ways than professionals; they detailed the gendered, emotional labor involved in raising a child with a disability, depicting it as a process that entailed rewards and struggles, dedication, ambivalence, and doubt, rather than simply a call to action.[13]

Preconditions for Overcoming

The Child Welfare League of America (CWLA) opened the door to the adoption overcoming narrative when it broadened its definition of adoptability in 1958. The CWLA recommended that adoption be considered for "any child who is deprived of care by his natural parents, who is or can be made legally free for adoption, and who has the capacity to form a relationship with new parents and develop in a family."[14] Although the CWLA standards stated that "there are no hereditary factors that should automatically rule out adoption," the organization did not recommend adoption for children who needed care in a "facility other than a family home" or who social workers believed could not emotionally function in a family setting.[15]

The CWLA revised its 1958 standards from those in 1948, which stated that an adoptable child must be able to "benefit from normal family life" and have a family found that would "accept him with his history and capacities."[16] The CWLA's more liberal 1958 stance on adoptability reflected what the organization's director stated was the ability of adoption leaders to recognize "the strength, the courage and the fiber of families in America to accept what comes and also to be really accepting of less than perfect children. In essence, we have recognized the power of love."[17]

Agencies variously interpreted and implemented the CWLA standards in the years that followed. But the new standards prompted them to reconceptualize children with diagnosed "handicaps" as potentially adoptable, particularly those with correctable impairments or children whom social workers thought of as having mild or moderate impairments.[18]

The CWLA's reconfigured concept of adoptability aligned with a broad challenge to traditional notions of the American family in the 1960s and 1970s. As both parents in a middle-class family increasingly entered the national economy, so too the American family economy changed, helping to reshape relationships and obligations. These developments resulted in a new concept of family as a unit "based on ties of affection and the actual performance of the child-rearing role," not just one based on biological ties.[19] Emotional labor became a measurement of good parenting, particularly of good maternal practice.[20] As Americans reconceptualized family in more permissive ways, they increasingly accepted adoption as a legitimate form of family.

The CWLA's new stance on adoptability also reflected the changing demographic characteristics of children in adoption. Whereas postwar social work attitudes sanctioned white women's decision to relinquish their child as a solution for their out-of-wedlock births, as time went on, transformations in women's reproductive rights and in adoptive practice left fewer and fewer white "normal, healthy newborns" available for agency adoption as compared to applicant demand.[21] Already in the mid-1960s, there were an estimated 182 parent applicants for every one hundred available white "healthy" infants.[22] Once the birth control pill became available to married and then unmarried women, the number of unwanted white births diminished even further.[23] In addition, as the stigma of out-of-wedlock births decreased and the number of children living in single-parent homes increased, white unmarried women were less likely to place their children for adoption. By 1975, agencies throughout the country started telling prospective applicants that they might be waiting between three to five years for a white, nondisabled infant.[24]

To have enough children for the number of parent applicants—like they had done in the immediate postwar period with children with pathological heredity—many agencies considered marginalized children who had yet to be included in adoption. Zelma Felten, associate director of the foster care project of the CWLA, remarked in 1959 that although most applicants still wanted able-bodied infants, "We have also found that adoptive parents are willing to take certain so-called risks and will assume responsibility for children who are handicapped." As adopters considered raising handicapped children, adoption professionals began to believe that "these children are not 'seconds.' "[25]

Felten questioned whether what agency workers and physicians deemed the risks of older children or children with handicaps in adoption were real or imagined; it all depended, she suggested, upon the family's perspective. Anita Colville of the Child Adoption Service of the State Charities Aid Association agreed, citing parents' need to freely decide about "the risks they will take."[26] Leaders like Felten and Colville introduced an idea of risk as a fluid concept—contingent upon parents' perceptions— rather than the previous dichotomous one where social workers deemed a child risky or not. The latter view, associated with earlier notions of individualized risk, often led social workers to determine children with impairments as "unwarranted risks for successful adoption." They refused to place children with "even minor medical conditions" until the "defects were improved or corrected." The notion that risk was contingent upon parents' perceptions also challenged the prior casework precept that agencies "should take every step to minimize risk, to protect applicants, and to assure success."[27]

Many adopters continued to believe, however, that they should avoid taking any risk to a successful adoption and that disabled children were much less desirable than other children. They conceptualized a "successful adoption" as a secure placement that brought satisfaction to *both* parents and child. Many parents still wanted children that resembled themselves. Adopter-child ratios seem to bear this out. In 1964, as in 1959, there were seven applicants for every one "white, normal infant." The opposite was true for marginalized children, including those social workers described as handicapped. Some experts therefore suggested that long-term boarding care with caring foster parents could be the best option for many children deemed "hard-to-place."[28] These trends transpired alongside a steady rise in adoption in general: from 96,000 adoptions in 1958 to 166,000 in 1968.

The disparity between applicants and available, healthy, "normal" children led agencies to move away from applying traditional matching criteria toward using more flexible child and applicant eligibility standards. Using the same logic to address a growing number of children of color needing adoption, agencies increased the number of transracial place-ments, especially for Native American and African American children.[29] Together, concerns about adopter-adoptee ratios, civil rights activism, and identity politics movements compelled adoption leaders to rethink how much of a "difference, difference actually made" when it came to building and sustaining families. By the mid-1960s and later, these leaders began to eschew notions of the disabled adoptee as a quintessential stranger and started to more fully acknowledge difference within and among families.[30] Adoption researchers, adult adoptees, and some adoptive parents also forcefully argued that adoption itself, and adoption records in particular, should no longer be shrouded in secrecy.[31] Within the context of these "adoptions revolutions," adoption professionals reappraised the capacity of a "handicapped child to provide satisfactions to an adoptive parent, the willingness of adoptive applicants to take risks, or the desire to adopt a child because of *his* need for parents."[32]

In the late 1950s and early 1960s, CWLA leaders, like Zitha Turitz and Joseph Reid, both of the CWLA, specifically challenged agency assump-tions that children with "severe" or "irremediable" disabilities were only receivers of pleasure and "satisfaction" in a family relationship and not givers; they newly conceptualized family as a relationship where parents and children should derive satisfaction equally and where the "desire to rear a child, to love and be loved as a parent can be satisfied by children with a wide range of characteristics."[33] Researchers like David Franklin (research director of the Children's Home Society of California) and Fred Massarik (associate professor in behavioral science at UCLA) questioned the concept of limited adoptability by invoking the same language of love and acceptance as their social work counterparts. They asked: "Who is 'the adoptable child'? Essentially it is the child whom parents can accept, who can give and receive love, who can benefit from family life." These re-searchers pointed out that although an adoptable child in the past would have meant one in "sound physical condition," their 1969 study on adopt-ees with impairments showed that "none of the defects, from minor to severe," precluded eligibility.[34]

Severity, Cure, and Overcoming

Even in this period of newly expansive thinking about what kind of chil-dren qualified as adoptable, most agencies limited adoptability to children diagnosed with "remediable" or "correctable" impairments. In 1968 and then again in 1971, the CWLA affirmed that "no child should be denied consideration for adoption because of . . . a handicap that does not prevent him from living in a family" with the caveat that children must have the "capacity to become an *integral part* [my italics] of family." Social workers indicated whether an impairment was remediable as a way to define the edges of adoptability and acceptability. Besides weighing the risk of an unsuccessful placement, agencies also considered their available time, effort, and money to place disabled children. Some agencies continued to argue that it was simply impractical to try to place older and disabled children.[35]

By the mid to late 1970s, however, opinions began to change due to a variety of developments. Social workers' discourse about risk had shifted to consider social barriers, adoption leaders established specialized adoption agencies catering to children with disabilities, and deinstitutionalization was underway.[36] As a result, a growing number of professionals and parents became open to the idea that children with "irremediable," "severe," and even multiple impairments should be afforded the opportunity for adoption, though consensus on what "irremediable" or "severe" meant proved elusive.[37] Still, by dividing children's disabilities into categories of severity (irremediable and remediable; minor, moderate, and severe) social workers engaged in an even more precise form of risk coding than the kind that had started in the immediate postwar period; that is, they parsed children according to a more specific relative scale of risk to determine the likelihood of what they considered a successful or unsuccessful placement.

By distinguishing between children with remediable and irremediable impairments, social workers considered the practical consequences of accepting child candidates who had impairments with different levels of severity. These consequences could impact the potential for parents and children to successfully overcome disability. So, for example, even as Felten argued that children with disabilities weren't seconds, she explained that social workers had to consider the "implications of the handicap" when placing such a child through adoption. She reiterated the need for thorough medical examinations and contended that the severity of the handicap, whether or not it was progressive, what it meant to the child's maturation, and the extent of necessary medical care should be of utmost concern to social workers.[38]

Agencies instructed staff to assess the social, financial, and cultural impact of bringing a disabled child into a family and the extent to which parents could overcome their fears in order to deploy love and acceptance. An agency intake form in 1968 bears this out. It directed the social worker to check off whether or not a child's impairment was remediable and the estimated cost, in time and money, to address it. The social worker had to note whether the impairment affected the child's appearance or physical and social functioning.[39] If Americans viewed children with "irremediable handicaps" as perpetually socially incapacitated, then it was not a leap for social workers to deem it impossible for such children to "benefit from family life" and to have the "opportunity for healthy personality development."[40] As Viola Bernard explained in 1964, adoptability depended upon a social worker's assessment that a child could become part of a family: "that is, on his emotional capacity to benefit from family relationships, and in turn to contribute to the happiness of his adoptive family." These conditions were not unlike those articulated by social worker Lucie Browning a decade earlier and by the attachment expert John Bowlby.[41] Yet in this period, it also depended upon an agency's ability to persist in finding a suitable family for the child, and in "helping to *overcome remediable defects as well as to allay groundless fears*" [my italics].[42]

Adoption leaders' commentary on the relationship between (un)correctable impairments and the ability to overcome fit squarely within extant vocational rehabilitation and medical definitions of disability that emphasized capabilities and limitations on physical functioning.[43] Rehabilitation practitioners focused on having clients gain economic and social independence by maximizing normative ability. Vocational rehabilitation professionals utilized the somato-psychological "whole man theory," which, as a deficit model, pathologized people with disabilities. Adherents of whole man theory assumed disabled people were emotionally maladjusted and abnormal as a result of their impairments. They argued that people with disabilities suffered from loss and therefore lacked the motivation and ability to cope in society.[44] Instead of civil rights, political and social equality, and fighting against discrimination, rehabilitation professionals emphasized breaking down "barriers in the minds of disabled people." They believed that a client had to compensate psychologically for her losses, to overcome social, physical, and emotional obstacles, and to conform to society, rather than the other way around.[45] To increase their success rates for these goals, rehabilitation counselors employed "creaming"; that is, they selected less severely disabled, and more socially acceptable, clients to more readily rehabilitate or cure them.[46]

Although adoption workers never explicitly used the term "creaming," they employed the same logic when they differentiated children's adoptability according to correctable or irremediable impairments. Social workers looked for ways to place a growing number of children with disabilities, but only those who they thought had the potential to fulfill what they conceptualized as belonging in families.

As in the prior period, adoption professionals' discussions about whether an impairment was remediable reflected the state of American medicine when correcting, or managing, certain impairments was increasingly possible. Novel medical technologies in this period, like surgical procedures, new pharmaceuticals, and modern assistive devices, tried to mitigate the effects of some physical, psychiatric, and behavioral impairments.[47] Social workers embraced society's enthusiasm for the promises of medicine and expected that parents would prefer a child who could benefit from those gains; they assumed that after overcoming their fears of risk, parents would avail their child of medical advancements to facilitate the child's *own* journey of overcoming. That is, if a physician deemed a child's impairment correctable, social workers expected parents to pursue rehabilitation or cure for their children as part of the praxis of overcoming; they believed that working toward these aims testified to parental dedication and love.

Social workers' focus on a child's capability was rooted in a cultural moment of democratization and equal opportunity that stressed the "dignity and worthiness of the individual," even as it based those values on ideas of normalcy. Applying this sentiment to the adoption overcoming narrative, social workers urged adopters to focus on a child's potential and abilities. Their and a physician's assessment of a child's adoptability would determine her functional capacities. Disability scholar Harlan Hahn has explained that this kind of framing often led to the "questionable assumption that there is a close relationship between a person's physical capabilities and his or her capacity to engage in . . . significant activities in life."[48] One such activity was the ability to engage and develop in a family. Indeed, adoption workers (and leaders) believed a child's development "for life in a democratic society can best take place in a family."[49]

Social workers who demarcated an impairment's remediability therefore opened up a space for a child's rehabilitation and recuperation; they made room for the "flexible normalization" of the disabled body via the family wherein a child could move from the "boundary areas of abnormality and return to the center of society" even as social workers ultimately reinforced the able-bodied family.[50]

From "Hard to Place" to "Special Needs"

As the boundaries of adoptability shifted, adoption professionals replaced the term "hard-to-place" with "special needs." "Special needs" underlined the social work principle that every child had the right to the best home possible, although the choice of best home depended upon the ability of parents to fulfill each child's special needs. Besides referring to a child's special needs *after* placement, the term "special needs" also indicated adoptions involving children having special needs *for* placement. Such placement needs often included specialized services, agency financial outlay, extra efforts to find prospective parents, and postplacement services. More often, adoption professionals used the term special needs to refer to children who required certain casework (e.g., "special needs children") as a shorthand, with "for placement" implied. Depending upon the adoption professional who defined "special needs children," the population could include older children (two or older or five or older, depending upon the state), members of minority groups or mixed race (terms used in the sources), and children who had "atypical patterns of needs and responses."[51] Many children of color were disabled and/or older, yet adoption professionals generally separated out these categories, thus eliding intersections as well as in-group differences.[52] Often, professionals considered sibling groups as having special needs for placement too. The term usually referred to both foster and nonfoster care children.

The term "special needs" itself first appeared during the Progressive Era in discussions about dependent children. It denoted children needing special care to achieve an optimal home life to protect their "right to childhood." These included mentally or physically disabled children, delinquent children, and dependent children.[53] In most early 1960s adoption discussions, the term appeared alongside "hard to place" but then largely replaced the latter; if social workers used "hard-to-place" thereafter, "so-called" often preceded it, eliciting skepticism about its claims.[54] The internal subcategories, however, remained intact.

The critique of the term "hard-to-place" began around the 1950s when scholars like Henry Maas, Bernice Boehm, and Donald Chambers began to question who was responsible for creating the label. Instead of espousing the belief that some children were inherently hard to place, these researchers asked whether agency practices themselves had contributed to the problem of the hard-to-place child. Maas wrote in 1960: "One wonders whether it is not only the role of adoptive parents which agencies set, but also to a larger extent that we have thus far realized the image of an unadoptable child."[55] After discovering in her 1958 case-control study, "Deterrents to the Adoption of Children in Foster Care," that there were "no children of less than average intelligence" in her sample, Boehm asked, "Do we really believe that children in the dull-normal group do not need or should not have permanent adoptive families of their own? If so, do the adoptive families share this opinion, or is this practice based on our own anxiety?"[56]

Why did this shift in language occur? Historian Veronica Strong-Boag has argued that post–World War II social workers in Canada used the term "special" for such children to attract "normal" families to no avail.[57] In the US, different parties tended to utilize a variety of terms, although there was no exact rule. According to Christopher Unger, a psychologist and the agency Spaulding for Children's research director, social workers commonly used the labels "hard-to-place" and "unadoptable." Parent and professional groups used the terms "waiting," "parentless," and "special needs," to increase awareness of children who remained unplaced, some of whom languished in foster care.[58]

Parent adoption advocacy groups that emerged in the late 1950s, 1960s, and 1970s helped propel the rhetorical shift from "hard to place" to "special needs" into professional and public discourse. Advocacy groups pushed this language shift to address agency prejudices and public stigma that had left large numbers of children without permanent families. These groups felt "the use of their terms will help to remove some of the stigma traditionally suffered by the unplaced child."[59] Advocates drew from trends in the fields of psychiatry, psychology, and sociology that analyzed the social dynamics of constructing marginalized identities.[60]

For their part, professionals working in the field of what was called mental retardation during this time emphasized the term "special" to describe their constituency (especially special education) while parent disability advocates with intellectually disabled, biological children stressed the "needs" part of the equation; it does not seem that parent disability advocates put the two terms together at the time. Instead, parent disability advocacy groups who addressed mental retardation (e.g., National Association of Parents and Friends of Retarded Children; NARC), along with other disability organizations dealing with cerebral palsy, autism, and epilepsy, developed the umbrella term "developmental disabilities" in the late 1960s. This term was later officially enshrined in the Developmentally Disabled Assistance and Bill of Rights Act (P.L. 94-103) of 1975 (DD Act).

By using the term "special needs," parent adoption advocates tried to discard the idea of burden affiliated with earlier framings of disability risk. Instead, they emphasized an individual child's needs and the necessity that parents and adoption workers accept difference.[61] Despite the influence of such ideas, social workers only gradually and unevenly integrated the term "special needs" into professional discourse.

In the mid to late 1960s, many adoption thinkers who accepted this shift in terminology began to explicitly argue that children themselves weren't necessarily hard to place, but that racial and disability prejudices that shaped parental desires made them so. Instead, parents were "hard-to-find."[62] Elizabeth Cole, director of the North American Center on Adoption (NACA), argued in 1975 that using the term "hard-to-place" actually blamed the victim. "The terms reflected less on the true characteristics of the child and more on the attitudes and experiences of those using the term."[63]

By applying the label "special needs" to children they categorized as handicapped, minority, older, or siblings, adoption professionals reconfigured the notion of risk as something inherently located in the child to something instead based upon her external needs. Such needs included a loving family, a home, adequate services, and medical treatment.[64] Adoption professionals solidified the term "special needs" in the late 1970s and 1980s. By 1982, the CWLA implored workers to view the "disabled child" as one who "has a problem needing special help, rather than seeing the child as the problem."[65]

Special Needs and the Praxis of Overcoming

With time, more adoption workers agreed that children with special needs deserved to be valued, acknowledged, loved, accepted, and placed.[66] They believed that parents' ability to fulfill a child's special needs implied the capacity to overcome their fears, embrace acceptance, and perform the caring labor of love.[67] These were the essential steps of the adoption overcoming narrative. Parents' ability to overcome their fears about what disability could mean for their family signified their ability to fully accept such a child. In this way, they made the "double stranger" their own. A focus on needs in the adoption overcoming narrative established a locus for parents' efforts in the praxis stage of overcoming. These acts mirrored the classic overcoming narrative in that disability was assumed to be something to fear or pity and the act of overcoming was figured a source of inspiration.[68]

A similar appeal for love and acceptance occurred in the field of mental retardation in the early 1960s. Through a confessional literature, parents endorsed "true acceptance" of a child so that they could furnish her with a promising future and fulfill the necessity of satisfactory parenthood.[69] Love and acceptance provided a socially sanctioned way to lift the veil of shame and guilt that caregivers with intellectually disabled children felt in earlier years. As one journalist stated in a parent advice manual on children with mental retardation in 1959, "An intelligent parent of a retarded child must have a tremendous reservoir of courage, endless patients [sic], staunch faith and enduring love if she (or he) is to help the child adjust to a world for which he is poorly equipped."[70] Other experts, however, used "acceptance" to push parents with disabled children to apply blunt realism when raising their child. According to these experts, parents (i.e., mothers) needed to acknowledge that cure was unlikely. Instead, the parent needed to try to secure the present and future welfare of their disabled child.[71] They cautioned mothers not to neglect other family members to provide too much care their disabled child because the latter could keep her child dependent.[72] By contrast, Americans expected a father to train his disabled son in tasks deemed culturally appropriate for boys, rather than to be a caregiver like a mother.

In adoption, love and acceptance followed from adopters' deliberate act of overcoming their fears of risks about the assumed "burden" of children with disabilities to attain a route to familial belonging. Displaying love and acceptance formed the praxis phase of the overcoming narrative; that is, the parents' caring labor and emotional work, seen as particularly integral to expressions of mothering, was necessary to promote a child's development and integration. Adoption professionals used the overcoming narrative to assuage adopters' fears, bolster and sustain their parental resolve, and provide a route for optimism. The gendered hard work of parental love and acceptance, they argued, would all but guarantee the social and emotional adoption that ideally accompanied the legal adoption.[73]

Furthermore, parents' overcoming enabled the *child's* overcoming. This dual overcoming reflected the connectedness between parent and child and formed an essential way to reap the rewards of family life. Mrs. Neville Weeks of the Brookwood Child Care Agency in Brooklyn, for instance, argued in 1956 that agencies should not necessarily correct a child's physical impairment (which also lengthened the child's time in foster or custodial care) because that act may "deprive the child and his prospective parents of the mutual satisfaction and pleasure they might find in working towards these ends together."[74] She urged social workers not to measure a child's "potential for love" unless they were given a chance to meet potential parents willing to take a "'calculated risk.'"[75] For her part, Anita Colville of the State Charities Aid Association argued that one way to become a parent was to help manage a child's overcoming; parents would solidify their love for their disabled child by supporting and caring for her through her challenges.[76] Drawing from success stories of overcoming, adoption professionals argued that both the parent and the child should engage in overcoming efforts to all but guarantee the child's belonging.[77] Moreover, overcoming could offer adopters a pathway to rehabilitate any marginal characteristics of their own identities. All of these overcoming acts would ostensibly create a socially validated adoptive family much like an assumed intact normal family.

Writers on adoption contended that love and acceptance would help overcome disability's trials and deliver hope and inspiration.[78] They represented parents as heroes. Media stories of the time, for instance, featured adopted children who had experienced so much love and commitment by their new parents (especially mothers) that they had either fully or partially recovered. Alice Lake's "Babies for the Brave," published in the *Saturday Evening Post* in 1954, is one such story.

The article describes the "courageous band" of American parents who adopted "blind, deaf or even dwarfed." Through stories about couples "willing to risk greatly," Lake portrayed how the tireless, mostly gendered dedication to home medical treatments or intense emotional support demonstrated how acceptance and love could restore a child to normalcy: "Sometimes a nearly miraculous recovery of health can result from the adoptive placement of a handicapped child."[79] Helen Hallinan, administrative supervisor of the adoption service of the Catholic Home Bureau in New York City, added, "We ask how much love can really do. . . . It can do almost anything."[80]

Journalists reiterated this message in other newspaper articles, like "Adopting a Multi-Handicapped Child," published in the *New York Times* in 1976. Stephanie, a child with intellectual and physical impairments transformed once placed in the Rossow household: "When Stephanie came to the Rossow family," stated her physical therapist, "she could not hold her head up, roll over in bed, or come to a seated position by herself. She was a very withdrawn and unresponsive child." Because of the love and understanding of the family, the physical therapist argued, "Stephanie is a different person. . . . Stephanie can now hold her head high and is proud of her many accomplishments."[81]

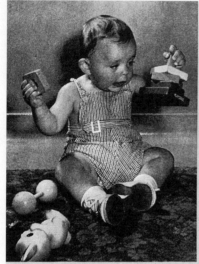
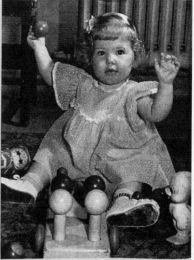

Eleven-month-old "Tim" hopes to find a home of his own—even though he's deaf. Adoption workers once considered such tots hopeless risks.

Bright-eyed little "Susy," nearly blind, is looking for a family. As many as eighty thousand "hard-to-place" children may be available for adoption.

Babies for the Brave By ALICE LAKE

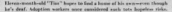

"Unadoptable" was the label once put on crippled babies, blind babies, babies with "bad heredity." But now thousands of childless couples are discovering happiness in adopting the children nobody wanted — and the babies are getting loving parents of their own.

BARELY a half-dozen years ago, a baby eligible for adoption through a reputable agency carried a gilt-edged guaranty, much like that of a purebred Holstein calf. A cloudless heredity and a little body unblemished by defect were assured as a matter of course. Less risk than in natural parenthood was the keynote of the transaction.

Yesterday's adoption workers would have recoiled in horror from the gambles which they are now asking childless couples to take. The unadoptables—children who are blind, deaf or even dwarfed; babies whose parents are epileptic or mentally ill; older children with severe emotional damage—are, by a miracle of faith, gaining parents of their own.

Although nine out of ten childless couples still ask for a normal healthy infant of good stock, a surprising number of brave Americans are settling for much less, and finding great joy in their choice.

Jean and Paul Talmadge, a Connecticut couple, belong to this courageous band. (Their names and the names of other adopting couples have been changed for this story.) After nine barren years of

marriage, Jean and Paul adopted a little boy and then a girl. These were old-style, unrisky adoptions. When they asked Ruth Taft, adoption supervisor of Children's Services of Connecticut, in Hartford, to find them another baby, she told them about Donald.

Donald was born in January, 1951. His birthplace was a state mental hospital. His mother had been committed to the hospital a year earlier with a diagnosis of schizophrenia, most serious of the mental diseases. There she had become pregnant. The father was also a patient and a schizophrenic.

When he was a month old, Donald was placed in a foster home. Danger signals consistent with his unstable heredity appeared almost immediately. An angry eczema of nervous origin flared up on his face, arms and body. The psychologist who tested him at three months found him unusually tense. At eight months, a report on Donald read: "Nervous and unstable."

What kind of adoptive parents could take the risk that Donald entailed? Looking at him, one saw a tense weepy baby, ugly with the red splotches of

eczema. Behind him lay the shadow of a mental hospital. Ahead there was only a question mark.

The pediatrician caring for Donald told Miss Taft bluntly that she was "completely crazy" even to consider adoption for the baby. Nevertheless, she persisted. When he was ten months old she consulted three prominent child psychiatrists, seeking to clarify heredity's role in such a case.

The first answer she received was discouraging. "It would be my own impression," the psychiatrist reported, "that such a combination of factors would weigh heavily for the possibility of this child becoming schizophrenic."

The two other doctors were more hopeful. "My own feeling," one of them wrote, "is that the character of the emotional relationship to parents is the main keystone to the personality development of any individual. Under proper care the child would be expected to develop and progress normally."

If any couple represented "proper care," it was Jean and Paul Talmadge. The Talmadges are warm and unruffled. They live in the country in a hundred-year-old farmhouse with ten acres of ground.

26

FIGURE 4. Alice Lake, "Babies for the Brave," *Saturday Evening Post*, July 1, 1954. *Babies for the Brave* article and photos © SEPS licensed by Curtis Licensing Indianapolis, IN. All rights reserved.

Movie writers and directors also featured stories about the therapeutic value of love and acceptance. *Room for One More* (1952), starring Cary Grant and Betsy Drake, was a Hollywood adaptation of Anne Perrott Rose's 1950 memoir with the same title. Mr. Rose resists fostering the emotionally disturbed adolescent Jane and the brace-wearing (because of polio) Jimmy John, but the humanitarian Mrs. Rose insists on exercising patience.[82]

Like many other families in real life, the Roses foster instead of adopt because they cannot afford the medical expenses and need the board payments. Mrs. Rose's love and dedication as central components of her performance of mothering enable both children to become integral members of the Rose family; they "touchingly" overcome, according to one review of the film, the "resentments of unwanted children."[83] In the movie, Jimmy John also overcomes in the classic sense; he abandons his combative behavior, rides a bike, hikes a long distance, and wins the Boy Scout Eagle badge where he accepts that honor without his leg braces—he is cured.

The Academy Award–winning 1977 documentary "Who Are the DeBolts?" conveyed a similar trope. In that movie, eighteen of the nineteen DeBolt children have various impairments. The film, which featured both international and domestic adopted kids, shows how the parents embrace the attitude that "nurturing children doesn't mean coddling them." The movie reveals how several children with mobility impairments have to learn how to navigate stairs and how the DeBolts are "spared" the guilt feelings of birth parents because they did not give birth to a child with a disability. It also displays how children with physical impairments "have to take a look early on" at themselves and say "'this is who I am.'" As Dorothy, the mother who helps her children overcome their disabilities, remarks: "Most people think we are nuts, but around here are incredible highpoints." The narrator adds: "Getting to know Karen DeBolt [a girl with no arms or legs] gives all of us a new idea of what a whole person is." Speaking to the capacity of children with disabilities to give satisfaction to their parents, the narrator continues: "If a handicap means limitation," what about a handicapped child "can't laugh, can't give, can't love?"[84]

In the adoption overcoming narrative, the acts of accepting the risks of raising a disabled child and imparting love embodied the caring labor of adoptive parenthood, especially adoptive motherhood.[85] This type of motherhood entailed the hard work required to fully integrate a nonrelative child into one's family and make her one's own. Adoption professionals, the media, and the public believed that "special" parents who adopted children with disabilities, though still in the minority, "affirmed full responsibility for parenthood with all its inherent satisfactions and risks."[86] As overcomers, they mastered their fears and mobilized personal agency in a way that Americans usually considered above and beyond the average parent.[87] Mothers, in particular, showed resourcefulness, courage, and resilience. Their "acceptance of risk, [and] the struggle against odds on behalf of a child, seemed to call forth unexpected adaptability and yielded significant personal social rewards."[88] By definition, they were superparents. To adoption professionals, these women were heroes.

Because it was inherently an idealized narrative, professionals' call for love and acceptance in adoption overcoming glossed over the emotional and financial vulnerabilities of some families who either gave birth to or adopted children with disabilities. Yet in its intention, the adoption overcoming narrative offered an answer to the needs of dependent children with disabilities and to potential parents within the sanctioned unit of family.

Kathryn and Tanya's story

Although in-depth parent accounts of the adoption of children with disabilities are rare for this period, one memoir deserves mention for its consistency with and distinctions from the adoption overcoming narrative. The memoir even grabbed the attention of Elizabeth Cole, the director of the NACA. Cole praised the memoir as a chronicle "filled with sentiment but devoid of sentimentality"; Tanya's story was "more than an account of the adoption of one little girl . . . Tanya is Every Child."[89] Tanya's symbolic status as "every child" reflected adoption leaders' efforts during this time to "reconcile difference with equality" in adoption practice. In its connection to the adoption overcoming narrative, the memoir exemplifies not only the caring labor of love and acceptance but also the intense, conflicted feelings that sometimes accompanied that labor.

Kathryn Wheeler, a mother who adopted a daughter through Lutheran Child and Family Services of Illinois detailed her experiences in a piece called *Tanya: The Building of a Family through Adoption.* Less lofty than the adoption leaders', media's, or researchers' formulation, the adoption overcoming narrative's basic elements are still present in *Tanya.* The text, however, is more nuanced than the former formulation as it explores the rewards, pains, doubts, and persistence involved in adopting and raising a child with a disability.[90] Like other parent advocates of the time, Wheeler offers a stinging critique of expert opinion, a rebuke of disability stigma, and a challenge to the idea of the foreignness of the adopted disabled child. As a parent, Wheeler felt the stigma associated with disability intensely. She replaced stigma and prejudice with her account of love and acceptance.

Before her adoption at age seven, Tanya went through several foster homes, surgeries, and medical treatments. This was typical of dependent

children with disabilities. Physicians diagnosed her with "multiple skeletal and muscular anomalies" at birth and later incorrectly diagnosed her
with Morquio's disease and then again with spondyloepiphyseal dysplasia.
Ultimately, the diagnosis of scoliosis held (although it is unclear from the
text whether even scoliosis is a full or accurate diagnosis).[91]

Wheeler decided to adopt a disabled child because she encountered
a description of Tanya in a newspaper column. She read books on the
subject which, she noted, were "terrible: either grossly maudlin or coldly
antiseptic." She also worried that her own marginal status could potentially disqualify her as an adoptive applicant: her financial situation, her
interfaith marriage, and her intention of working after adopting.[92]

Wheeler critiqued the paternalism that doctors exhibited and instead
privileged the value of caring labor. She described the frustration she felt
because of a series of misdiagnoses she received from experts she relied
upon. Her growing distrust of doctors caused her to depend even more
upon her own research.[93] In this way, Wheeler's account demonstrates
scholar Chloe Silverman's observation that acts of love are part of biomedical work. Parents like Wheeler were "expert amateurs"; they drew
from an intimate "situated knowledge" of their children, questioned doctors' advice, and sought their own solutions based in love.[94] Even more,
parents who wrestled with professional opinion and chronicled those
struggles took part in a larger move to reject the idea that an objective
notion of disability risk existed. Instead, parents personalized the experience of disability and demanded that they have input into the assessment
of risk.[95]

Some physicians exhibited insensitivity, discourteousness, and disapproval to Wheeler. Others were arrogant and condescending. Unaware
that Wheeler had adopted Tanya, one doctor invoked the "fetal rights"
debate of the time, which held women responsible for birth defects, especially pregnant women and those addicted to drugs. In line with this
thinking, he accused Wheeler of taking drugs while pregnant as a possible
reason for Tanya's medical problems.[96]

Wheeler attributed such behavior to a disapproval of disability in general and of the adoption of disabled children in particular. When her relatives condemned her for bringing Tanya into the family, for instance, they
claimed they were trying to "protect" the Wheelers from heartbreak and
shield the Wheelers' biological son from "injustice," embarrassment, and
resentment. But Kathryn saw through their excuses, concluding, "They
feel such adoptions are doomed."[97]

Throughout her writing, Wheeler challenged prevailing ideas about disability, parenting, childhood, and family.[98] When she described strangers' problematic responses to and stares at Tanya, Wheeler exposed feelings of frustration and dismay. She questioned the social norms surrounding disability, citing people's reactions to a disabled child as "sometimes strange." She described an instance when "one day, an elderly lady walked up to us in the grocery store and said, 'I once knew a blind lady.' 'Oh, really?' I replied. What was I supposed to say?" Wheeler noted that a year later, she was no longer aware that people stared at her and her daughter. "Is it because they no longer stare, or have I grown blind spots?"[99] Here Wheeler reappropriated the woman's absurd comment about a "blind lady" to relocate it outside of medical descriptor and mark it as her own. Her word play was a strategy to disarm the social stigma, the spectacle of difference, so often directed toward people with disabilities.[100] This "myopia" can be read as a reflection of what adoption sociologist David Kirk observed: that adopters become oblivious to the differences that outsiders see. In the process of acceptance, he argued, adopters become unaware of difference; a physically or mentally disabled child, therefore, will "come to appear normal to them." Though Kirk acknowledged adoption difference, and refrained from equating difference with damage, he nevertheless saw this strategy as double-edged in that it both obscured the "reality of difference" but also facilitated belonging.[101]

In addition to her discussion of doctors and strangers, Tanya's mother critiqued the devastating opinions of psychologists and the grave consequences of IQ testing in school. "I firmly believe IQ tests tell us practically nothing about a child's intelligence. . . . They [the testers] don't know her, How can they measure her?"[102] Her indignation at psychologists served as an expression of her love.

As her account reveals, Tanya didn't fit into a neat box, nor did the Wheeler family feel pity for their daughter/sister. Instead of seeing Tanya as subsumed by her disability—a common representation of people with disabilities often perpetuated by the overcoming narrative—Wheeler captured Tanya's personality, dreams and difficulties. These descriptions displayed Wheeler's love and acceptance of her daughter and challenged extant cultural scripts of disability.[103] According to Wheeler, Tanya was a charming girl who quickly won the Wheelers' hearts. Upon their first meeting, for instance, Tanya greeted her soon-to-be mom with cheer: "Hi! . . . My boyfriend says my nose is very soft, would you like to feel it?"[104] At the same time, Tanya keenly understood her own difference and expressed her deep frustration with it: " 'It's not fair! Everybody in the world can run and jump and tie shoes except for me!' . . . What can I say?," Wheeler sympathized. "She's right."[105]

Wheeler's honest assessment of the ups and downs of raising Tanya, the inaccessible places they encountered, her need for social support, the lack of necessary services, and her realization that the taunts of children "reflect their parents' attitudes toward people who are different" pointed to a new parental reproach of stigma and discrimination against people with disabilities at this time.[106] In contrast to the idealized calls for love and acceptance in professional adoption overcoming accounts, Wheeler captured the nuances of love and acceptance in action. She expressed the pride she felt for her daughter, the Girl Scout Brownie who wanted to be a famous actress with two husbands and twelve children; her "little social-ite."[107] Wheeler not only debunked stereotypes about disability, but also challenged firmly accepted ideas about biological kinship and the claim that attachment and bonding at the moment of birth were imperative to develop a loving relationship with one's child: "I don't believe it," she says. "Tanya was ours from the moment we saw her, whether she knew it or not."[108] Kathryn Wheeler's account showed that adopting a child with a disability involved an ongoing praxis of care, of love, and of acceptance.[109]

Reconciling Agency Barriers with the Overcoming Narrative

Evidence of parental overcoming indirectly impelled agencies that had failed to pursue disabled children's permanent placement to take steps to overcome their own attitudinal barriers. These agencies began to reassess their procedures to enable parents' pathways to overcoming. Starting in the mid to late 1950s, adoption leaders argued that children were not hard to place in and of themselves but that agencies *made* them hard to place by practices that "denied thousands of parentless children the chance of permanent homes."[110] Leaders' calls to examine the "conscious or uncon-scious attitudes on the part of caseworkers" as key nonclient barriers to these children's adoption confirmed that special needs children faced deep-seated prejudice and stigma, even by workers who were supposed to be serving their best interests.[111]

In 1956, for instance, Mrs. Neville Weeks asked whether agencies ra-tionalized their failure to place children "who happen to have been born with very dark skins, slanted eyes, unruly hair, crooked limbs or other

characteristics which do not appeal to the majority of adoptive applicants?" Weeks questioned whether agencies had exhausted all options
to find homes for noninfant children: "Do we tell ourselves that some
circumstances are beyond our control?"[112] Weeks argued that placing a
disabled child was possible, even though many social workers expressed
surprise that there were applicants open to adopting disabled children;
these social workers assumed such children had too many marks against
them.[113] She argued that workers' hesitation could be explained by attitudes about who was a worthy child candidate for adoption and by their
need to express professional authority. Some parents' attitudes were not
dissimilar: "If our applicants cannot accept some differences and idiosyn-
crasies in children, we may be right in drawing the conclusion that they are
unconsciously rejecting the adoption of a child."[114] Adopters' inflexibility,
she concluded, signified deep repudiation of adoption itself. These types
of parents would not be overcomers.

In the following decades, other leaders critiqued agency practices as a
step towards reforming them. They implored social workers to seek applicants who would love and accept children with disabilities, despite risks
and limitations. As Colville stated, "If we conclude that the handicapped
infant will best be served by adoption placement, we as agencies are responsible for finding parents for him; parents who, knowing the elements
of risk, are willing to accept them as part of their child." Invoking the idea
of dual overcoming, Colville remarked, "There are families who can find
happiness in meeting the challenge of these children, in developing their
potentialities."[115]

Despite calls to expand opportunities, barriers to the adoption of children with disabilities reflected the difficulties of squaring agency procedures with the adoption overcoming narrative. Why did some agencies
hinder such adoption? Besides the fact that social workers assumed that
handicapped children were extremely hard to parent and therefore less
desirable, researcher Katherine Nelson, like Weeks, contended that issues of professional authority were at stake. She asserted that such cases
often involved parent-child relationships that had been established *prior
to* agency involvement. These relationships "usurped" the agency's traditional role in deciding which parents were matched with which children.
Thus, agency workers could have seen these types of adoptions as akin
to independent adoption, with its sour historical relation to agency adoption. Nelson argued that posing obstacles was one way to reestablish
agency control over the placement process.[116]

Agency impediments very often had to do with workers' negative attitudes towards disability; in essence, who social workers thought were worthy of family. These workers enacted "scripts of normalcy" that created struggles between workers and adopters.[117] Take the Osborns, who met Bruce while volunteering at an institution for the severely mentally retarded. The Osborns reported that their agency told them to leave Bruce alone because it felt he was a "hopeless case" who would "never be normal."[118] After several years, the agency agreed to place Bruce in foster care with the Osborns, but the arrangement required bimonthly visits to the institution (rather than providing home care). The Osborns "thought (the institution) was a horrible place for Bruce." So they fought to take him out. Rather than place Bruce with the Osborns, however, the agency placed him in a residential care facility and denied his family visitation rights for two years, claiming that the move to the facility had been traumatic for Bruce. After two years of prodding, the agency finally allowed the Osborns visitation rights after Bruce himself requested them. Nine months later, it gave permission for Bruce to move into their home. Two years after that, they officially adopted him. Such agency behavior made parents extremely resentful, though the parents' persistence and dedication paid off.[119]

Struggles like these tested parents' resolve to overcome their fears of risk and proceed with adoption. Parents who wanted to adopt children with disabilities had to go to great lengths to do so, showing the tenacious labor of parental love and proof of acceptance, a hallmark of those who could and would overcome. When the Janis family went to their agency to adopt Melinda, a child with cerebral palsy, for instance, the social worker "thought [Ms. Janis] was the martyr type" because of how she was pursuing intensive treatment for her biological son's physical disability. "The worker thought because we'd done this . . . we didn't like the kid the way he was and couldn't accept a handicapped kid. That was contrary to the case." The worker turned the Janises down. The agency sent another worker, who offered the family Joann, who the social worker described as "a second Helen Keller, like a wild animal. They offered us Joann [an autistic child] and told us that Melinda at the time was having seizures, [that she was] hospitalized and unadoptable." The Janis family visited Joann and "decided that the kid would know I loved her if it took my entire life and even if she didn't love me back. . . . After Joann did so well with me I guess they figured I wasn't a kook."[120]

When faced with agency obstacles, some parents explained that they played the game to achieve their goal of adoption. Social worker power plays were often no match for parents' counterstrategies. According to Nelson, parents "overcome agency obstacles" by "wearing the agency down" through repeated calls to the social worker or surpassing the worker and calling on the supervisor.[121] For instance, Mrs. Frye, a social worker, wanted to adopt Ed, a child on her caseload. When the agency told her she could not request a specific child, Frye requested a child with exactly his description: "a blonde boy, deaf, about one year old, who is from [the city]. And then drew Ed without naming him."[122] These innovative tactics exhibit adopters' deep commitment to their soon-to-be children, a dedication integral to the adoption overcoming narrative.

Relaxing Eligibility Requirements

During this time, agencies more amenable to placing special needs children began to reconsider their applicant eligibility standards. This change allowed social workers to consider different types of parents who could potentially overcome beyond those traditionally considered as adopters.[123] Beginning around the 1960s, agencies started to deemphasize objective "functional" measures of parenthood such as income, age, whether or not a couple already had a biological child (most agencies in the 1950s preferred childless couples), proof of infertility, religious affiliation, or ethnic similarity. Rather, they assessed whether a particular set of parents—still largely imagined as couples—was emotionally stable and could meet the needs of a particular child.[124] One judge working in child welfare critiqued the stringent applicant requirements that agencies had applied, arguing that they needed to give up the idea of the "mythical Anglo Saxon family of two parents named Prince Charming and Cinderella."[125]

With remarkable prescience, Eleanor W. Gordon of the State Charities Aid Association in New York City, had suggested this kind of thinking already in 1945. Gordon argued that social workers often failed to acknowledge the "range of adaptability of people" and parents' "wider range of acceptance" due to agency standards of taking "as little risk as possible." Instead, she advised agencies to consider parents' flexibility when they explored "special opportunities for children"; they had to summon their imagination and focus on the child's needs.[126] Against the backdrop of a growing number of children in foster care and fewer "white, healthy infants," agencies finally began to do so at midcentury.

While some agencies continued to disqualify applicants with children, many others began to recognize that such parents were actually better equipped to parent a disabled or other special needs child because of their parenting experience. They could "extend their love and care to children who need them."[127] Similarly, adoption leaders acknowledged that foster parents, many of whom had shown love to their foster children, should be recognized as eligible adoptive candidates for marginalized children.[128] The 1973 Child Welfare League of America Revised Adoption Standards reflected this shift. Still, in 1974, many agencies and states prohibited foster adoption.

Two years later, social worker Patricia Kravik, whose words opened this chapter, argued that when it came to finding parents for children with disabilities, many existing restrictions acted as excuses, rooted in the belief that applicants for disabled children had to be "super-human, saint-like parents" because the child already had too many problems of her own. These agencies effectively used the overcoming script as a screening device. Instead of asserting an *opportunity* for overcoming, Kravik observed that these agencies required adopters to already *be* overcomers; they needed to be superparents in order to adopt. She described agencies that were "perplexed" by parents willing to adopt children with disabilities and were suspicious of their motives. These agencies even frequently disqualified such parents because they were "too" something: "too old, too young, too single, too divorced, too low in income, too religious, too uneducated, too well-educated or they have too many children or too many problems already."[129]

At the same time, adoption professionals described parents who adopted children with disabilities as heroes and inspirations; they were the overcoming superparents that caseworkers expected them to be. As Joseph Reid said in 1956 at the National Conference of Social Work, "And who would question that parents who will go to great expense to correct a serious physical defect in a child or knowingly struggle through several years of difficult adjustment with a seriously disturbed child are not worthy of praise and are not doing something for their fellow men?"[130]

Instead of shared physical, intellectual, and demographic characteristics, new matching criteria between adopters and children put stress on both a child's "potentialities" and on parents' "capacity for parenthood." Social workers had to now assess parents' ability to give love to a child "as an individual in his own right."[131] They had to evaluate parents' flexibility, adaptability, and adjustment as adults; that is, whether parent applicants had the necessary "coping" mechanisms to deal with the ups and downs of life, especially those parents who considered raising a disabled child.[132] As part of a larger challenge to traditional notions of the American family, the, CWLA published new guidelines by the 1970s that stated: "Adoptive parents should be adults who can give and receive love, who can assume responsibility for the care of another person, who can cope with problems and frustrations and who are willing to accept normal hazards and risks."[133] Love became a primary requirement for adopting.[134]

By 1980, agencies accepted divorced women and men, couples without children or those with large families, families with low income, older applicants, and single applicants in greater numbers. Single applicants could have included gay and lesbian individuals, although this is never mentioned or probably asked. Gay and lesbian couples were not allowed to adopt because same-sex marriage was not yet legal.[135]

Still, this sea change had been a long time in the making, with some agencies along the way willing to place children with nontraditional parents if they would not be adopted otherwise. In 1965, for instance, the Los Angeles County Bureau of Adoptions, a public agency, introduced the first program targeting single African American parents to find homes for "hard to place" children of the same race for whom married couples could not be found. By 1968, the CWLA admitted that a single parent was better than no parent at all.[136] Whereas agencies had previously experimented with "trial adoptions" for disabled children who had a strong relationship with their foster parent, agencies now welcomed foster parents willing to adopt their foster children.[137] Foster mother Mrs. Last, for instance, eventually adopted Denny. She remarked that she adopted because "the people [the agency] wanted him to have a home, and I didn't figure nobody else would want him because of his handicap."[138] As she explained, "People don't want no children with anything wrong with them," and she and Denny were used to one another.[139]

Changed eligibility requirements reflected the idea that family was more than, or even unrelated to, biological kinship. While David Kirk argued that Americans should acknowledge adoption as a different form of family, Clayton Hagen, supervisor of the adoption unit of Minnesota Lutheran Social Services, argued for a new vision of parenting. In 1969, he wrote that parents should "see their purpose and function as helping another human being to develop as a unique individual."[140] Once parenting could be based on something beyond one's physicality, adopting a disabled child or a child with a different colored skin was possible; a child did not have to look like one's parents (social workers viewed biological parents as largely white and nondisabled).

This new notion of parenting involved accepting unpredictable situations and therefore risk. As Hagen continued, "This concept is just as important for the biological parent as the adoptive parent in our culture. Our children must enter a world that we can neither prepare them for or protect them from because we can't know how it will be."[141] Hagen concluded that adopting the child "who is different from the average" meant that parents must be able to accept one's own differences and separate their ego from that of their child. It also meant that parents had to acknowledge that they were responsible for developing a positive identity in their child. Such a reframing of parenthood, Hagen argued, could bring about changes in parents' lives such that these children, once called hard-to-place, "may be the most desirable of all."[142]

Two years later, in a 1971 keynote address at the First Colorado Conference on Adoption, Kenneth Watson of the Chicago Child Care Society also embraced a new kind of parenting: "If we begin to perceive the adoptive family as not having to be like the biological family, we are free to do all sorts of wonderful things."[143] One of those things was agencies' ability to recruit nontraditional parents to adopt special needs children, including children with disabilities.

Agencies' freedom to consider other types of parent candidates enabled the Little People of America organization, for instance, to inquire about being considered as suitable parents for certain disabled children.[144] On October 30, 1961, Anna Dixon, coordinator of the national convention of the group, wrote a letter to the CWLA, explaining that "just like the average couple, the 'little couple's desire to have children but most often are incapable of having any of their own. We imagine that there must be children, dwarfs and midgets, who are sometimes put up for adoption." Dixon added that "we have a long list of 'little' couples who have expressed a very strong desire to adopt children with handicaps like their own"[145] and requested that if the CWLA had children "of this type" and had difficulty placing them, they should inform the Little People of America so that they could advertise this prospect at their upcoming national convention. If not, she continued, "please keep our organization on file so that in the future when you have cases of placing midgets and dwarfs you can give our people a chance to make application to adopt these children."[146]

There seems to be no follow-up to this request, but the letter reveals both an interest by "little people" in adopting children with their same disability—reflecting a belief in a seemingly automatic bio-affiliation through resemblance—and an opening by the CWLA to pass the request along to its constituent agencies.[147] For years to come, many other parents would seek children to adopt that had their same disability or the same as their biological children.[148] To these parents, such children were not strangers at all.

Identifying the Overcomers

As parent eligibility requirements relaxed, researchers and adoption leaders tried to discern a profile of parents who adopted a disabled child in order to facilitate the active evidence-based recruitment of future parents. Researchers in the early 1960s through 1980 explored which factors could predict the parents that would excel at overcoming. They examined the qualities of parents who *had already* adopted children with disabilities to identify those factors.

Researchers generally found that "marginal families" tended to adopt hard-to-place children more often than parents who social workers traditionally considered most suitable for adoptive placement. Experts found that blue-collar families, parents of mixed religion, divorced individuals, those with health problems, those who were over forty, and those with children were more accepting of children labeled hard-to-place than families social workers usually screened in for adoption.[149] Researchers also concluded that parents who already had children had the ability to "weather the unexpected"; they could overcome "developmental obstacles and physical deviation" in their adopted children.[150]

Furthermore, applicants who realized that their eligibility could be jeopardized because of a particular demographic characteristic often accepted a broadened spectrum of difference in the children they were willing to adopt. As researcher Alfred Kadushin argued in 1962, by trying to reduce the effect of their own marginality, applicants increased their flexibility and lowered their "hierarchy of preferences," to accept a "less desirable child," even a "medical[ly] disadvantaged child lest they not otherwise qualify for adoption."[151] "Less desirable" parents could be matched, therefore, with "less desirable" children.[152]

Twenty years later, researchers confirmed the correlation between parents' marginality and eligibility, finding that the *appearance* of the parents correlated with their decision to adopt a disabled child. "Families who look 'unusual' themselves," adoption experts Judith DeLeon and Judy Westerberg noted, "were more likely to adopt children who look 'unusual' as well, or who are limited intellectually." "Unusual appearance" included: "a) observable physical handicap, such as blindness; b) severe dental problems (e.g. missing teeth); c) wife significantly larger than husband (not just a little taller or heavier); d) one parent at least 100 pounds overweight or 25 pounds underweight."[153] Acknowledging the subjective nature of the term, yet still applying it unproblematically in their study, the researchers defined unusual appearances as those that most social workers would not have imagined as eligible, even in 1980, since applicant appearance had played a role in previous eligibility standards.[154] Instead of denying nontraditional parents' access to adoption, they argued that these parents were the *exact ones* that agencies should recruit. These families may not fit social workers' "traditional middle-class image of adoptive parents but . . . may, nevertheless, be able to provide the love, security and commitment" that a child needs.[155]

Besides eligibility, the complex interplay of applicant preferences, class, severity of a child's "handicap," social workers' attitudes, and notions of family belonging all produced decisions to adopt a child with a disability and to engage in overcoming.[156] Researchers cited love and acceptance as priorities for those parents who made a positive decision. Experts identified class, education, and motivation to adopt as particularly important in parents' decision to bring a child with a disability into their family.

In 1969, Franklin and Massarik cited two profiles of parents who typically adopted children with medical conditions. The first profile consisted of less well-educated parents (those who had dropped out of high school or had one to two years of college). The father was a blue-collar craftsman, skilled or semiskilled; the family was financially comfortable but "not achievement oriented." The parents went to church and believed that "a child is a child." The second profile was of a more affluent family. The father was a professional, an official, or in the corporate world. The parents of the second profile "wanted to do something special; they were motivated more by humanitarian sentiments than by personal ones."[157] Although agency workers hesitated to place a disabled child into a middle-class or upper-class family, "believing that a child who deviates from physical or health norms may not 'fit in' with the more highly achieving, better-educated couple," parents of both profiles described themselves as "close to the norm of the American family."[158] As overcomers, these parents could see the "child's worth, undiminished by his defect; they were undaunted by his developmental uniqueness; they took a hopeful, nurturant attitude toward his achievements; and they accepted his special pattern and tempo of learning."[159] They displayed love and acceptance.

The interplay between class and ideals of physical perfection also influenced decision-making, with less well-educated, older, and longer-married couples tending to adopt older children with disabilities as compared with younger, well-educated, and wealthier parents who most often adopted nondisabled preschool children.[160] Concerns about upward mobility for the latter group certainly also played a role. A white-collar, middle-class family was "perhaps too preoccupied with its own upward mobility to enlist fully its resources to cope with the problems of the medically impaired child."[161] Whereas well-educated and wealthier applicants focused on physical perfection, researchers found that parents who adopted "different" children recognized and accepted human imperfection and considered love and care as principal considerations.[162]

Religious parents seemed to fit that bill, adopting children with intellectual disability, especially those with Down syndrome, more often than nonreligious parents by 1980.[163] That religious parents expressed more open attitudes toward adopting children with intellectual disability was in keeping with the messages of Christian parental memoirs of the time. Much like the overcoming narrative, these Christian memoirs mobilized notions of rescue and salvation, portrayed intellectually disabled children as a moral lesson and inspiration for others, and elevated a mother's sacrifice and caregiving to the level of a spiritual calling. Insofar as these testaments stressed a child's symbolic import, they also posited the children as having value for the family at a time when many professionals recommended institutionalization.[164]

The severity of a child's impairment, their age, and the adoptive parents' marital status also factored into adopters' profiles during this period. Franklin and Massarik found in 1969 that older parents, fertile couples, and larger families tended to adopt children with moderate or severe conditions while more than a fifth of their study parents who adopted "severes" had been divorced. "Severes" in their study included children with: blindness, deafness, cleft palate, noncorrectable skeletal deformity, and other congenital anomalies. "Moderates" included congenital cataract, hearing impairment, and urogenital defect. "Minors" included inguinal hernias, hydroceles, minimal clubfoot, and skin issues. But ten years earlier, Henry Maas and Richard Engler had found that whereas a middle-class set of parents would accept a child with a remediable physical impairment, an intellectual or psychological disability would not be acceptable; "matters of the mind were mysteriously troublesome."[165] Later, DeLeon and Westerberg found a similar pattern to that of Maas and Engler, with professionals "less likely to adopt a child who appeared retarded or functioned lower in the retarded range."[166]

Unlike studies that examined parents who had adopted a child with a disability to predict likely future adopters, a 1970 study looked solely at applicant *willingness* to adopt these children. Social work scholar Donald Chambers found that when asked about their willingness to adopt "atypical" children (over five years of age, minority-group parentage, or "mentally retarded, physically handicapped or emotionally disturbed"), responses similarly depended upon the type of attribute in question. Applicants by far only desired *one* atypical attribute. Encouragingly, half the respondents indicated a willingness, at least in theory, to adopt a child with an irremediable physical impairment. Chambers defined irremediable conditions as paralysis of the left arm and shoulder, blindness, deafness, a repaired congenital heart defect with functional limitations, severe food allergies, and a large birthmark. Twenty-two percent of parents were willing to accept a child who was a "slow learner," and seven percent expressed a willingness to adopt a child with an emotional disability.[167]

There could be several reasons for parents' parsing of acceptable types of disability. First, the enduring equivalence between normal intelligence and adoptability in social work practice could help explain this finding. Second, the typical social and cultural hierarchy of disabilities (physical, intellectual/psychological, emotional—in that order) or unfamiliarity with children who were commonly institutionalized for the earlier studies could also explain parents' differential reasoning. Third, limits to which children parents found acceptable may have also reflected persistent mental matching ideas among agency workers and parents that had operated so explicitly in the early decades of this period.[168]

Despite similarities and differences, all of the studies tried to identify parents who could overcome their own fears and marshal love and acceptance to develop and establish familial belonging. These studies' findings helped solidify a profile of parents willing and able to adopt children with disabilities. Moreover, this profile reflected a new form of adoptive family that had developed over two decades: people who were middle- to low-income, individuals less concerned with their social status in the community (considered "downwardly mobile" as a result of adoption), applicants who had been exposed to people with disabilities through their extended families or work environment, individuals who were comfortable with differences, religious individuals, people who already had children, those who were able to handle crises, and those who were family oriented.[169]

This profile featured parents who did not engage in conditional parenthood; they did not place preconditions like the health status of a child on their desire to parent. They "require no support of [a child's] background, of appearance of intellectual potential, no guarantees."[170] According to Palo Alto pediatrician Joseph Davis and social worker Patricia Montgomery, these parents were neither typical of parents in larger society nor typical of parents who adopted normal children. Instead, these parents emphasized the "standpoint of the child as an opportunity to do something for someone else, to nurture children already living."[171] They recast the notion of parenting itself; they centered the child's needs in their parenting, rather than envisioning parenting as the opportunity to propagate parental appearances, needs, and desires first. According to Davis and Montgomery, in their ability to see the child, these parents had the capacity to express accepting, attentive love.[172] These were the most probable candidates to embrace the overcoming narrative. Recruitment efforts needed to target them to be overcomers.

Conclusion

In its idealized form, and in its inspirational mode, social workers' call for love and acceptance offered a major shift in addressing the needs of dependent children with disabilities and in responding to the desires of potential parents to raise a child. While changes to the definition of adoptability enabled overcoming, adoption professionals framed parental eligibility and family life as contingent upon it. In this way, the overcoming narrative opened up a culturally accessible and sanctioned pathway for previously excluded children to become part of families who intended to make them their own.

Substantial changes to professionals' and many parents' attitudes between 1955 and 1980, however, were not enough to place special needs children with parents who would overcome. Overcoming also required new institutional arrangements and programs to support parent recruitment and an adoption's sustainability. Changes in agency practice, parental screening and approaches, adoption exchanges, social work training programs, and financial assistance were all required in order to materialize overcoming.

CHAPTER FOUR

From Overcoming to Programmatic Solutions

As adoption professionals reconfigured adoptability, risk, and parent eligibility between 1955 and 1980, they also pursued strategies aimed at the permanent placement of heretofore-marginalized children, including children with various disabilities. Their efforts involved changing adoption practices and establishing mechanisms to achieve this goal, such as creating new forms of casework, establishing specialized adoption agencies, launching a national adoption exchange, and forming a national adoption center.

The thrust underpinning these efforts—promoting a more inclusive adoption system that attended to children's specific needs—was consistent with the push by American grassroots movements to address the rights of previously marginalized persons on the basis of gender, race, ethnicity, and disability.[1] Acknowledging that children with developmental disabilities waited the longest in foster care, the Child Welfare League of America established a developmental disabilities adoption project whose specific objective was to place these children in permanent homes. Adoption professionals established training programs intended to help social workers destigmatize disability and to learn new, suitable casework skills. States began to offer subsidies to help families afford medical and other care needs. By the end of this period, the federal government was providing financial assistance to families and restructuring incentives so that states would permanently place these children. All of these initiatives underscored professionals' emerging belief that children with disabilities deserved families. They helped bring social work ideas about parental overcoming to fruition.

Foster Children "At Risk"

A changing demographic landscape in adoption drove professionals to respond in specific conceptual and programmatic ways. Cultural shifts in reproduction and child-rearing, as well as child welfare policy changes that promoted out-of-home placement, changed the types of children available for adoption during this period. Adoptees slowly but increasingly came from the foster care system, especially towards the end of this period, from the 1970s on.

As the numbers of white healthy infants gradually shrunk, the foster care population began to grow. In 1962, 272,000 children—sometimes called "orphans of the living"—lived in foster care in the United States, which was double the number in 1933.[2] By 1972, the number grew to approximately 319,800 children, many of whom passed through multiple homes in succession. Social workers identified these children as more likely to be minority or mixed-race, older, emotionally challenged, or physically or intellectually disabled. By 1977, more than half a million children were in foster care. By the late 1970s, the problem was so significant that three-quarters of child welfare funding went into foster care.

As we saw in chapter 3, amid the changing picture of child welfare during the years from 1955 to 1980, adoption workers urged parent applicants to overcome their prejudices and embrace love and acceptance to adopt foster and nonfoster children with disabilities alike. In the 1960s and 1970s, however, most parent applicants still desired "normal, healthy newborns." Adopters' typical desires are not surprising given that common stereotypes of the time depicted children with disabilities as "devastating burdens who made their families socially abnormal and shattered their parents' dreams."[3] This stereotype undeniably applied to foster children with disabilities. In response to the imbalance between these desires and needs, social work leaders began to respond to the particular circumstances of the foster population.

Many factors contributed to the rise in the foster care population. In the 1950s, most children who ended up in foster care came from white families, but two decades later, the majority of children in foster care came from poor African American families.[4] Children ended up in foster care for multiple reasons, ranging from parental illness or disability to incarceration or death, financial hardship, and poor housing. Deinstitutionalization also contributed to the growing number of children with intellectual disability in foster care. Their higher rates of entry into, rather than discharge from, the foster care system exacerbated the problem. Discharged children from mental health and juvenile justice institutions also increased the numbers of those in foster care.[5]

The greatest driver of poor children's entrance into the foster care system in the 1960s, however, was changes to child welfare policy. During that time, Congress extended Aid to Families with Dependent Children (ADC) assistance to foster children. It funded a program called ADC-Foster Care, which gave matching funds to states for out-of-home placement. Medicaid became available to foster children while Congress also authorized emergency payments to families in crisis. Congress shifted funding from family preservation to out-of-home placement, in part because child welfare leaders increasingly perceived a growing crisis of child abuse, neglect, and abandonment. This led to child welfare workers' removal of children who were suspected of being abused from homes during the late 1960s and early 1970s. Certainly neglect and abuse caused disability in children exposed to such environments, but child welfare leaders also considered children with disabilities at high risk for being neglected or abused.[6] In essence, a growing awareness of abuse and neglect made child welfare leaders reassess the traditional principle that children should, if possible, be returned to their birth families.

In 1976, a reported 100,000 children with disabilities experienced extended foster care and a phenomenon that child welfare experts called "foster drift"; that is, the placement of children in a series of temporary homes in succession.[7] This phenomenon contributed to child welfare and adoption leaders' focus on foster children's need for permanent placement. In addition, professionals often tied foster drift to discussions of disability and risk. They specifically identified the foster care system itself as a risk factor that created the conditions for children to acquire emotional disabilities.

Henry Maas and Richard Engler first made the field of child welfare aware of foster drift in 1959. Other academics studied the issue thereafter. These scholars argued that foster drift put all children, with or without impairments, *at great risk* for emotional and behavioral issues. Many of these children could not be reunited with their birth families, but they were also not legally free to be adopted. They therefore faced impermanency (the state of not having a secure, legal, permanent family) for unforeseen lengths of time.[8] Child welfare experts expressed intense anxiety over these children's predicament. They believed not only that these children were at risk for various disabilities, but also that foster drift threatened their experience of childhood.[9]

Experts also worried that foster children lacked consistent medical care, including needed psychiatric counseling and treatment, putting them at risk for disability and complicating their overall poor health status. Impermanence, foster drift, large social work caseloads, a lack of resources, and high rates of social work turnover combined to interfere with foster children's already sporadic and inadequate access to medical care. As a result, foster children had three to seven times as many chronic health problems as their counterparts in the general population.[10]

In the mid to late 1950s, many adoption leaders tried to address what they saw as the interrelated problems of disability and foster drift by suggesting changes to the idea of adoptability. Employing psychodynamic explanations that located risk in a child's psyche, Joseph Reid, executive director of the CWLA, declared in 1956 that "some psychiatrists believe that many children's ability to love and be loved has been so severely damaged that _they_ _are very poor risks for adoption_ [my underscore and italics]."[11] To Reid, these foster children's emotional problems made their adoption a risk to adopters because they would likely threaten the integrity and unity of the adoptive family. Yet the CWLA director also acknowledged that adoptability, functioning as a measure of risk, was not solely a static attribute of the child; social work efforts could help "_make_ [my italics] those children left behind in foster care adoptable" to facilitate permanent placement.[12] His line of thinking was consistent with the slow expansion of adoptability starting in 1955 for both foster and nonfoster children.[13]

Bernice Boehm's 1958 study, "Deterrents to the Adoption of Children in Foster Care," did not frame foster children as very poor risks for adoption. Instead, she, like Maas and Engler, explicitly linked the intensity and incidence of waiting children's emotional and behavioral problems to external factors like the length of time spent in foster care.[14] She argued that adoptability was not "readily measurable"; it depended upon an interaction of many factors, some of which related to the child, some to the birth family, and some to the agency's degree of service. She offered a vision of adoptability in transition, one that still incorporated pre–World War II criteria denoting specific attributes of the child and family, but also one that began to identify social and institutional barriers to placement. This new vision relocated the onus of risk and adoptability from the child to factors external to, but impinging upon, the child. Boehm argued that adoption professionals could increase adoptability and reduce any risks to adopters by avoiding delays in casework and IQ testing, addressing or removing adoption deterrents, and relinquishing the idea of reuniting foster children with their "real" families.[15]

From the middle to end of this period, child welfare experts continued to posit foster care as a significant risk to children, but they also offered new interpretations of parenthood, children's needs, risk, and the chain of events that led to impermanence. In their influential 1973 publication, *Beyond the Best Interests of the Child*, for instance, Joseph Goldstein, Anna Freud, and Alfred Solnit reinforced Boehm's insights and explained risk as a function of foster care delivery. They blamed the foster care system for having a hand in producing impermanence and posited impermanency as a significant risk to the child's emotional health. Following psychological trends that stressed nurture over nature, the authors argued that child placement law and practice should prioritize the essential need of a child for a sustained relationship with a nurturing adult; they contended that a child needed a "psychological parent." A psychological parent could be a biological, adoptive, or any other caring adult, but they had to provide "day-to-day interaction, companionship and shared experiences."[16]

Goldstein, Freud, and Solnit argued that this secure, supportive relationship produced positive effects upon children's development and growth. They deemphasized the primacy of blood ties and contended that by disrupting a child's relationships and environment, foster drift produced "inevitable internal difficulties" for the child.[17] They argued that save those intended for brief temporary care, all child placements should be seen as permanent.

Like these psychologists, parents and child welfare workers in the late 1950s promoting what they called permanency planning held that a child had the right to a stable and permanent relationship within a family unit, whether biological or adoptive. They defined permanency planning as a process that laid out "goal-directed activities" to move children into permanent families with nurturing parents within a brief amount of time.[18] As more marginalized children lingered in foster care indefinitely, these advocates contended that children, rather than childless parents, were the principal clients of adoption services. They emphasized the autonomy and needs of the child for a permanent family, even for a child whom social workers deemed hard to place.[19]

Permanency planning advocates addressed the specific problems associated with foster care by demanding new casework procedures and services. In practice, this meant providing social work services to biological families to care for their children in order to prevent their entrance into foster care in the first place, promoting family reunification when appropriate, and advancing adoption for children who could not return to their birth families. Child welfare agencies offered counseling, crisis intervention, and other services to keep families intact. Social workers asked biological parents who voluntarily put their child in foster care to specify an amount of time after which the child would return home so as to avoid unlimited delays. Permanency planners also encouraged arranged visitations by birth parents, when possible, while the child was in foster care. Advocates worked to change laws to enable the termination of parental rights so that children could be legally free for adoption. Permanency planning demonstration projects, like the federally funded Oregon Project of 1973, showed that, with intensive services and planning, children could either be returned to their biological families or placed through adoption.[20]

By 1980, child welfare experts had fully transitioned to the idea that the responsibility for all foster children's risks now lay in *the failure of society* to deal adequately with the foster care problem.[21] They suggested that children no longer embodied a risk to adopters; they were neither hard to place nor inherently psychologically damaged or maladjusted. Adoption leaders explained that long-term foster care *created* the prejudices and barriers associated with placing these children, putting children at risk for psychological problems, which, in turn, made it harder to find families who would adopt them.[22]

Deinstitutionalization and Access to Family

Parents and social workers who focused on the particular needs of children with disabilities contended that the idea of access to permanent family should inform all new adoption practices intended for this population. Their position not only reinforced permanency planning principles, but also harmonized with a broad public consensus emerging in the 1970s that supported deinstitutionalization. Advocates for deinstitutionalization argued that persons diagnosed with mental retardation and other developmental disabilities should live in the community. Disabled residents had suffered from abuse and neglect; they had lived in unsanitary and crowded conditions in large custodial warehouses, all at costs significantly higher

than community care. As formerly institutionalized children moved to living in the community, some went back to their birth families while others
moved into group homes or entered specialized family foster care (which
merged family foster care with access to community-based needed treatments). Others were adopted.[23]

Deinstitutionalization grew out of rights-based movements, judicial
rulings, and parent advocacy that argued that people with disabilities had
a right to full and satisfying lives.[24] These efforts had particularly profound effects on persons with intellectual disabilities, the vast majority
of whom had lived in institutions since the 1940s. Bengt Nirje and Wolf
Wolfensberger proposed that people labeled "retarded" should be treated
as normal people, with the opportunity to live as close as possible to the
conditions of mainstream society; they should be served and live in the
"least restrictive environment."[25] Allies argued that people with mental
retardation had the right to privacy and deserved to engage in what they
called the "dignity of risk"; that is, the dignity that comes from having the
ability to decide to take reasonable risks, to succeed or fail, rather than
being overprotected and segregated.[26] Proponents of deinstitutionalization considered the ability to engage in risk taking a fundamental part of
being human.

Adoption professionals, researchers, and parents in the 1970s embraced the notions of normalization, least restrictive environment, and
dignity of risk when thinking about the adoptive placement of disabled
children. They applied these concepts to programmatic solutions to facilitate such adoptions. By challenging adoptability criteria, focusing on
the special needs of children with disabilities, identifying social barriers
to placement and impermanency as central drivers of making children
at risk, and rectifying extant casework practices, they acknowledged that
children with disabilities were not afforded the same opportunities to ex-
ercise dignity of risk as other children.[27]

These leaders effectively extended the principle of dignity of risk to
adopters. They repudiated social workers' tendency to overprotect parents by foreclosing certain children from their consideration. They encouraged social workers to offer more comprehensive medical information to adopters to enable informed decision-making. Along with the
overcoming narrative, these advocates for the placement of children with
disabilities promoted a more holistic approach to treating the child with
a disability in casework settings. They posited children with disabilities as
the same as nondisabled children in their basic needs for love and family.[28]

These leaders sought practices that would allow children with disabilities to experience a "happy and secure childhood, enabling them to make full use of their inherent capacity."[29]

Several initiatives aimed at moving institutionalized children into family settings showed positive results. For example, under the auspices of the Alaska Easter Seals Society, the Alaska Developmental Disabilities Program and the Northwest Regional Center for Deaf-Blind Children granted funds to the Alaska Vision/Hearing Impaired Program in 1977 to provide, on an experimental basis, a least-restrictive environment for deinstitutionalized children. Whereas many professionals still hesitated to place what they called severely handicapped children into adoptive homes, the Alaska program identified three severely handicapped youth who did not need extensive medical treatment. Although the pilot program's goals fell short of direct permanent placement, the Alaska Vision/Hearing Impaired Program worked toward that goal. It provided family foster homes and educational programming, counseling, and other ancillary services for these children. Social workers trained the foster families, all of whom had experience with children labeled severely handicapped, to address the children's needs.[30] This experiment proved quite successful, with child participants showing marked improvements in their behavior, communication, language, and play skills.[31]

Parent Advocacy and Specialized Adoption Services

As agencies and adoption leaders assessed their own culpability in failing to place children with disabilities, parents who had navigated the system provided their own interpretations of the problem. Instead of focusing on the physical, emotional, or intellectual issues of the children per se, parent adoption advocates emphasized the need to remove social, economic, structural, and institutional barriers to permanent placement. They also repeatedly challenged stigmatizing attitudes that kept children with disabilities from adoption.

Adoptive parents in groups like the Council on Adoptable Children (COAC, founded in 1967; renamed the North American Council on Adoptable Children, NACAC, in 1974) and the Open Door Society of Montreal (started in the late 1950s by three white families who had adopted Black children; devoted to cross-racial placements) helped prospective parents navigate agency policies that obstructed children's adoption.[32] Deeply concerned that a substantial number of children were growing up in foster care and experiencing foster drift, parent adoption advocates, like their professional counterparts, argued that children needed permanency planning.[33] Parents trained other parents, used the media, lobbied, and sued to achieve their goals. They also suggested a new collaborative model that positioned adoptive parents and private and public agencies as casework partners.

Parent adoption advocacy operated alongside other parent and self-advocacy groups in the US at this time, including those involved in the child advocacy movement. General parent advocacy for biological children with disabilities, for example, emerged in the 1950s, with local parent groups banding together to address the barriers families faced in attaining services.

Public discourse on the family at midcentury elevated it to the center of American life. Even though this discourse implicitly and explicitly promoted a vision of the ideal family as able-bodied, white, and middle class, parent disability advocates built on Americans' focus on the family to argue for their legitimate place within it.[34] They challenged societal and professional norms that posited their children wholly as burdens upon their family, a view borne out of the historical social isolation experienced by families with disabled children during a time when health care providers recommended accessing services through institutionalization. These parents actively contested the notion that their children were defined solely by their disabilities. Like parent adoption advocates, parent disability advocates stressed love and acceptance, railed against stereotypes of their children as defective, and argued that, invisible or visible, disability should neither be feared nor shunned. In essence, they pushed for a radical shift in the way Americans conceptualized disability.

There is no clear evidence that the disability parent movement involved some of the same people as parent adoption advocates. The two groups, however, used similar rhetoric to advocate for the value of their children's lives and for the services they needed, whether in education or through adoption. For their part, adoption professionals tried to translate parents' ideas about acceptance, worthiness, and the inclusion of children with disabilities into programs whose goal was to facilitate the adoption of special needs children.

The emergence of agencies specializing in permanently placing children with special needs, including children with disabilities, responded to strong parental demands. One, Spaulding for Children, created in Ann

Arbor, Michigan, in 1968, was touted as a model.[35] Led by Kathryn Donley, Spaulding was the outgrowth of a conference called Frontiers for
Adoption that included scholars from the University of Michigan as well
as officials from the Michigan Department of Social Services (MDSS),
private child welfare agencies, and parents who sought to change the
adoption system. Spaulding explicitly dropped "perfection" as a goal for
either parents or children and embraced the notion that all children were
valuable and worthy of family.[36] Spaulding's inclusivity spanned both its
definition of adoptable children and the types of families it made through
adoption. The Spaulding model "believed, and [has] proven, that parents
do exist who are interested in and capable of parenting older and handicapped children."[37]

To find families, Spaulding introduced a weekly newspaper column
called "Wednesday's Child," which featured profiles of children waiting to
be adopted. Spaulding also offered indefinite postplacement services to
support adoptive parents and connect them with the services they needed.
By doing so, Spaulding sought to change the context of adoption by providing access to support.[38] Its staff aggressively worked to "overcome the
chaos, madness and unpredictability" of the legal and child welfare systems in order to permanently place children.[39]

As Spaulding successfully placed greater numbers of "special needs"
children, both the agency and the MDSS revised the profile of children
who they considered "hard-to-place," shifting it to older and more severely impaired children. In 1968, for instance, MDSS defined a child as
"hard-to-place" if they were over two years old, a racial minority, or had
"minor handicaps or deformities." By 1977, the same department had altered its definition to only include white children over age ten, minority
children over age eight, and children of all ages who were "moderately
retarded, severely or multiply handicapped, emotionally disturbed, or terminally ill."[40] Age, race, and disability intersected here in determining the
category hard to place. Younger able-bodied or mildly disabled minority
children were no longer categorized as hard to place, for instance, presumably because more prospective parents were open to adopting these
children. But they were not as amenable to adopting children of the same
age with moderate to severe disabilities. For its part, Spaulding used a
slightly different definition; it referred to children as "hard to place" if
they were older than eleven, siblings, had moderate-to-severe physical,
educational, or emotional disabilities, or had multiple disabilities.

The MDSS's changed definition reflected a positive trend toward placing
children deemed as having minor disabilities. With successful placement,

those children no longer needed Spaulding's preadoptive specialized services, so agency workers no longer considered them hard to place. But the state's decision to recategorize these children had the inadvertent effect of shifting the profile of children now under Spaulding's care to even more marginalized (sub)groups, sometimes even leaving children with "severe multiple handicaps" without families. Spaulding was unable to find a family, for example, for a fourteen-year-old boy who was a "trainably retarded child (functioning on a first-grade level), poorly coordinated, and small for his age. He blinked frequently, had a head twitch, speech defect, and an explosive temper."[41] It is likely that he grew up either in a group home, an institution, or a foster family.

Overall, however, professionals and parent advocates alike heralded Spaulding as a leader in specialized agency work. Inspired by the Spaulding model, groups in New York, Ohio, Maine, New Jersey, and Pennsylvania created their own agencies and parent groups.

Strategies to Recruit Parents

Agencies dedicated to the adoption of children with disabilities used new recruitment strategies to attract parent applicants. "Waiting child" columns, usually titled "Sunday's Child" or "Wednesday's Child," television and radio spots, adoption week campaigns, flyers, and newsletters all became staples in agencies' attempts to find families to adopt children with disabilities.[42] A typical newspaper article described Shirley, "a tiny 8-year-old with huge problems," who needed parents who could nurture her to her fullest potential, "whatever that may be."[43] The story of an unmarried father, who saw a picture of a child in a newspaper, demonstrated the effectiveness of these recruitment strategies: "There was Pete, in his Scout uniform, staring up from the Sunday paper with that 'tough guy' look of his. I didn't know anything about adoption or spina bifida and mental retardation. I didn't even know that a single person could adopt. But something about Pete just made me make that first call."[44]

In the mid-1970s, a combination of intensified recruitment efforts via television and print media, a new attitude among social workers, and a revised philosophy among agencies willing to find parents for children with disabilities helped locate permanent homes for a "blind baby, a deaf twelve-year-old boy, a four-year-old mongoloid girl, a ten-year-old boy with cystic fibrosis," and "eight-year-old Billie who is quadriplegic and will never walk." If they searched hard enough and looked to "draw a different kind of adoptive family," agencies found they could identify parents for emotionally and physically disabled, minority, and older children.[45]

To facilitate the adoption of special needs children, social workers deliberately described a specific, rather than an abstract, child to applicants. A caseworker often gave a picture of the child to establish an attachment.[46] They took their cue from adoption leaders and researchers who argued that abstractness enabled prejudice when it came to the placement of children with disabilities. In contrast, they argued, offering a specific portrait of a child, via a picture or a newspaper description, promoted a child's humanity. Adoption leaders contended that when a social worker described a child's unique personality, she allowed parents to see the child as *more* than, and not only, their "handicap" (physical, social, or otherwise).[47] They recommended that agency workers allow applicants to explore the "range of difference" they could accept, stressing "not in the abstract, but in relation to a specific child. . . . With the focus on a particular child, with its appealing potential as a human being, the medical condition may be clearly seen, but in perspective, with its relative importance better understood."[48] By emphasizing specificity, adoption leaders and researchers tried to temper the fear and trepidation they presumed many adopters might have when considering a disabled child.

Sometimes, however, parents came to agencies wanting to adopt a particular child they had seen in a specific media forum. These adopters' initiative was consistent with an idea percolating in the 1970s called "client self-determination," which removed family building decisions from the social worker or medical professional and placed it into the hands of the parents.[49] Many experienced adoption professionals opposed this strategy because it reduced adoption agencies' decision-making powers. But client self-determination also allowed families who were waiting for a younger healthy child, for instance, to consider an older child with a disability. Proponents argued that client self-determination allowed parents to make an informed decision about their family, including understanding the responsibilities involved in raising a child with a disability.

Many adopters wanted very specific information about a child or about parenting before placement in order to understand what her adoption would mean to them. Katherine Nelson explained this preference as a desire for preparedness: when social workers provided less abstract depictions of a child, they helped parents make a decision to adopt a disabled child and to cope with its practical consequences.[50] One downside of this approach, however, was that it tended to replicate two operative yet incongruous American constructions about children with disabilities at the time. As Gliedman and Roth explained in 1980, a child with disabilities was defined simultaneously "as a complex, growing child who, among other things, happens to have a handicap" and as "a handicap, a freak." They added that such children "are usually treated as persons in the home and almost always defined as handicaps elsewhere."[51] Adoptive families could not have missed this public-private disparity after adoption.

Attesting to Gliedman and Roth's keen observations, even parents willing to adopt special needs children desired certain characteristics above others. A 1972 report stated that "a family may be quite ready to adopt a physically handicapped child but only if he is unusually bright. Or a family may be interested in adopting a black child but only if he is under 5 years old and free of intellectual and physical handicaps."[52] Only one in ten families surveyed would consider adopting a "slow" child, and only one in ten would find a child with an "irremediable" handicap acceptable. Children with irremediable handicaps had the lowest proportion of infant adoptions of any group.[53]

By 1974, a handbook for child welfare workers acknowledged that adopters willing to parent "children with handicaps are not waiting on the doorsteps of adoption agencies." Neither were many social workers able to handle the demands necessary to recruit families, to adequately assess adopters' interest in parenting disabled children, and to help children acclimate to their new families.[54] Despite these challenges, the existence of new parent recruitment strategies did indeed reflect child welfare's newfound commitment to placing these children. These recruitment strategies are particularly compelling when read within a context where the number of children needing placement outstripped the number of willing homes.

Adoption Exchanges, Centers, and Training Projects

Adoption resource exchanges, centers, and training projects were broad institutional mechanisms that helped facilitate special needs adoptions on a national scale. Broadly speaking, these projects paired parent applicants with children needing placement across state lines, created a network of agencies that serviced disabled children, and trained social workers and social workers-in-training about best practices in special needs adoption, respectively. Each project significantly transformed the ways agencies thought about and placed children with disabilities.

Adoption resource exchanges enabled recruitment and placement by cross-referencing waiting children with interested applicants. A national adoption exchange had its roots in state exchanges established at midcentury. Between 1949 and the late 1950s, state exchanges focused on placing hard-to-place children, including children with certain disabilities.[55] Based on the success of state exchanges, the Child Welfare League of America created the Adoption Resource Exchange of North America (ARENA), first as a demonstration project in 1966 and then as a full-fledged program a year later.[56] Based in New York City, ARENA was the first national adoption resource exchange that incorporated children serviced by U.S. public and private agencies and those in Canada. It facilitated interstate adoption, which had started before 1960 but gained needed protections with the Interstate Compact for the Protection of Children, which had passed that year. The U.S. Bureau of Indian Affairs, the American Contract Bridge League Foundation, the Field Foundation, and private contributors funded ARENA.

Although ARENA descended from the Indian Adoption Project, which had usually placed Native American children in white homes since 1958, it went beyond this mission.[57] It sought to eliminate barriers to the placement of 60,000 children without permanent homes, including those children that applicants considered "imperfect" (e.g., with "serious" physical handicaps) and "difficult" (e.g., with emotional disturbances).[58] In its first year, it helped place more than a hundred children of various ethnicities, disabilities, and ages.[59]

With a national reach, ARENA addressed the uneven geographic distribution of potential adopters and children waiting for placement. In 1966, for instance, there were more babies for adoption on the East and West coasts, but more potential parents in the Midwest and Rocky Mountain states.[60] As Joseph Reid, director of the CWLA, commented with regard to these regional differences: "We are betting we could demonstrate that local prejudice might work *for* a child instead of *against* him [my italics]."[61] Rejecting stigma, one ARENA pamphlet stated that "people adopt children—not problems."[62] Notably, the pamphlet separated out healthy minority children and disabled children, showing that adoption professionals conceived of minority children as healthy. The term "handicapped" presumably applied to all children with disabilities, no matter their race. The pamphlet noted that whereas ARENA helped place healthy African American, White, and Native American children and siblings, whose "only problem has been that for one reason or another no adoptive homes had been found for them," it also assisted children with "very 'special needs,' such as the physically disabled, 'mentally retarded' and emotional disturbed, who also 'deserve families.' "[63]

The staff of ARENA performed seven main activities. They recruited homes on a national scale; published a monthly index or bulletin about the exchange's activities; registered children and kept a list of waiting children and families throughout the United States; helped establish new exchanges; worked to eliminate laws that prevented interstate placement; developed standards for agency cooperation; and provided field consultation to state exchanges.[64] Its staff left casework and placement decisions to agencies. Instead, the exchange facilitated agencies' recruitment attempts within a cooperative framework.

In dramatic contrast to earlier practices, ARENA set no restrictions on the age, race, marital status, socioeconomic status, or lifestyle of applicant families who wished to be registered on the exchange. Applicants merely needed to demonstrate the ability to appropriately meet the needs of a child.[65] Even with such expansive criteria, however, adoption workers found recruitment difficult and acknowledged that placing special needs children required different skills and more time, staff, and money than placement of normal children.[66] ARENA's efforts nevertheless demonstrated that with these assets, it was possible to place such children. By 1975, ARENA had facilitated 1,500 placements.[67]

In the late 1970s, ARENA became part of the North American Center on Adoption (NACA) program.[68] The Child Welfare League of America established NACA in 1975 to increase national adoption services while "removing the barriers to adoption" for special needs children.[69] In addition to its partnership with ARENA, NACA organized a national network of agencies, called Family Builders by Adoption. Whereas ARENA was an exchange for all special needs children, Family Builders, founded in 1975, specialized in older and handicapped children, many of whom were in long-term foster care and had a persistent need for families. Like ARENA, Family Builders accepted a wide range of applicants to parent these children.[70]

Under NACA, ARENA and Family Builders operated successfully throughout the 1970s. Thereafter, the U.S. Children's Bureau, the Department of Health and Human Services, and the Office of Human Development Services awarded NACA a contract to establish the National Adoption Information Exchange System (NAIES) to operate a national adoption exchange, publish materials to support special needs adoption, and train the staff of local, state, and regional exchanges to improve their participation in the national exchange.[71] ARENA became the outreach unit of NAIES.[72] By 1983, NACA no longer provided the exchange component of its service but continued to advocate on behalf of "older, minority and 'special needs' children."[73]

Under NAIES, the process of the national exchange worked like an ever-expanding geographic circle. A caseworker first referred a child to a local agency. If she was not placed within approximately ninety days, the agency would register the child on a state exchange and circulate the child's photo within the state and sometimes regionally. If the agency could not find a family on the state exchange within a certain time frame, it referred the child to the national exchange.[74] Agency workers automatically referred certain categories of children, particularly those who were terminally ill or "severely" disabled, minority children, or children older than five years, to all levels of exchanges because of the usual difficulty of finding families.[75]

NACA also initiated the Developmental Disabilities Adoption Project (DDAP) in 1978. The DDAP functioned as a unit under ARENA and lasted two years with federal funding. It was the first program to specifically address the adoption needs of developmentally disabled children as a separate and distinct population from other marginalized children. Drawing on the Developmental Disabilities Assistance and Bill of Rights Act (P.L. 95-602; 1978), the DDAP defined a child with a developmental disability as having substantial functional limitations in three or more major life activities, including "self-care, mobility, learning, receptive and expressive language, self-direction, capacity for independent living, [and] economic self-sufficiency" (see appendix 2).[76]

NACA leaders established the DDAP because they noticed that children with developmental disabilities waited the longest of all child populations on the national exchange. Staff found it easier to find families for African American children, older children, and siblings than for children with developmental disabilities. Yet almost half of the children registered with ARENA in 1978 had an emotional, physical, or intellectual impairment.[77] Staff observed that the younger the child, the easier it was to find a home.

To resolve the particular issues facing children with developmental disabilities, NACA leaders realized they needed to actively recruit social workers as well as families. They therefore articulated DDAP's two main objectives: (1) identifying skills and attitudes among social workers that impeded the placement of children with developmental disabilities; and (2) developing the professional expertise necessary for their permanent placement.[78] In the DDAP's first year, staff disseminated a survey of agency practices and conducted interviews with both public and private agencies.[79] The survey and interviews revealed that mental retardation was the most common disability (73 percent) among developmental disabled children waiting for placement, that 9 percent of the children had more than one disability, and that 39 percent of the children were from minority backgrounds.[80] In its second year, DDAP staff provided training for agency workers at ten demonstration sites, child welfare projects, and advocacy groups to change workers' knowledge of and attitudes about developmentally disabled children in need of placement.[81] They also operated a Developmental Disabilities Unit within ARENA to facilitate adoption planning for twenty children with developmental disabilities listed on the national exchange. The outreach unit served as a model for adoption staff on what skills, support, and attitudes it took to place "these special children." Finally, the DDAP developed training and resource materials for agencies.[82]

The DDAP also served as a liaison between the Department of Health, Education and Welfare and other agencies, citizens, and organizations relating to issues concerning children with developmental disabilities.[83] The project pursued outreach to the National Association for Retarded Citizens, United Cerebral Palsy, the American Association on Mental Deficiency, and the North American Council on Adoptable Children, all of which were interested in partnering with the DDAP to address the serious needs of children who could not return to their biological families after deinstitutionalization.[84] DDAP staff also developed educational materials for judges and physicians, some of whom still considered "a developmentally disabled child as 'unadoptable' and likely to be a burden to a family," thus hindering placement.[85]

A significant thrust of the DDAP's training work was transforming agencies' negative attitudes towards children with developmental disabilities, which included conditions that fit with the Developmental Disabilities Assistance Act definition, like cognitive delays or diseases related to failure to thrive. Staff exposed demonstration sites to resources from developmental disabilities councils, universities, and advocacy groups, sent families with children with developmental disabilities to speak to select agencies about their experiences, enhanced "workers' appreciation of the adoptability of children with disabilities to encourage them to recruit and

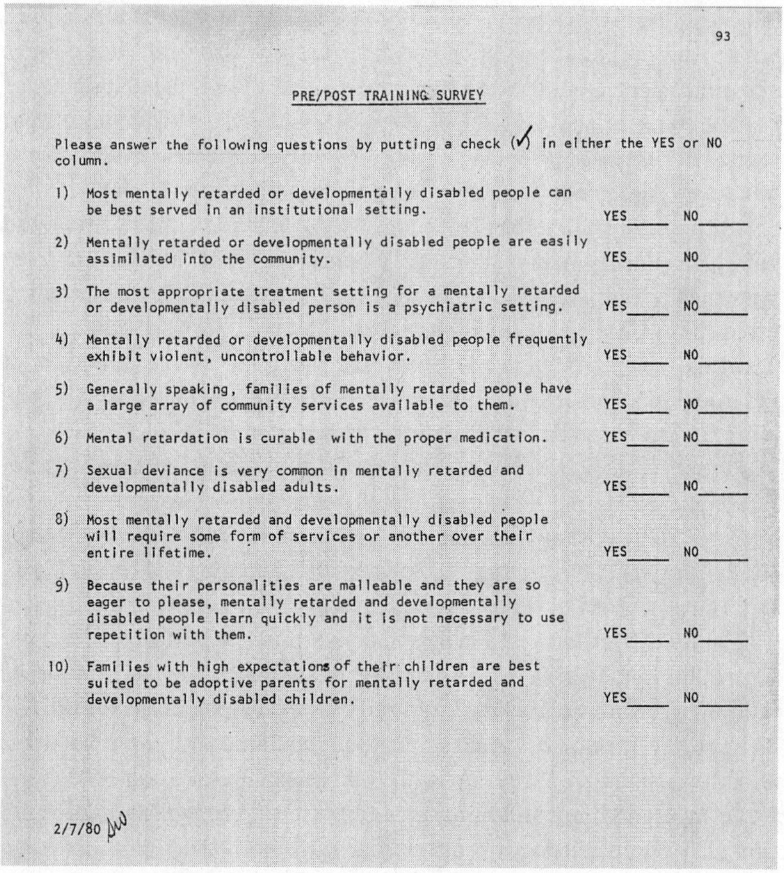

93

PRE/POST TRAINING SURVEY

Please answer the following questions by putting a check (✓) in either the YES or NO column.

1) Most mentally retarded or developmentally disabled people can be best served in an institutional setting. YES_____ NO_____

2) Mentally retarded or developmentally disabled people are easily assimilated into the community. YES_____ NO_____

3) The most appropriate treatment setting for a mentally retarded or developmentally disabled person is a psychiatric setting. YES_____ NO_____

4) Mentally retarded or developmentally disabled people frequently exhibit violent, uncontrollable behavior. YES_____ NO_____

5) Generally speaking, families of mentally retarded people have a large array of community services available to them. YES_____ NO_____

6) Mental retardation is curable with the proper medication. YES_____ NO_____

7) Sexual deviance is very common in mentally retarded and developmentally disabled adults. YES_____ NO_____

8) Most mentally retarded and developmentally disabled people will require some form of services or another over their entire lifetime. YES_____ NO_____

9) Because their personalities are malleable and they are so eager to please, mentally retarded and developmentally disabled people learn quickly and it is not necessary to use repetition with them. YES_____ NO_____

10) Families with high expectations of their children are best suited to be adoptive parents for mentally retarded and developmentally disabled children. YES_____ NO_____

2/7/80

FIGURE 5. Pre/post training survey. Carol E. Smith, MSW, project director, Final Report: Developmental Disability Adoptions Project, North American Center on Adoption (December 1981), 93. CWLA Collection, Box 57: Developmental Disabilities Adoption Project, Folder 1 of 3, Social Welfare History Archives.

prepare families," and provided pre- and postplacement services to families.[86] Pre/post training surveys given to demonstration site staff evaluated the project's ability to instill more inclusive attitudes about the placement of children labeled mentally retarded.

Some agency workers initially resisted the DDAP's inclusive approach because they were either unfamiliar with developmental disabilities or had a general "discomfort" toward children with a developmentally disabled label. As Shelly Wimpfheimer, field consultant for the DDAP, wrote in her initial assessment of the Chicago site, "For the most part, children with 'special needs' remained in foster care or residential institutions since they were a mystery to many workers." Before the DDAP intervention, for instance, the only children with developmental disabilities placed for adoption in Chicago's Cook County were those who happened to come to the attention of an interested social worker.[87] By 1979, however, it was clear that the DDAP's work had begun to change agency attitudes toward the adoptability of children with developmental disabilities. A DDAP survey of 199 agencies nationwide showed that the agencies placed approximately 1,600 developmentally disabled children in adoptive homes.[88] The survey's principal investigators, Ann Coyne and Elizabeth Cole, defined "developmental disabilities" as mental retardation (IQ of 70 or below), autism, uncontrolled epilepsy, cerebral palsy, cystic fibrosis, muscular dystrophy, spina bifida, sickle cell disease, and terminal illness. They queried directors and supervisors on their attitudes toward the potential for successful adoptions involving these children, asking them to agree or disagree with such statements as "I don't think an adoptive family should be burdened with the lifelong care of a DD child"; "you can't make adoptive plans for a child until you know how disabled he/she is going to be"; and "I have objections to placing severely disabled children in adoptive homes."[89] Although social workers' individual responses are not detailed in the DDAP's final report, the researchers found that, after training, most agency workers began to believe that children with developmental disabilities were adoptable and that parent applicants could raise them.[90] The investigators also discovered that the type of agency (public or private) and caseworkers' level of knowledge about disability predicted which placements of these children would succeed.[91]

The DDAP's findings were not universally positive. The group found that many structural issues prevented parents from adopting children with developmental disabilities. Some agencies lacked the apparatus to identify and move children from institutions to adoptive families or lacked the mechanism to recruit parents.[92] In Colorado, for instance, a social worker could prevent a legally freed, developmentally disabled child from being photo-listed in newspapers or pamphlets for several reasons, including "limited life expectancy"; profound retardation; inability to attach; or "medical, developmental or emotional problems which are not sufficiently clarified."[93] To remove the "mystery of diagnostic labels," DDAP staff recommended that agencies adopt certain best practices to mitigate stigma in special needs adoption: getting to know the child, finding the right family for that child, identifying financial subsidies, connecting the family to community services, and finding sources for respite care. As one Texas agency worker reported: "I remember the first time I saw Kelly's record. Those labels just jumped out at me—cerebral palsy, speech impaired, mental retardation—and I guess I felt really overwhelmed. But during visits with Kelly at her foster home and at her school, she became a real child to me. That's when I became committed to find her a family."[94]

Whereas the DDAP targeted practicing social workers, university training programs focused on social workers in training. The University of Michigan's Project CRAFT (Curriculum Resources in Adoption/Foster Care Training) and programs at Columbia University and UCLA taught social work students to identify families, recruit parents, assess children, train parents, and provide postadoption counseling.[95] Taking a radical position for the time, CRAFT faculty pushed adoption workers in training to consider adopters with disabilities as valuable applicants for special needs children. The CRAFT handbook stated, "An adoption worker who places a multiply-handicapped child with a family in which the father is confined to a wheelchair is pressing on the boundaries of what many members of the community will accept gracefully. Workers must become advocates for these families and children."[96] In the years to come, adoption professionals would increasingly identify adults with disabilities as a key group to parent children with disabilities.

Through programs like the DDAP and CRAFT, social workers became increasingly aware of the challenges facing adoptive parents of children with disabilities. Such programs tried to reorient social workers' preconceived perceptions and give them the tools to support and facilitate the adoption of children with disabilities.

Removing Financial Barriers

In addition to establishing institutional mechanisms, states and adoption professionals offered critical forms of financial assistance and support to enable parents to adopt children with disabilities. Providing subsidies and other types of aid helped remove parents' financial concerns as a major obstacle to adopting many children with disabilities, particularly those with medical needs. Offering services after adoption also helped parents optimally care for their new disabled child.

Still, several federal policy disincentives hampered foster families from adopting their foster children during this period. First, Title IV-A of the

Social Security Act (Aid to Families of Dependent Children, AFDC) only reimbursed maintenance expenses related to foster care, not adoption. So foster families who wished to adopt an AFDC-eligible child would lose that benefit if they adopted her. They would also lose their foster care payments.[97] Second, Title IV-B, which gave funds to states for child welfare services like day care and salaries of welfare workers, dictated that the bulk of those funds go to the foster care system.[98] Medicaid (1965), which Congress established through Title XIX of the Social Security Act, covered the costs of medical treatments for *all* foster children, regardless of foster parents' financial status, since they were legally state dependents. But once they were adopted, foster children lost their eligibility for Medicaid unless their adoptive parents were poor enough to qualify for the program. Although agencies typically required applicants to have a certain level of income to adopt, most adopters were neither poor enough to qualify for Medicaid nor rich enough to fund a child's expensive medical treatment, especially given that private medical insurance plans generally excluded people with preexisting medical conditions during this time. This discriminatory practice was only later rectified with the Patient Protection and Affordable Care Act (2010). Parents might be able to obtain durable medical equipment, like wheelchairs, through telethons or private donations, but charity work did not extend to medical treatments evenly. Some diseases and conditions were covered; others weren't.[99] Furthermore, Congress did not pass the Supplemental Security Income (SSI) program, which made many disabled children eligible for Medicaid, until 1972. The program began operating in 1974. This left many families for at least half of this period without access to guaranteed medical care once they adopted a disabled foster child. Adoptive parents could apply for SSI (after 1974), but they could fail to qualify because eligibility criteria depended upon a wide variety of factors, including family income and the number of children already in the family.

The Child Welfare League of America acknowledged that trends like the growing number of children in long-term foster care, the incurred state costs, and the lack of federal funds for postadoption care were not sustainable. It recommended in 1968 that states offer some form of assistance to adoptive families to increase the "number of adoptive homes for children for whom there are inadequate resources including . . . handicapped children."[100] New York followed suit, enacting a subsidy law in the same year that provided assistance to families to pay for a child's medical needs and other costs. A year later, California granted children with disabilities continued eligibility for Crippled Children's Services after their adoption. While other states also considered subsidies for special needs children around this same time, eligibility criteria differed by state; some states required that adoptive parents prove that supporting a child would lower the families' standard of living, while others limited subsidies to parents from lower economic groups.[101]

To encourage more uniform laws, the US Children's Bureau gave the CWLA a grant in 1974 to develop a Model State Subsidized Adoption Act. The model act explicitly made adoption subsidies available for children who had, or were considered to have, a "physical or mental disability, emotional disturbance, recognized high risk of physical and mental disease, age disadvantage, racial or ethnic factors, sibling relationship, or any combination of these conditions."[102] By the late 1970s, more states had passed subsidy legislation. Finally, by 1981, in response to a new federal law, all states except Hawaii had passed subsidy legislation.

Until Congress authorized federal subsidies in 1980, state adoption subsidies facilitated special needs adoptions in real ways. One adopter reported: "Without a subsidy, we couldn't have made it. It would have killed me to have to give them back, and them too, I think."[103] Following permanency planning principles, state subsidies focused on "the child and his needs, rather than on the financial ability of the adoptive parents to meet those needs."[104] Considered one of the "service linchpins of special needs adoptions," 8,579 children in twenty-seven states received subsidies by 1977.[105] State subsidy laws not only helped families but also created substantial state savings in foster care and institution dollars. By 1977, for instance, states that provided subsidies saved an average of 36.9 percent of their foster care expenses.[106]

States offered two types of subsidies: medical subsidies and maintenance subsidies. Medical subsidies allowed the state to continue to pay for all of the treatment expenses related to the child's medical condition at the time of her adoptive placement. These subsidies paid for services like counseling for the child and the parents, physical and occupational therapies, surgeries like shunt installations or the correction of clubfoot, other medical treatments, and tutoring.[107] Legislators and adoption professionals widely acknowledged that these state medical subsidies helped increase the number of families willing to parent a disabled child. Maintenance subsidies, usually an amount less than the state would pay for foster care, reimbursed parents for the nonmedical financial costs of raising a disabled child. According to many adoption leaders, both types of subsidies made a "crucial difference in allowing the family to provide a home for a handicapped child."[108]

One drawback of state subsidies was that both eligibility criteria and payment amounts varied from state to state. The result was an imbalanced

Table II – Purposes

	A	B	C	D	E
MODEL ACT	X	X	X		
Alaska					
Arizona	X				
California	X	X		X	X
Colorado	X		X		
Connecticut					
Delaware					
Dist. of Col.			X		
Georgia				X	
Idaho			X	X	
Illinois					
Indiana			X		
Iowa					
Kansas	X	X	X	X	
Kentucky	X				
Maine					
Maryland					
Massachusetts		X	X		
Michigan			X		
Minnesota					
Missouri					
Montana	X	X	X		X
Nebraska	X		X		
Nevada			X		
New Jersey				X	
New Mexico	X	X			
New York					
North Carolina		X			
North Dakota					
Ohio			X	X	
Oregon			X		
Pennsylvania		X			
Rhode Island					
South Carolina			X		
South Dakota	X		X		
Tennessee			X		
Texas		X		X	X
Utah					
Vermont*					
Virginia			X		
Washington		X	X	X	
Wisconsin					
TOTALS	9	9	17	8	3

27 states with stated purposes
14 states with no stated purpose
*Vermont – to protect and promote the welfare of children in the state.

Legend

A – Establish a program of adoption support
B – Promote adoption of "hard-to-place" with special needs
C – Authorize payments for "hard-to-place" with special needs
D – Benefit "hard-to-place" in foster care and save state money
E – Make information available to prospective adoptive parents

FIGURE 6. From Sanford N. Katz and Ursula M. Gallagher, "Subsidized Adoption in America," *Family Law Quarterly* 10 (1976): 47.

system across the US for children and parents.[109] States could differentially include cash payments for daily maintenance costs or could cover such medical expenses as occupational training, prostheses, braces, crutches, wheelchairs and other devices, dental treatments, and speech therapy. Some, but not all, covered legal fees for the adoption. Subsidies could be long-term, or they might be provided only for a limited time, or until the child reached a certain age. In Michigan, for example, the State Subsidized Adoption Act made a subsidy available only "if the risk [for physical or mental disability] was recognized at the point of placement," and if the agency could prove that no other family could be found without the subsidy.[110]

Still other forms of public and private assistance helped lift the financial barriers of special needs adoptions in concrete ways. Expenses paid as a result of a special needs adoption, for example, became tax deductible. Some employers offered adoption benefits to employees who sought a special needs child, while some agencies waived fees to encourage applicants. Though not limited to adoptive families, the Home and Community Based Medicaid Waiver Program, created in 1981, also helped families by paying for community-based services for people with disabilities who had previously received institutional care and needed help transitioning into the community.[111] This waiver program was particularly important given that the insurance industry's discrimination against people with preexisting medical conditions was commonplace.

Agencies expanded postplacement services in the late 1970s to support adoptive families and try to keep them intact. Adoption professionals strongly recommended that agencies provide such services for families who adopted children with disabilities. Agencies helped families obtain financial assistance or find community resources that provided durable medical devices like eyeglasses or adaptive equipment like wheelchairs. Some agencies identified and helped navigate the network of state and local organizations that offered special education or day care services to these children, offered in-house counseling, helped families find respite care programs, or created a directory of community resources listing clinics, schools, churches, advocacy groups, and treatment centers that served children with disabilities.[112] One parent remarked that when she and her husband adopted their child Tyrone, they felt they could handle things: "We aren't super-parents but we just kind of take things one day at a time." But they realized that they needed a "breather," especially once Tyrone reached eight years old and needed help with activities of daily living. The agency helped the family find a respite care family to take care of Tyrone one week every two months. "He's adjusted well and it's a big help to all of us. But I can tell you, when Ty comes through that door on Sunday night, there are six happy people in this house!"[113]

While many agencies delivered valuable postplacement services, others had limited human resources, especially given the increasing caseloads and turnover as this period proceeded. Tight human resources and time constrained these agencies from providing consistent support to families. Some agencies refused to provide assistance if they did not agree with the treatment plans or parenting styles of certain families. Still others failed to carry out promises to enroll families in financial assistance, perhaps because they still adhered to the traditional idea that adoptive families' ability to parent was dependent upon taking total financial responsibility for the child's needs. A related enduring public belief that subsidies were like welfare could not have helped matters because many Americans assumed welfare was bad.[114]

Two examples from the 1970s bear this out. One involved Ms. Blake, a single woman who made $16,000/year, adopted a "severely brain damaged four year old boy who 'is blind, doesn't speak, can barely sit up and is like a baby, he is so limp.'" Ms. Blake felt that the agency did not want to grant her an adoption maintenance subsidy because they did not agree with her plan to enroll the child in a controversial treatment program. In the end, she received the subsidy but only after suing the agency and incurring debt. Although the agency arranged the financial maintenance subsidy retroactively, she did not receive a medical subsidy. Similarly, an agency worker promised Mrs. Last, who adopted Denny (a child with a hearing and speech impairment) that she would receive "Medicaid or Medicare, or whatever it was. I could send him to the dentist or take him to the doctor whenever anything happened." But the adoption agency never helped Mrs. Last fill out the forms, most likely due to insufficient postplacement services and intensive caseloads. Mrs. Last was therefore left with no insurance after she adopted Denny.[115] Rather than posing outright obstacles, some agencies simply did not offer to help out of negligence or mistaken information; they may have not discussed financial assistance options with prospective families because they incorrectly thought the family was ineligible or may have underestimated the extent to which parents needed help and services.

A Federal Commitment

By the end of this period, the federal government had, at long last, fully recognized the need to include children with disabilities in adoption. Lawmakers had enacted statutes like Section 504 of the Rehabilitation Act (1973; regulations written in 1977), the Education for All Act (1975),

and the Developmental Disabilities Act (1975), which expanded the
rights of people with disabilities. These laws, in turn, helped support governmental efforts to grow opportunities for disabled children's adoption
(appendix 2).

Certain legislative steps led to a fully developed federal commitment
to special needs adoption. For example, the 1978 Adoption Opportunities Act made model adoption legislation available to states with the goal
of removing obstacles to special needs adoptions. It also developed an
information exchange system that matched families to foster children legally free for adoption.[116] The law funded regional adoption resource centers and expanded interstate adoption exchanges. It implemented social
worker training programs to help agencies prepare prospective adoptive
parents to adopt foster children, and it established demonstration programs to recruit adoptive families from minority groups and to provide
postadoption legal services for families with special needs children. Although the act's programs were limited in scope, this law created a federal
role in the adoptive placement of marginalized children, including those
with disabilities, for the first time.[117]

But 1980 was the year that lawmakers significantly changed the play-
ing field for the adoption of children with disabilities.[118] The Adoption
Assistance and Child Welfare Act of 1980 (P.L. 96-272) was by far the
most noteworthy expansive federal policy to date. Enacted during the
Carter administration, the act amended Title IV of the Social Security
Act to enshrine preserving the birth family or permanent placement as
the primary goal of child welfare services. The act endorsed the idea that
children develop best in their birth families and that family preservation
is possible for many families; adoption should only be considered when
all else fails.[119] Despite its commitment to family preservation, the act also
propelled child welfare professionals to move special needs children from
foster care into permanent adoptive families.

First and foremost, lawmakers wanted to reduce the number of children entering foster care in the first place in order to prevent foster drift
and stem the rising costs of foster care. To achieve those aims, the federal
government began to monitor how foster care services were financed. It
restructured how state services, child welfare, foster care, and adoption
services were delivered. To receive federal payments, a state was required
to develop a plan for foster care and adoption assistance, had to track
every child, and had to create an individualized case plan for each child
in the foster care system to lessen foster drift.[120] When designing the case

plan, a caseworker had to ensure that the child was placed in a "least restrictive setting" (much like "least restrictive environment" in disability legislation).[121] To qualify for additional funds, the state had to create a system that would prevent family breakup, try to reunify birth families, or otherwise place children in adoptive homes. It had to review foster care cases every six months and assess whether adoption was appropriate for children in long-term foster care. Courts had to determine a child's future status (to return to birth parents, continue in foster care, or turn to adoption) within eighteen months after the child's initial placement in foster care.

Perhaps most significantly, the 1980 act provided states with the first federal financial incentives to develop an alternative to foster care, including adoption, for children with disabilities. It did so through the use of federal subsidies. Prior to the act, the federal government only reimbursed families for foster care; state and local funds paid for subsidized adoptions. Because states would lose federal foster care dollars when a child was placed into a subsidized adoption, most states had an interest in maintaining foster placements over subsidized adoption. With the exception of Democrats' 1977 attempt to provide federal subsidies for disabled children, "administrations never would listen to the argument that a mentally or physically handicapped youngster adopted by a private family ought to receive the same kind of federal money for care and treatment that was being spent on his or her behalf in an institutional setting."[122] Both President Carter and his secretary of Health, Education, and Welfare, Joseph Califano, had, in fact, at first opposed federal subsidies. Their position changed in July 1977, perhaps not coincidentally three months after sit-ins by disability activists against the administration, which pressured Califano to sign the 1973 Rehabilitation Act regulations.[123] Even with their limited support, the federal government did not officially back adoption subsidies until the Adoption Assistance and Child Welfare Act.

To reverse adoption disincentives in states, the law created a new provision, Title IV-E, the Federal Payments for Foster Care and Adoption Assistance. This title guaranteed subsidies to families who adopted children with special needs when the child was on Social Security Income or Aid to Dependent Children (ADC). Title IV-E required states to create an adoption assistance program to continue the children's participation in ADC.[124] Title IV-E also provided federal monies to states for the administrative costs needed to carry out special needs adoptions. The federal government paid a percentage of the adoption subsidy cost. To limit state welfare agencies' use of foster homes and to decrease foster drift, Title IV-E reduced federal support for foster care costs.[125]

The state had to classify a child as having special needs for her to be eligible to receive subsidies under the new law. The federal government encouraged states to define the term broadly; it supported child profiles that adopters typically did not choose outright and for children who could not return to their birth parents' home. Children had to have a "special condition" that *required assistance* (the "need") to be placed; without that assistance, placement would not likely occur. States consistently defined children with physical or mental impairments as belonging to this newly configured special needs category.[126]

One condition of Title IV-E was that states had to first make efforts to find a home where subsidy was unnecessary, except for cases of foster adoption where the child had emotional ties to the foster family but the parents needed subsidies to adopt the child.[127] By federally reimbursing states to promote adoption from foster care (fost-adopt), the act removed previous barriers and decreased foster care costs.[128]

Most importantly, under the law a child on ADC could continue to receive these payments and also receive Medicaid even after her adoption, *no matter the income level of the adopting family*. If interstate adoption occurred, benefits followed the child. The law's Medicaid provision removed a "tremendous barrier to adoption" for children with disabilities, and Congress hoped this would increase the likelihood of their adoption.[129] Henceforth, caseworkers used subsidies as major recruitment tools for these children's adoption: besides gaining Medicaid coverage for medical expenses, adopters could receive funds for the adoption's legal expenses and obtain a one-time adjustment payment for expenses incurred by bringing the child into the family. They could also receive assistance payments until the child reached eighteen.

Federal adoption subsidies heightened the chances that disabled children would be adopted. Although subsidies did not completely resolve the great need for adoptive families, Title IV-E tried to increase the number of "'special needs' adoptions," both through fost-adopt and otherwise. Though some states were initially reticent to take advantage of this federal assistance, those that used the program saw decreases in their foster care loads and substantial increases in their adoption rates. After an aggressive special needs adoption campaign in 1982, for instance, Illinois saw a 70 percent increase in such adoptions and a 132 percent increase in the number of subsidized adoptions.[130]

Subsequent federal actions tried to resolve persistent placement issues facing marginalized children. The Department of Health and Human Services issued a Model Act for the Adoption of Children with Special Needs, for instance, to address concerns about the estimated 100,000 special needs children in the foster care system.[131] Although it uses the word "act," the Model Act (as distinct from the Model State Subsidized Adoption Act) was a set of HHS recommendations directed at states to append to their existing adoption laws to facilitate children's adoption, including providing assistance to adoptive families to pay for medical and other needs, giving full genetic and medical histories of the children to adopted parents, and offering a timely family assessment to adopters interested in bringing a special needs child into their family. Like the Adoption Assistance Act, the model act showed the federal government's commitment to moving special needs children into adoptive homes.[132]

Possibility of Inclusion

From 1960 to 1980, adoption professionals and organizations, parents, and the states increasingly saw that it was possible to include children with disabilities in adoption. They translated this potential into action in conceptual and programmatic ways.

Conceptually, adoption professionals reconfigured risk from a trait inherent in children with disabilities to something located in social and structural barriers. As the demographic characteristics of adoption changed and the numbers of children in foster care grew, many children—especially those experiencing foster drift—became at risk for disability and impermanency. These new circumstances shifted the onus for permanent placement from children to advocates, agencies, and states. Adoption professionals focused, in turn, on devising programmatic solutions.

Compared to prior decades, these solutions were numerous and consequential. With parent advocates stressing the inherent value of these children, casework practices and recruitment strategies reflected a holistic picture of the child, rather than one primarily focused on the child's impairment. Professionals' move to relocate risk and instead emphasize barriers led them to establish specialized agencies, adoption centers, adoption exchanges, and social work training programs that tried to destigmatize disability and facilitate disabled children's permanent placement. For their part, state and federal legislators enacted laws that provided subsidies to help remove the financial barriers to placement that had, until this point, proved exceptionally tenacious in preventing applicants from adopting children with disabilities. These laws similarly showed a commitment to placing disabled children.

It is difficult to overstate the impact of professional and parent efforts to transform agency adoption to include children with disabilities during this period. An increasing number of disabled children gained access to permanent and secure families. Yet there were also limits to the ways professionals and parents framed the possibilities for inclusion. Although most of the initiatives were badly needed, they were confined solely to the realm of adoption; they generally did not address the interface between adoption, disability, and broad social change. Professionals framed the adoption of children with disabilities as a personal and private mission for parents rather a broader societal concern. Save for state and federal subsidies, programmatic responses like changing individualized casework practices or addressing social worker prejudice, stigma, or limited parental acceptance did not push the limits of national social, financial, or medical support for *all* individuals with disabilities. Neither did it offer a broad political solution to the question of the status of people with disabilities in American life, like more sweeping demands for equal citizenship and structural justice that activists at the time increasingly presented as needed for minorities and women. Moreover, adoption initiatives did not address the fundamental issues of inequality specifically facing children with disabilities in society.[133] Adoption professionals' work to include children with disabilities therefore remained largely dependent upon distinctive, specialized (and therefore segregated) agencies, programs, and strategies that, perhaps by necessity, eluded mainstreaming in adoptive practices. This reliance upon individualized practices therefore made inclusionary programs somewhat tenuous and particularly susceptible to shifting political and cultural conditions. As we will see in part 3, these limited gains failed to keep certain structural, institutional, and cultural barriers at bay in the face of a deepening foster care crisis.

PART III

Continued Obstacles: 1980–1997

Institutional and Structural Barriers to the Adoption of Children with Disabilities

In the spring of 1996, the *New York Times* ran a story on the growing serious problems in child protection services which prompted court supervision in at least twenty-one states. With very high caseloads of foster children, child welfare officials were slow to investigate reports of neglect and abuse and failed to provide adequate services for family reunification and adoption, thus jeopardizing foster children's legal rights of protection from psychological abuse and physical harm. Kevin E. had been under the custody of the District of Columbia for nearly a dozen years, and the district had no plans for his adoption or for psychiatric care. A judge found that he "told hospital staff that he hated himself and then climbed into a trash can and asked to be thrown away."[1]

Sadly, by the end of the 1990s, situations of long-term foster care like Kevin E.'s were not uncommon. Despite the fact that agencies had begun to address the need to revise attitudes and practices to promote disabled children's adoption, such placements turned out to be more complicated and difficult than adoption professionals originally anticipated. Even though social workers had some tools in place to facilitate placement, and the rate of special needs adoption increased compared to earlier decades, several tenacious institutional and structural barriers thwarted agency efforts. There were never enough parents to meet the overwhelming need of children with disabilities for permanent placement. By the end of the twentieth century, both the discrepancy between the number of applicants and children and intractable barriers produced a situation where disabled children had only partial access to the adoptive family.

Four main factors limited access to adoption for children with disabilities. The first was simply the magnitude of the problem. By 1980, the number of children in the foster care system had swelled to epidemic proportions.[2] Their sheer numbers made it difficult for child welfare workers to keep up with the need for permanent placement. During the 1980s and 1990s, case backlogs in the foster care system, particularly concerning children exposed to abuse and neglect, created "outrageous deficiencies" in state child protective services across the nation. Child welfare workers labeled many of these children disabled. Such pressures put children with physical, intellectual, and emotional disabilities and "special needs adoptions" at the center of foster care and adoption professionals' attention.[3]

Second, social worker bias and agency practices at times undermined the claim that "all children are adoptable." Though necessary, the special programs that professionals began adopting in the 1970s for recruiting parents and managing casework for children with disabilities reflected an underlying prejudicial vision of separate services that hindered these children's full inclusion in American adoption. Despite training programs like the Developmental Disabilities Adoption Project, some social workers continued to consider these children unadoptable.

Third, the grind of trying to find families taxed agencies' resources. Although adoption exchanges tried to facilitate placement, a lack of families undermined their purpose. Some social workers were also ambivalent about the kinds of families that might adopt these children. Given their other responsibilities, agencies had little time to offer robust postplacement services, itself a situation that threatened the success of the placements. Collectively, these strains threatened agencies' ability to place children with disabilities in anything resembling a sustained way.

Fourth, policy failures abounded. In particular, government cuts to child welfare and community care for people with disabilities in the 1980s tested the resolve of the "love and acceptance" discourse. It put families under great strain and exposed a set of societal priorities that jeopardized adoption placement. Court delays and legislative cutbacks further weakened the gains in special needs adoptions of the previous period.

Certainly, some halting progress in the area of adoption and children with disabilities had been made during this period. But serious institutional and structural challenges remained that ultimately led to an incomplete and partial inclusion of disabled children in adoption by the end of the twentieth century.

A Foster Care Surge

Beginning in the late 1970s, an increase in the number of children in the foster care system fundamentally altered the adoption sector and brought a new sense of crisis. The surge in the number of foster children caused adoption professionals to give intense focus to special needs adoptions.[4]

The demographics of children in the foster care system had also undergone major shifts. By the 1970s, the average age of children in the system had risen, and more children displayed behavioral and emotional problems than had previously been the case.[5] In 1975, the number of children in foster care reached the unprecedented level of 500,000, largely as a result of welfare policies, including the expansion of AFDC, which added federal funding for foster care, and child abuse laws.[6] During the 1980s, the numbers dropped but then rose again to 323,000 by the end of 1988.[7] Children available for adoption now mostly came from the foster care system, rather than from hospitals or maternity homes.

These changes engendered a new set of adoption agency practices and heightened anxieties about whether a given child would be disabled, traumatized, neglected, or all of the above. Even as the foster care population swelled, the rate of adoption slowed. The 31 percent rise in completed adoptions between 1990 and 1994 could not keep up with a 90 percent increase in foster children waiting for adoption during the same period.[8] By 1992, an estimated 429,000 children were waiting in foster care, of whom 85,000 were classified as special needs (which included children with disabilities, minority children, siblings, and older children—or the intersection of these groups).[9] In places like New York, Illinois, and Michigan, one third of them would never be adopted. Children of color made up more than half of those children in 1993.[10]

The crisis had numerous sources: attacks on welfare, increased rates of incarceration, rising levels of drug addiction, and the AIDS epidemic all contributed to the dramatic increase in foster care caseloads between 1986 and 2000.[11] But child welfare professionals honed in on two alternatives to address the crisis: biological family preservation and adoption reform, by which they meant reducing barriers to terminating a biological family's custody rights for a child who was languishing in the system. Until 1997, policymakers tried to strike a balance between these two approaches through federal legislative reforms, but each option had its own problems. Because of the lack of both sufficient foster care caseworkers and available resources to help biological families, attempts at preserving or reunifying families often faltered. Temporary placements could go on for years; a child could be reunified with her birth parents after years of no contact.[12] As a result, all children, with or without disabilities, were often left in legal limbo; either the child's biological parents were not ready to relinquish her for adoption, the child never became reunified with her birth parents, or the child moved in and out of foster care. None of these was in the best interests of the child. At the same time, faster adoption processes hindered efforts to keep biological families together and failed to address the social and structural issues that led to most foster care placements in the first place.

The deficiencies and incompatibility of these two options left special needs children particularly vulnerable. Leaders in the permanency planning movement defined special needs adoption as "furnishing a service to children deeply in need of a parent or parents who can provide them with nurturing despite atypical patterns of needs and responses, their old ages, or their minority or mixed biological heritages."[13] Like "hard to place" before it, the "special needs" category brought age, disability, and race into a collective category. In this case, the key word was "need," meaning the need for parents. For children with disabilities, major social changes like deinstitutionalization demanded more professional and legislative action to address the specific needs of these children and their prospects for adoptive placement. These pressures often left agencies in the 1980s and 1990s floundering.

It is unclear exactly how many children with disabilities were in the entire system at the beginning of this period. The National Center for Social Statistics stopped collecting this data in 1975, and neither public nor private agencies seemed to have maintained aggregate statistics on how many children awaited placement. Estimates of adoption rates for these children in 1974 and 1975 point to lower than a one-in-ten chance of permanent placement for these two years, while about 40 percent of waiting children in 1977 had an impairment of some kind.[14]

The lack of uniform national adoption reporting practices made it difficult for child welfare professionals and the government to adequately address the foster care and adoption problem.[15] In response, in 1984, the Administration on Children, Youth and Families formed the Adoption Information Improvement Workgroup. This workgroup made recommendations to the assistant secretary of the Department of Health and Human Services (HHS) to improve adoption information, including adding the descriptor "handicapped status of the child" to a new data system.[16] Given the increased need for quality data on adoption and foster care, three years later Congress amended the Social Security Act to address this problem. For its part, the Advisory Committee on Adoption and Foster Care submitted a report to Congress in 1988 in which it proposed best practices for collecting and reporting foster care and adoption data. The proposal resulted in the Adoption and Foster Care Analysis and Reporting System (AFCARS). Until this system began reporting in 1995, it was nearly impossible to grasp the magnitude of the problem of disabled children's adoption.[17]

Lacking national statistics, researchers in the 1980s attempted to fill in the gaps. One researcher reported that 35 percent of foster care children in 1982 had "marked or severe psychiatric impairment," while the American Public Welfare Association noted that as of 1985, 20 percent of the children in foster care in twenty-nine states had one or more disabling condition.[18] Adoption researchers Penny Deiner, Nancy Wilson, and Donald Unger described a typical child in foster care in the mid- to late 1980s as nine years of age and having emotional, mental, or physical impairments. They noted that in 1980s Delaware, for instance, the average time a child with an impairment spent in foster care until her biological parents terminated their rights was four years, while the average time from her placement until finalized adoption was almost six years.[19] For its part, the CWLA's 1988 *Standards for Adoption Service* noted a slightly but not altogether different profile: "The 50,000 waiting children [in 1984] were primarily minority; severely handicapped; slightly more boys than girls; age 12 or over; and in foster care for four or more years."[20]

Specialized agencies aggressively sought parents for these children. But even among children with disabilities, certain children were less likely to be adopted. As early as 1978, David Fanshel and Eugene Shinn observed that "the child *remaining* [my italics] in foster care was more likely to have a severe physical handicap which affected his social functioning, and he was more prone to be of a dull-normal intelligence or mentally retarded."[21] Some judges hesitated to terminate parental rights for a child with a mental, physical, or emotional disability if they were convinced that no family would choose to parent her.[22]

In the 1980s and 1990s, child welfare professionals differentiated between two subsets of children with disabilities in the foster care system as potential candidates for special needs adoptions: children who acquired emotional and behavioral disabilities through trauma (meaning abuse and neglect) and "children in need of chronic care." Although many did, not all handicapped children came from the foster care system. Parents also surrendered children to voluntary agencies or through independent placement, but child welfare professionals mainly focused on disabled children in foster care, who were then usually placed on the adoption exchange or through a specialized agency. Social workers deemed most children with acquired disabilities neglected, delinquent, abused, abandoned, or dependent.

A main contributor to the increase in children with acquired disabilities was the Child Abuse Prevention and Treatment Act (CAPTA) of 1974. Intended to facilitate children's placement in adoptive homes, CAPTA also "strengthened mandatory reporting of child abuse."[23] Often, social workers labeled children abused or neglected because a biological parent used drugs or alcohol, but they also categorized children that way because they thought there was an unstable living arrangement or an absence of a functional and caring parent.[24] CAPTA vastly expanded child welfare workers' abilities to remove children from their birth families if they suspected abuse or neglect; the workers did not have to offer a basis for their suspicions or bring a case to court. As such, CAPTA enabled social workers to label a child abused without ever having to prove that she had in fact experienced such abuse.

CAPTA resulted from a shift in social and political thinking in the 1960s that saw abuse and neglect as "intergenerational, pathological problems" akin to, and consistent with, the findings of the Moynihan Report about the Black family.[25] As Dorothy Roberts has pointed out, CAPTA did not address structural inequities like poverty nor did it decrease child mistreatment. Rather, reflecting stereotypical ideas about "Black female immorality and Black family dysfunction," child protection decisions to remove children from their biological parents under CAPTA disproportionately affected minority families on welfare.[26] The uneven effect of the law was so large by 1993 that three times as many Black, Hispanic, and Native American children were in the foster care system as their percentage in the general population.[27]

In 1996, Congress amended CAPTA to define child abuse as a parent's or caregiver's act, or failure to act, that resulted in serious physical or emotional injury, sexual abuse, and imminent risk of harm or death. Intended to tackle procedural issues that contributed to the influx of children into foster care, the new CAPTA required states to expedite the termination of parental rights for abandoned infants and established community-based programs to prevent child abuse and neglect. Congress believed the new CAPTA would alleviate problems in child protective services and foster care proceedings, including false reporting of abuse and neglect, a general lack of oversight of child protection, and delays in parental rights termination.[28]

Despite minority children's increased presence in foster care in the 1980s and 1990s, agencies were limited in where they could place these children. In 1972, the National Association of Black Social Workers (NABSW) declared their opposition to the ongoing discrimination against African American adoptive applicants in adoption recruitment and to the assumption that Black children would be better off in white families. The organization challenged the pursuit of transracial adoption, claiming that it threatened the racial identity and psychological well-being of Black children and that it threatened the integrity of the Black family. This stance was understandable given that within that historical moment Black Americans saw the sterilization of poor Black single mothers, vigorous debates about and actions related to the "illegitimacy" allegedly caused by these women, claims about the "pathology" of Black families, and an increase in the foster care placement of Black children.[29]

The Indian Child Welfare Act of 1978 (ICWA) applied NABSW's to Native children. It gave jurisdiction over child placements to individual Native American tribes as a corrective to programs that placed Native American children into white homes through the Indian Adoption Project (1958–1967); the struggle for ICWA started in 1968. It was also an attempt to redress the pattern of state efforts to break up Native American families and send children to boarding schools.[30] ICWA posited that Indian nations should govern themselves through their tribal courts, rather than through the courts of the states that surrounded them.[31]

These two communities intended, first and foremost, to preserve the integrity of communities of color and to challenge adoption's orientation toward satisfying the needs of white families. One of ICWA's consequences was that it curtailed transracial adoptions until the late 1990s.[32] From the 1970s on, efforts to place minority children from the foster care system were highly sensitive to transracial arrangements as a last option. In 2018, however, some states questioned the constitutionality of ICWA and threatened to overturn the ability of Native American tribes to self-govern, including in areas of family law, and to restructure American federalism.[33] As of April 2021, the Fifth Circuit Court of Appeals issued an en banc ruling in *Brakeen v. Haaland* that ICWA is constitutional in terms of sovereignty but struck down several provisions, including the "active efforts," expert witnesses, and record keeping parts of the law. Active efforts require timely and comprehensive attempts at parent reunification; qualified expert witnesses provided an extra layer of oversight if a child welfare agency intended to place a child in foster care or to terminate parental rights; and record keeping obliged states to record their efforts to maintain a placed child's bond with her tribe.[34] At the time of this writing, experts expect the case will be appealed to the Supreme Court.

CAPTA also significantly affected children with disabilities, including those who were minority children. Child protective services removed children with acquired disabilities involuntarily from their birth parents and placed them in foster care. Often, child welfare workers believed that these children had little chance of reuniting with their birth parents. The children usually stayed in foster care for several years (in 1991, between three and six years) before becoming adopted, exposing them to considerable foster drift. This caused child welfare workers to consider children in foster care at high risk for emotional, behavioral, and learning disabilities (if they didn't already have them).[35] If they were adopted, parents frequently noted that they required a multitude of specialized psychological, medical, and educational services that were not readily available to adoptive parents.

A second, new group of disabled children in the 1980s and 1990s were children in need of "chronic care." They largely came into the foster care system because of deinstitutionalization and the AIDS crisis.[36] Deinstitutionalized children who were rejected by their biological families or were not yet placed into an adoptive family spent years in the foster care system. They had a variety of physical and cognitive impairments and had experienced traumatizing conditions while institutionalized. Children who had contracted HIV/AIDS through mother-child transmission required expensive medical treatments and care.

Although children with varying degrees of intellectual disability had the most pressing need for adoption, those children who were Black, older, *and* intellectually disabled were hardest to place. Agencies discovered that finding homes for children who were "older or who have physical or other handicaps has for a variety of reasons been fraught with difficulties."[37] Despite these foster care demographics, thousands of prospective parents were still holding out for several years to adopt a "much-preferred healthy infant."[38]

Agency Impediments to Adoption

These demographic changes in the foster care population led adoption professionals to frequently and repeatedly state that "no child is unadoptable"
(or "every child is adoptable"), no matter what the "special" characteristic of the child. Adoption professionals started to make this claim in the
1970s but intensified their position in the 1980s. Their insistence reflected
the new adoption landscape, but it also showed they really meant it.[39]

The position that no child is unadoptable was consistent with the support for children's rights in child welfare circles in the late 1970s and into
the 1980s.[40] Child welfare workers embraced the idea that every child
should have an equal opportunity to be permanently placed in the best
home possible, no matter how "hard to place" a child was or how many
"special needs" she might have.[41] In an approach reminiscent of Helen
Hallinan's claim in 1951, child welfare professionals now contended that
although children might be unplaceable, "no child is unadoptable."[42]
These professionals implicitly argued that human worth and adoptability
were conceptually inseparable; if social workers truly believed that a child
was worthy of family, they would deem her adoptable.

Of course, this refrain did not mean that all social workers translated
the idea into practice, nor did it resolve the procedural delays that functioned to undermine those needs. Agencies' persistent residual prejudice
against placing disabled children, especially those with intellectual disability, led to an uneven integration of the idea that no child is unadoptable. They assumed children with "handicapping conditions" could not
live in a "normal family setting, develop normal relations with parents
or function adequately in a family."[43] When asked at a Senate committee
hearing in 1985 if it was common for some social workers to discourage
interested families from adopting severely handicapped children, adoptive mother Mrs. Ashton Avegno testified, "Yes, it is quite a common
practice. This happened to us with Matthew, and it has happened to us on
a number of other occasions also."[44] Matthew, three at the time, was diagnosed with cerebral agenesis and other congenital disabilities. From New
Orleans, Avegno and her husband had adopted two of her seven children
through the State of Louisiana's Department of Health and Human Services. Six of her children were labeled as having special needs.

Social workers discouraged applicants for a variety of reasons, some explicit, some implicit. Some social workers discouraged applicants because

they did not see particular types of children as being able to function within family life. In her testimony before the Senate, Avegno stated that social workers had a hard time believing that parents could actually want to adopt a physically, mentally, or emotionally disabled child, making statements like "Why in the world would you want to adopt a child like *that*? Are you sure you want to adopt *him*? Why don't you not adopt him—just keep him in foster care. He won't know the difference anyway."[45] Other social workers had a more benign motivation; they believed that caring for children through the foster care system, rather than through adoption, gave parents better access to the financial and material resources their children needed to survive and flourish. Still others felt that spending any money or time on these children was a futile effort and a waste of "precious resources."[46]

Procedural delays also posed major barriers to disabled children's adoption. The process by which a child was placed in a permanent home usually followed three steps under the foster care system. First, child welfare workers would try to reunify the child with her biological family. If that effort was unsuccessful, a court would terminate parental rights. Adoption planning could only commence after these steps had taken place. Slowdowns at any of these stages could delay the child's return to her birth family or adoptive placement.

Several kinds of bureaucratic issues resulted in delays. First, the Child Welfare Act's family preservation and reunification guidelines were often vague, leaving agencies to interpret what constituted "reasonable efforts." In some states, like Illinois, the court could take up to a year after the initial petition to formally rule on any findings of abuse or neglect. This timeline contributed to further delay in reunification or adoptive placement.

Second, only specialized adoption staff could undertake the process of terminating parental rights, meaning that a case would often have to move to a new caseworker who would need to take some time to get familiar with the case. In some states, like Michigan, foster care workers had control over the case until termination, achieving greater consistency. During the termination phase, judges could and did raise questions about the adoptability of the child, often challenging some of the agency's affirmative claims. Until the Adoption and Safe Families Act (ASFA) of 1997, in fact, some states would not allow termination to occur until a permanent family was found.[47] Court delays or a lack of sufficient documentation could also cause delays.

After termination, agencies had to commence adoption casework, which included assessing the child, recruiting families, training parents, and then finalizing the adoption. This part of the process could take a year or more, depending on the agency's caseload. Adoption planning could take place only after child welfare workers had made attempts to reunify the child with her biological parents or when the state terminated parental custody rights.

As time passed, the children aged, contributing to a vicious cycle that made them less desirable to prospective adoptive parents. In 1980s Delaware, for instance, the average time in foster care for a child with an impairment was four years; the average time from placing the child until finalizing her adoption was almost six years. Most children were originally placed in foster care by age two. Once legally free for adoption, a child could spend an additional two years waiting to be adopted because of the state's slow bureaucratic process or because of agency procedures. These time lapses made the moniker "waiting children" very accurate.[48]

Thus, despite the rhetoric of adoptability, that status was actually conditional upon social workers' support of children's eligibility, the removal of bureaucratic barriers, and, of course, the willingness of certain parent applicants to welcome such children into their homes. These conditions made the inclusivity of disabled children's adoption only partial rather than unequivocal.

The Quest for Hard-to-Find Families

To fulfill the pledge that "no child is unadoptable" and to respond to the foster children's overwhelming need for permanent placement, adoption leaders broadened the criteria of parental eligibility. Yet challenges remained, even for agencies who placed foster care children in adoptive homes, and which made finding these "hard-to-find families" a priority. Social workers who used the term "hard-to-find families" deliberately turned the concept of "hard-to-place" children on its head. "Hard-to-place child" implied that the child was a placement burden or inherently to blame for her status; "hard-to-find family" moved the onus from child to parents.[49]

But, as in years past, families were harder to find for some children than for others; a disabled child's likelihood of adoption in the 1980s and 1990s often depended upon her condition, the community in which prospective parents resided, and the state and social worker dealing with the case. An unintended consequence of the understandable efforts to curtail transracial adoption during this time to counter the breakup of families of color was that these efforts further limited agencies' ability to find enough families for disabled children of color.[50] Yet no matter what their race, children with Down syndrome, multiple disabilities, and emotional disabilities faced more placement challenges than children with visible physical disabilities, usually either because of social worker prejudice or because of applicant reticence.

In 1988, a CWLA survey, "The State of Adoption in America," found that the primary barrier to timely adoption placement was simply a "lack of parents willing to take special needs children"; certainly not enough to meet the urgent need.[51] Parents' reticence generally stemmed from several different but related factors: fears about disability and a child's different appearance or behavior, a lack of knowledge about particular impairments, friends' and relatives' disapproval, fears about emotional and financial demands, and concerns about other children in the household.[52] Given many prospective parents' hesitations about community, family, and finances, adoption networks that served older, disabled, and minority children explicitly welcomed a wide variety of parents, an even broader group than in the past.[53]

Agencies' openness to older, single, African American, and lower-income parents, which had started in the 1970s, only grew during this time. By 1984, for instance, about two hundred single-parent adoptions occurred per year. But because agencies continued to prioritize couples over single parents for healthy babies, single parents' choices remained limited; they either had to adopt "special needs" children or to adopt from abroad.[54] More agencies also organized recruitment efforts for Black parents to encourage adoption, often working alongside Black churches.[55] Some states allowed agencies to consider gay parents. Half of the states by this time allowed each person in a gay or unmarried relationship to adopt a child, but it was generally still difficult to jointly adopt as a couple.[56] Toward the end of the 1990s, gay and lesbian couples from New Jersey won the joint right to adopt a child, but only from state custody. New Jersey was the first state in the nation to take such an action; advocates at the time saw it as a first step for gay and lesbian couples to eventually adopt children outside of state custody.

Perhaps the most notable change during this period was that agencies grew more open to two new sets of prospective adoptive parents: foster parents and disabled applicants. The child welfare world promoted fost-adopt as an important new avenue to fulfill the desperate need for adoptive parents. In contrast to earlier constraints to fost-adopt—particularly the financial criteria for adoptive applicants that many foster parents could not meet and the taint of accepting state money for an endeavor that was supposed to be about love—many agencies now saw foster parents as preferable applicants. By the mid- to late 1980s, foster parents adopted about 70 percent of older child placements. Researchers at the Special Needs Adoption Project in Delaware (SNAP) found that the typical fost-adopt family in Delaware was white, very active in their church, older (an average of forty-two years old for mothers and forty-five years old for fathers) and had an annual median income of $19,000. Most foster parents were not originally looking to adopt, but they established an emotional bond with the child in their care and changed their minds.

Though disabled people had expressed a desire to adopt children for decades, agencies had often turned them away. But beginning in the late 1970s, agencies began to consider this applicant pool more seriously.[57] There were, however, important limits to disabled parents' eligibility. The 1978 CWLA Standards, which remained operative in the 1980s, noted that "couples where one mate is physically handicapped may be considered, provided that they meet the foregoing health requirements and are *emotionally well-adjusted* to the handicap" (my italics). These health requirements included medical evidence that both parents had a reasonable life expectancy (reasonable was not defined) and that they had the physical and emotional ability to care for the family.[58] Those caveats had real consequences for parent applicants with disabilities. For example, Jane Zirinsky-Wyatt, an adoptive mother with cerebral palsy, initially worried that adoption agencies would presume that she was unfit. This assumption led her to first try fertility treatments rather than adoption. It turned out that she was right. The first private adoption agency she went to rejected her because it thought she and her disabled husband "would present an extensive risk to the overall best interest of the child." She then turned to Family Focus, a specialized agency for "hard-to-place kids," where she and her partner first fostered and then adopted Sara, a child who was born preterm and exposed to drugs.[59]

Like Family Focus, Spaulding for Children in Michigan took disabled parents seriously as applicants. They did so in the case of Marty, a child diagnosed with cerebral palsy and intellectual disability at age two. Marty was referred to Spaulding at five years of age because his adoptive parents terminated the adoption before they had finalized it. Although they reportedly felt very attached to him, they also felt unable to deal with his disabilities. He became a ward of the state; by the time he was referred to Spaulding, he had been moved among seven foster homes. Caseworkers' assessments ranged from "severely retarded" to "reasonably intelligent."

A newspaper article featuring Marty led to several couples expressing an interest in him, but an older couple, Donald and Mary, with older bio-logical children caught the agency's attention. They had previously ap-plied to a private adoption agency, but social workers there rejected their application because Donald was paralyzed from the neck down due to multiple sclerosis. His income derived from Social Security and Veterans Administration payments. Donald and Mary had an interest in adopting children with major physical or mental disabilities because of their "famil-iarity with handicaps and their realistic appraisal of a handicapped child's opportunities for adoption."[60]

Like Donald and Mary, many of the families with and without disabilities who sought a special needs adoption were familiar with disability through work or a child in the home. These families felt they had unique qualities that were suited to this kind of adoption. As Grace Sandness, a woman who had had spinal and respiratory polio as a teenager and then became quadriple-gic, stated about her own desires, "We wanted to take 'special' children—those who were from minority groups or had physical problems—since we felt that with our personal experience with disability we had perhaps more understanding to give a disabled child than would the average parent."[61]

Increasing numbers of disabled parents not only began to offer parent-less children the opportunity for family during this period, but also helped dispel the presumption that disabled parents were neither competent enough nor able to be good parents. This prevailing attitude, for instance, led child welfare workers to remove children from the homes of disabled biological parents like Tiffany and Tony Callo. Tiffany, who had cerebral palsy, had her two sons taken from her because state child protective ser-vices believed she couldn't raise them simply because of her disability. Their rationale was that she could not pick up her children unassisted and so they assumed this hindered her ability to parent.[62] A lack of state funding for in-home baby care services and assistive parenting devices to support disabled parents compounded these child welfare workers' claim.[63] In this sense, they broadened parental love and parenting as integrally involving independent physicality, rather than solely deriving from an emotional commitment.

But activists in the disability rights movement and many social workers challenged the child welfare belief that disabled parents like Callo could not parent because of their disability.[64] Sandness, for instance, argued for a more inclusive attitude about this issue. "The successful disabled person is not dominated by his disability. He desires nothing more than to have normal responsibilities, duties and pleasures including, for some, a fam-ily." Throughout the US, she wrote, thousands of disabled, "but certainly 'adoptable'" couples had the necessary love to parent the "otherwise un-wanted children of the world."[65]

Donald and Mary's example showed adoption agencies that disabled parenthood could have positive outcomes. By the turn of the century, as discussed in the epilogue, other parents increasingly used their stories to reinforce this point. Although they described continued prejudice sur-rounding their candidacy to be an adoptive parent—especially within a context where the birth parent chooses the adoptive applicants—disabled parents' accounts emphasize that disabled parents could offer their dis-abled children pride and insight into the cultural and practical experience of living with a disability.[66] As disability activist, scholar, and adoptive mother Corbett O'Toole has observed, disabled adoptive parents could introduce their child to a strong disability community, in much the same way that adoptive parents of color did for their children of color.[67]

Agencies likely began to consider disabled parents not only because of their need to find more willing parents, but also because of a broader con-text in which the disability rights movement challenged society's invalida-tion of disabled people. Disability rights activists argued that civil rights and access to the public sphere needed to be extended to people with dis-abilities. The movement made many strides during this time, but it was the Americans with Disabilities Act (ADA; 1990) that enshrined legal protection for disabled parents. In the past, agencies commonly rejected disabled parent applicants outright; even judges felt that such adoptions should be "nipped in the bud" because homes with disabled parents were not "normal."[68] The ADA explicitly prohibited discrimination in parent eligibility criteria and casework, *as long as* the parent would not endan-ger the child.[69] Agencies could no longer ask prospective parents to un-dergo medical exams or to respond to health-related questionnaires in the evaluation process unless it was tied to the capacity to parent, and agencies had a much harder time rejecting applicants based on projected life expectancy. The agency could, however, ask for a medical exam once a parent was accepted. The ADA's purview was inclusive of all public and private agencies, no matter the number of employees.[70]

Stretching Applicants' Desires

Of course, many prospective families did not initially come to adoption agencies looking to adopt a disabled child. Faced with such a pressing need for adoptive families, agency workers began asking applicants to "stretch" their preferences; that is, to expand the idea of what they would accept in a child. In light of the decreased number of white, healthy children available for adoption, agency workers urged applicants to stretch in order to consider children with all kinds of disabilities. One child welfare handbook, for instance, cautioned agencies not to discourage applicants during their initial contact if they came seeking an infant or a nondisabled child. "All applicants to the agency must be seen as potential parents of a handicapped child. If applicants are abruptly informed that the agency is no longer taking applications for infants or that there is a long waiting list, many potential families for special need [sic] children will be lost and others will never call."[71]

Although some researchers described the idea of stretching in the 1970s, adoption professionals more commonly utilized this language in the 1980s and 1990s. To accomplish stretching, social workers played down the child's impairments and framed the child as an individual who "*happen*[s] *to have* certain needs and /or is of a certain age, rather than with a list of handicapping conditions" (my italics).[72] In some ways, this was a continuation of the 1970s strategy of using a child-specific recruitment approach that turned the notion of disability as inability into one where the child had unique qualities.[73] At the same time, however, social workers still tried to privilege normality; they sought to make more apparent "facets of a child who is more like a 'healthy and normal' child than one who is different."[74] These strategies, seemingly contradictory, worked together to achieve their goal. In their effort to recruit new applicants, agencies described families who adopted children with disabilities as typical families, too. Spaulding's booklet about placing special needs children in the late 1970s, for instance, described families who sought such an adoption path this way: "Families who adopt older or handicapped youngsters are not some form of exotic faunae found in remote forests. They are all around us, camouflaged among the ordinary people quietly going about the business of living."[75]

Florence Tillman, a single adoptive mother, followed this same descriptive logic when she described her life with her adopted daughter Marion. She portrayed the quotidian as different, but no less ordinary:

Having a wheelchair in the house means thirty-six inches of fresh grass clippings tracked in the house every time the lawn is mowed. It means having a thick rug by the door to park on while the snow melts from the spokes. . . . The peanut butter and jelly has to be on a low shelf. . . . It means having a place to tuck a purse and packages while shopping and meeting people who are willing to hold open doors.[76]

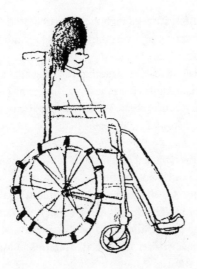

Self Portrait by Marion Tillman

FIGURE 7. Marion Tillman sketch. From Spaulding for Children, *Adapting to the Adoption of Special Children: The Stories of Five Special Families* (Chelsea, MI: Spaulding for Children, 1978), 11.

In their effort to achieve applicant stretching, agencies also emphasized typicality in order to humanize families who had adopted children with disabilities. However, they also tended to downplay the sometimes more demanding practical ramifications of fulfilling children's needs, whether educational, medical, social, or financial. These needs could include lifting and toileting, going to medical appointments, procuring and paying for physical or occupational therapy, finding an appropriate school, and experiencing higher health care costs. Of course, the needs differed from child to child, but the potential necessity of unpaid (and usually gendered) labor that was involved in fulfilling children's needs often posed emotional, financial, and time barriers for applicants.

Parents who adopted disabled children recognized the challenges related to the diligent planning, disability discrimination, the impact an invisible disability had upon receiving services, and behaviors that are "not always acceptable to society." But they also acknowledged the rewards and joy their children brought to the family, highlighting mental, physical, or emotional "difference" rather than "handicaps."[77] For instance, giving advice to other parents, adoptive mother Jo Ecarius reframed parenting a disabled child as a question of rights. She articulated three facts that she urged parents to remember when they felt discouraged:

> First, your child has an inalienable right to an education best suited for him no matter what his handicap. Second, he has a right to medical assistance so that he can function as a human being. Third, you, his parents, have a real obligation to fight for and obtain your child's rights.[78]

Ecarius stressed how a parent of a disabled child must also be an advocate for their child. But such advice often sat in tension with parents' questions about life-long dependence, educability, and quality of life, particularly after their deaths. To address these concerns, experts recommended that caseworkers give a complete and precise picture of the child's current functioning. The caseworker needed to "make some reasonable predictions of the child's future."[79]

The need for social workers to reassure applicants of a child's "competency" was, in effect, a desire to assess the degree of acceptable risk parents were willing to undertake to make a child their own. Toward that goal, social workers tried to address applicants' wishes by only making tempered predictions and by helping the family "understand WHO the child is and HOW he became that person," including disclosing part of the child's record. Sometimes caseworkers also introduced the child to the applicants, often without the child knowing it (e.g., having applicants observe a child), in order to allay applicant parents' fears. Other times, when appropriate, caseworkers would arrange for the adoptive applicants to actually meet the child. Dottie Blacklock of Spaulding described this attempt to strike a balance between addressing the fears of applicants and refusing to guarantee anything: "Risk is always part of the job, but risk must be balanced by cautious, shared judgments."[80]

New Mechanisms but Long Waits

Although the Adoption Resource Exchange of North America (ARENA) continued to be one of the main ways to address special needs adoption, the mere existence of this exchange was not enough to solve these children's placement issues. Thus, other organizations tried to fill children's unmet placement needs. The North American Council on Adoptable Children, a coalition of adoption groups, coordinated with groups like AASK (Aid to Adoption of Special Kids) and the National Foster Parents

Association to promote the adoption of children with special needs and to work to sustain these families' adoptions. Unlike ARENA, these organizations provided information and support to families, agencies, and children.

The Department of Health and Human Services also began a National Special Needs Adoption Initiative that worked with states and local communities to promote special needs adoption, including for children with disabilities. The initiative involved a public awareness campaign about children in foster homes, institutions, and group homes. It also publicized the need to recruit adoptive parents, especially minority parents. In addition, the initiative trained adoption workers to update their practices, addressed adoptions across state lines, and encouraged a review of state adoption laws. Among its many activities, HHS gave funds to the National Black Child Development Institute to sponsor a national special needs adoption conference for representatives of major Black organizations. Several governmental agencies also came together to promote special needs adoption, including the Administration on Children, Youth and Families, the Administration on Developmental Disabilities, the President's Committee on Mental Retardation, and the Administration for Native Americans.[81]

For their part, agencies created their own projects. The United Methodist Family Services of Virginia's two-year project (1987–1989), for example, addressed common barriers to recruiting parents for developmentally disabled children. By 1988, the agency had pinpointed 66 children and placed 41 (out of approximately 500 children legally free for adoption in Virginia) for adoption in 40 families. Twenty-four per cent of the children had learning disabilities, 20 percent were considered developmentally delayed, 17 percent were "mentally retarded," 15 percent had multiple disabilities, 12 percent were physically disabled, and 12 percent had emotional disability.[82] Although 686 families responded to the agency's recruitment efforts, only 6 percent actually went through with an adoption. The agency worked with Virginia's adoption exchange, volunteer adoption and foster parent organizations, foster parents of children with developmental disabilities, media, churches, and community service organizations across the nation to find potential families. Community outreach and awareness initiatives were key to the agency's recruitment success.[83]

Other agencies instituted community-based adoption practices, particularly for minority children. Projects like Homes for Black Children and One Church, One Child concentrated on finding homes for waiting Black children while projects like Spaulding for Children Southwest Hispanic

Recruitment Project in Texas looked to find Hispanic parents for Hispanic waiting children.[84] In 1985, the federal government granted funds to the national Spaulding for Children to create a National Resource Center for Special Needs Adoption to provide technical assistance to agencies in other states and to expand social work and parent training in special needs adoptions. The center provided training to over 25,000 professionals and parents from 1985 through 1990.

Despite all these efforts, developmentally disabled children still tended to be the least served, even in agencies with special needs adoption programs.[85] In Virginia, for instance, other procedural barriers to their adoption existed, like the inability of the local departments of social services to carry out home studies or do the intensive matching needed for children with special needs, even when a family was interested in such an adoption. United Methodist Family Services, for instance, found that caseworkers failed to place many developmentally disabled children on the Virginia exchange or feature them in photo-listing books because supervisors, directors, and child welfare workers did not consider the children adoptable and could not imagine parenting such a child themselves. Caseworkers also resisted transracial placement of children with developmental disabilities, despite a general policy that allowed agencies to place transracially after they had first made "reasonable efforts" to find a family of the child's race.[86]

To make matters worse, states offered uneven services and subsidies for adoptive parents of disabled children. Despite the 1980 Child Welfare and Adoption Assistance law, Virginia agencies did not offer postplacement counseling and services, nor did it consistently offer subsidies. In 1988, California passed a law requiring agencies to notify every family involved in special needs adoption about the difference between adoption subsidies and foster care benefits. Typically, subsidies for adoptive parents were about one-third of foster care rates, creating a financial disincentive to adopt.[87] In states where Medicaid was available after adoption, the program offered limited coverage for children with emotional disabilities, a major subpopulation of waiting children.[88]

Thus, despite a myriad of projects, initiatives and specialized agencies, agencies simply found it very hard to find families for these children and to fulfill the necessary social work processes to make their adoption possible. A 1982 inquiry found that boys ages eight or older "with some degree of mental retardation," children with multiple mental or physical disabilities, older children with Down's Syndrome, healthy Hispanic and Black children, and adolescents waited longest on the national exchange. Exchange consultants consistently specified the heightened need to find Black families and families for school-age children with "varying degrees of mental retardation."[89]

The persistent need to recruit families to adopt special needs children led adoption professionals to articulate best practices for special needs foster children. They recommended that states free children for adoption at a younger age; that agencies put in place permanency plans that delineated a specific timeframe for either returning children to their biological homes or making them available for adoption; that agencies place children in foster care environments that are *clearly promising* for adoption; that adoption agencies reevaluate potential adoptive parents according to the particular demographics of parents who adopt special needs children and changing the public image of who is eligible to adopt; that agencies inform those interested in adoption that foster care is a legitimate way to determine whether a placement might work out; and, finally, that agencies clearly provide information about the demands of the adoption process and provide postplacement referrals for therapy if needed.[90]

Legislation and Policy Failures

Legislative efforts in this period played a major role in promoting the adoption of children with disabilities by restructuring foster care and removing financial barriers to placement. But these policies were ridden with extensive bureaucratic issues and were never adequately funded. Furthermore, they did little to address the structural barriers that make it difficult for anyone with disabilities to survive and thrive in the United States. As such, these were piecemeal policies designed to address symptoms rather than underlying problems.

As we learned in chapter 4, the Child Welfare and Adoption Assistance Act, passed in 1980, tried to make biological family preservation the primary goal of child welfare services for special needs children. If that was not possible, the act promoted adoption as a solution to the foster care problem. The federal government tried to achieve these ends by transforming how child welfare services were delivered. It introduced planning and oversight procedures to track foster care children and to create plans for placement. It provided medical and maintenance subsidies to address postplacement needs. Still, because. the act had many layers to fulfill its multifaceted goals, it required the states to set up numerous bureaucratic mechanisms, including child tracking and reporting procedures, and an adoption assistance program to preserve children's enrollment in Aid for Dependent Children (ADC). While the Child Welfare and Adoption Assistance Act was the first, later policies would have similar bureaucratic and budgetary issues, especially as the politics of federal economic retrenchment became prominent beginning under the Reagan administration.

One of the largest hurdles for adoptive families with disabled children involved financial support for medical care since the US lacked (and still lacks) universal health care. As a result, a legislative patchwork to assist families was available but not comprehensive. The Adoption Assistance Act of 1980, for instance, excluded from Medicaid disabled children who had been placed through private agencies. Adoptive parents had to obtain medical insurance for their child through their existing medical policy, but since the Adoption Assistance Act was enacted thirty years before the Patient Protection and Affordable Care Act, some of these policies explicitly excluded adoptive children or family members with preexisting conditions.[91] If a disabled child did not qualify for her family's medical insurance policy, she had to qualify for SSI, which was not guaranteed. Some states, like Texas, routinely denied these claims.[92] These insurance gaps left a portion of disabled children uncovered or not adopted. Though later legislation, particularly the Medicare Catastrophic Coverage Act of 1988 (PL 100-360), tried to address one particular type of gap, the broader lack of guaranteed access to health care consistently deterred prospective parents from adopting children with disabilities.[93]

Another attempted policy solution was in the area of subsidies. As we saw in chapter 4, there were two types of adoption subsidies: one for medical care and the other for maintenance. We should remember that the Adoption Assistance Act provided federal subsidies (Title IV-E, for legal expenses related to the adoption itself and for maintenance) to adoptive parents and allowed children to stay on Medicaid if they were already on ADC.[94] It also gave states subsidies for the administrative costs related to special needs adoptions. The Model Act for the Adoption for Children with Special Needs (1981) offered guidance to states to govern subsidy payments for an adopted child's medical and maintenance needs.[95] These efforts reduced foster care loads and increased adoptions for states that fully participated.

But subsidy provision was not uniform across the country. In practice, as many as one-third of all states violated the intent of the Adoption Assistance Act by refusing to provide these federal subsidies. The states claimed that subsidies were conditional on the continued availability of state or federal funds. Moreover, the subsidy payments were not automatic; parents had to apply, and not all agencies provided this information to families. It is unclear why agencies would withhold this information; perhaps it reflected social workers' continued belief that prospective parents should be able to support their child without assistance.[96] For those families who did receive subsidies, states often delayed reimbursement for medical expenses, leaving some families waiting six months or more for a claim to be paid. These actions ran counter to the expressed intent of the law, which offered subsidies to remove disincentives from special needs adoption.[97]

Throughout the 1980s and 1990s, federal legislators introduced a series of other bills to address special needs adoption, to no effect. Senators Lloyd Bentsen (D-TX) and Bob Packwood (R-OR), for example, introduced the Special Needs Adoption Assistance Act in 1991 (S. 268) to provide a tax deduction of up to $3,000 to help families with the costs of adopting a disabled or other special needs child. They also proposed creating a demonstration project wherein federal employees could be reimbursed for up to $2,000 for any incurred expenses relating to a special needs adoption.[98] Even if this legislation had passed, however, a one-time $3,000 deduction would have done little to address the ongoing expenses of caring for children with disabilities in an adoptive family. Depending upon the child's needs and whether a child qualified for SSI, medical costs alone could exceed that amount for one year, and ongoing or intensified needs requiring additional support and assistance in subsequent years could potentially cause additional outlay. Furthermore, there were also invisible labor demands for which one could not put a price, and which could lead to a parents' need for respite care.

These needs and costs were surely replicated in families with biological children with disabilities. But the difference here is that adoption subsidies provided a way to incentivize states to move children from foster care to permanent homes. It did so by stimulating parents to adopt foster children with disabilities to provide such homes. Unlike the biological situation, subsidies addressed a major, national child welfare problem. They catalyzed a process whereby children who otherwise had no permanent homes to access them. Given that they were under state custody, the government had an interest in helping to alleviate barriers to placement.[99]

Or so one might have thought. Known for its cuts to child welfare, the Reagan administration tried but failed to repeal the 1980 Child Welfare and Adoption Assistance Act. Instead, the administration's policies of budgetary retrenchment frustrated family reunification efforts that were central to the law and would have reduced the number of children waiting for adoption. The administration shifted social service funding to block grants, a move the CWLA and North American Center on Adoption (NACA) vehemently opposed.[100] The Reagan administration also neglected to provide federal guidelines to states on qualifying for federal funds and family support services to preserve or reunify biological families. Accompanied by staff turnover, high caseload, and depleted resources, many states either did not try to reunify families or significantly delayed those efforts.[101]

Additional federal legislation tried to address a growing unsustainable foster care crisis in the 1990s. Congress passed laws offering assistance to states for child abuse and neglect prevention (1992) and for programs to preserve biological families and offer support services (1993). By 1993, about 17 percent of all abused children had disabilities, which was twice the rate for youth without disabilities. This rate contributed to their disproportionate presence in the foster system.[102] These laws confronted the foster care dilemma by establishing new mechanisms for both family preservation and adoption. However, the laws only addressed the immediate crisis of child abuse and saw the issues of abuse and neglect as individualized problems that were separate and distinct from other social problems. There was no legislation, for example, that was specifically designed to protect children whose parents were incarcerated. Neither did these laws address other reasons for the entrance of children with disabilities into the foster system, like relinquishment at birth because of the inability or unwillingness of a birth parent to care for such children or because of a biological parent's illness. Nor did these laws address trauma that incurred within the foster system itself.

Agency reluctance to make interracial placements in the 1980s led to the 1994 Multiethnic Placement Act (MEPA). MEPA required agencies to actively recruit families of color to reflect the racial makeup of children in foster care. It simultaneously attempted to reduce adoption planning delays by prohibiting agencies from delaying or denying placements because of the adoptive parents' race or national origin. At the same time, MEPA allowed an agency to consider the "cultural, ethnic or racial background of a child" and the ability of an adoptive or foster parent to meet the needs of the child when it made a placement. Concerned mostly with the dynamics of African American children, the federal government considered a violation of MEPA a violation of Title VI of the Civil Rights Act.

The Interethnic Placement Provisions Act (a 1996 amendment to the Multiethnic Placement Act) and an adoption tax credit tried to incentivize adoptive families (often white) to adopt minority foster children and other special needs children. The Interethnic Placement Provisions Act prohibited an agency from racially discriminating against prospective parents when it made decisions about placement. In fact, it emphasized the need for agencies to recruit different types of adoptive applicants. Yet there was a controversy around MEPA and the Interethnic Placement Provisions Act, which centered around the benefits and challenges of race-matching practices in adoption in the face of a larger context relating to the child welfare system's historical pattern of child removal and discrimination against families of color.[103] Those opposed to the law argued that transracial placements were harmful to children's overall well-being and identity. They claimed that Congress needed to try to address poverty as a reason for the foster care crisis and prevent the removal of children of color in the first place. They also wanted Congress to invest in recruiting adoptive parent applicants of color, rather than what it did—offering a supposedly "colorblind" policy, a racial rather than structural solution—to facilitate transracial adoptions.[104] Proponents, however, claimed that these children needed permanency, no matter what the race of the adoptive family was. They argued that one way to rectify the historical discriminatory mistreatment of these children was by providing them with more adoption opportunities.[105] Notably, the law did not apply to Native American children because they were protected under the Indian Child Welfare Act (ICWA), which itself was a statute that redressed the disproportionate fostering and adoption of Native American children in the 1960s and 1970s and earlier policies to separate and institutionalize them. ICWA created a political relationship of children to tribal governance, rather than a racial one; race was the key category featured in MEPA.[106]

Finally, the Adoption Promotion and Stability Act (1997; P.L. 105-89, HR897), otherwise known as the Adoption and Safe Families Act (ASFA), amended the 1980 Child Welfare Act to address the dramatic increase in adoption backlog during the 1990s. Congress intended to reaffirm early pieces of legislation that supported family preservation and family reunification (called the Safe and Stable Families Program) while simultaneously upholding adoption as the solution.[107]

ASFA was a major piece of legislation with significant ramifications for children. Scholars have vigorously debated its impact. To many of its critics, the law hastened adoption instead of supporting family reunification, and so it reflected a "dramatic change in the way the federal government deals with the overloaded foster care system."[108]

Framed as a way to address the safety and well-being issues inherent in child abuse and neglect cases, ASFA allowed states to waive the "reasonable efforts" provision for family reunification set forth in the Adoption Assistance Act of 1980 when a child's safety was at risk. It tried to clarify "reasonable efforts," a term that adoption agencies found vague in the Reagan years, by requiring states to note when services to prevent foster placement and family reunification were *not* required to facilitate adoption (called a reunification bypass). In the interest of child safety, ASFA required states to recognize that adoptions did not have to wait until reunifications failed.[109] But as Dorothy Roberts has pointed out, an accompanying 1996 federal welfare adjustment law that mandated that states protect children from abuse and neglect failed to supply basic support to poor families to mediate child neglect through structural reform. Instead, it used adoption as the primary way to solve an overcrowded foster care system. By shortening the time children spent in foster care and by quickening custody termination processes, ASFA made it particularly hard for birth mothers, especially those incarcerated with longer sentences, to retain custody of their children.[110]

One positive aspect of ASFA was that it guaranteed health coverage for adopted special needs children. But, according to Roberts, these policies effectively altered the delicate balance between family reunification and adoption since states could lower the foster care population, and therefore their cash outlay, while also receiving funds when they placed foster children in adoptive homes.[111] Indeed, the Safe Families Act provided financial incentives to states that successfully placed children for adoption. For every foster care adoption over the state's average number of placements, the government paid states $4,000; for every special needs case, the government paid states $6,000. The higher payment for special needs cases reflected the harder task of placing children with disabilities in adoptive homes. So that states would not put this money back into the foster care system, the federal government required that states show the steps they were taking to move children out of foster care.

To ASFA's advocates, like Elizabeth Bartholet, the act addressed the serious and continued problem of foster care drift and supported the notion that every child deserved a loving and stable home. ASFA advocates argued that the act put children's safety over parents' interests and therefore preserved children's rights.[112] To ASFA advocates, the statute was a serious way to address the limited pool of families willing to adopt children with special needs, to solve delays in making timely decisions about permanency, and to alleviate the high caseloads of caseworkers and judges. It also attempted to clarify the confusion about "reasonable efforts" that had, until then, complicated efforts to reunite a child with her birth family. To critics like Roberts, however, these arguments wrongly assumed that family preservation is only in the interests of parents and not those of children.[113]

ASFA's effects are difficult to fully disentangle from state adoption initiatives that were already in place to address long-term foster care, but scholars have noted the changes that have occurred in child welfare since its passage, a topic further explored in the epilogue. In short, the results have been mixed. In general, adoptions of children from foster care increased significantly, from about 37,088 in 1998 to 52,839 in 2002. In urban centers, there was a 25 percent increased likelihood of placement.[114] Although study results track general trends, ultimately adoption dynamics after ASFA, like those prior to it, have varied by state.[115] A decade after ASFA, children waited an average of approximately three years in foster care before their adoption.[116]

It is unclear whether the rate of adoptions of children with disabilities increased substantially after ASFA. One statistic suggests that a decade after its passage, twice as many children received adoption subsidies as received federally supported foster care. The overall dollar expenditures for adoption assistance also skyrocketed, creating unease among researchers about whether the assistance was actually going to pay for postplacement adoption and medical needs. As Richard Barth, a prominent child welfare scholar, remarked, "Subsidies were intended to ensure that families did not suffer a fiscal disincentive to adopt, not as a payment to those who would not otherwise adopt."[117]

ASFA's shortened timelines did not ease, and perhaps even exacerbated, the difficulties agencies faced when placing children with disabilities. Despite subsidy increases, children with physical and emotional disabilities, and those exposed to drugs or alcohol, still faced (and continue to face) significant barriers to adoption. At the end of the 1990s, for instance, of the 77 children who remained in New York State's foster care system the longest, 39 percent had learning or mental disabilities and

18 percent had multiple disabilities.[118] Even though some families are willing to adopt children with special needs, their attitude does not automatically translate into finalized adoptions.[119]

Conclusion

This period was an exceptionally complex time for foster care and adoption, with numerous new practices, programs, and laws to address (which sometimes aggravated) the growing child welfare problem in the United States. Child welfare and adoption professionals increasingly paid attention to special needs children and their adoption in the 1980s and 1990s, thus giving rise to an age of special needs adoptions. As a response to the number and type of waiting children with disabilities, agencies, parents, physicians, and policymakers intensified their efforts to place disabled children and to characterize them as unequivocally adoptable. Despite their work, the foster care crisis endured, and major barriers remained.

From 1980 to 1997, the characteristics of children with disabilities in the foster care system changed. Children often acquired disabilities from abuse, neglect, or years spent in foster care itself. Other children in foster care included waiting children with various physical, mental, emotional, and learning disabilities; medically fragile children, including those with HIV/AIDS; and children who had benefited from deinstitutionalization.

Although there were parents that either came forward to adopt children with disabilities or stretched their preferences to do the same, there were still never enough parents to fulfill the need. In response, the federal government took a more active role in child welfare reform by providing subsidies and increasing support services to incentivize parents. But numerous structural, bureaucratic, and budgetary obstacles frustrated these reforms, including a persistent shortage of adequate services, high medical costs, the uneven provision of subsidies across states, continued agency prejudice, and a paucity of sufficient funding. These shortfalls ultimately reflected a weak federal commitment and a lack of social responsibility to take care of society's marginal children.

CHAPTER SIX

The Limits of Inclusion

Each waiting child's future is limited only by our vision of him.[1] —Patricia Kravik

Agencies, states, and the federal government dedicated numerous efforts and funds during the 1980s and 1990s to placing children with various disabilities, and many of these efforts were indeed successful at recruiting a larger number of parents than before. But even if all the initiatives had achieved their aims, broad sociocultural forces (like cultural messaging about perfection and damage, and general social instability) worked against narrowing the gap between those efforts and the incomplete results agencies faced in practice. These contextual factors helped limit parents' ability to imagine children with disabilities as part of their families. Thus, these forces frustrated the full inclusion of children with disabilities in adoption during this time.

Five major developments during this period formed the social and cultural backdrop in which the reluctance of many families to adopt children with disabilities persisted. These are: the idea of foster children as damaged; an overlay of consumerist discourses about children; the emergence of the problem of what was called "crack babies" and infants with HIV/AIDS; the rise of reproductive technologies; and the question of withdrawal of treatment for disabled infants. The phenomena of adoption disruption and wrongful adoption cases emerged, in part, as a consequence of these trends. Besides the many practical and policy barriers, messages of damage, risk, limited futures, and perfection and imperfection inherent to these trends help explain why there were never enough parents to fulfill the need for placement. Children with disabilities continued to struggle to find permanent homes and a permanent family, although their access was limited and uneven. By the end of the twentieth century, children with disabilities faced a persistent need for placement, making them only partially included in adoption.

Stigma and Inherent Risk

Child welfare professionals tried to explain the gap between the placement requirements of children with special needs and the rate of their permanent placement by noting the heightened risk of incurring problems in an adoption involving a foster child. They cited the cultural stigma of damage to account for this discrepancy. Given that the special needs category also included children of color, the latter stigma was highly racialized and conflated with poverty and the drug crisis.

Adoption discourse during this period simultaneously formulated foster children as embodying risk and as "at risk." In the early 1960s, experts had already vacillated between constructing waiting foster children as both at risk and potentially risky to a sustained adoption. By 1980, they still formulated risk as based on disability—whether a child was risky *because* of disability or was *at risk* for disabilities. But in their critique of the foster care system, child welfare professionals now blamed institutional failures as the main producer of the disability risks foster children faced; these failures were the reason why children were considered "at risk" in the first place.[2]

As before, risk was acutely connected to ideas about damage, but the roots of damage during this time were different. Because the causes of out of home placement (neglect, trauma, abuse) often had a significant psychological impact on many foster care children, the public and some social workers saw these children as "damaged" or as "bad seeds." Child welfare professionals simultaneously portrayed the children's personal safety as being at risk because of abuse and neglect. Characterizing these children this way aligned with the public's wider resurgent application of damage imagery to African Americans and speaks to social workers' possible racial animus.[3] It also reflected the public's view of disabled children as "damaged goods," as "seconds," as "disposable commodities," and as "less socially marketable than non-disabled persons."[4]

The fact that many neglected and abused children were both in foster care *and* disabled only compounded notions of difference, damage, and the risk attributed to, and affiliated with, them. Their combined status called into question their ability to participate in family life. As one adoptive couple testified at a special hearing on barriers to adoption in 1985, social workers, health care professionals, prospective adoptive parents, and the public held deeply ingrained prejudicial attitudes about special needs children in foster care. Their perceptions hindered these children's adoptions.[5]

Indeed, the American public revived the question: could parents form a healthy family relationship with a "less-than-perfect child"?[6] One single adoptive father said it best when he remarked that most people could not imagine having a disabled child in their family, especially if it was by choice. He argued that most people

> feel that such a child would limit the types of outings and activities they could do, cause a strain on their budgets, affect the other children in the family, cause them to deal with uncertainties about the future and generally be a depressing influence on their lives.[7]

This adoptive father noted that many of these people felt uneasy around individuals with disabilities and just preferred to avoid the situation entirely. These feelings reflected a renewed decreased tolerance to uncertainty and risk in family making during this time.

Numerous child welfare professionals and the public applied the stigma of damage not only to foster care children but to adoptees writ large. The rise in the foster care population and the stigma social workers applied to adoptees were probably not coincidental and were definitely not new. This stigma was rooted in a long history of viewing dependent children and adoptees as socially inferior. It resurrected the stigma of illegitimacy and the targeting of the poor that we saw in the early part of the century. It also reignited the 1950s notion of maternal deprivation. Finally, it solidified the tie social workers, experts, and the public made between adoptees and damage after the 1970s.

Child welfare professionals and experts continued to tweak this association into the late 1980s. Because of their different kinship status, psychologists claimed, adoptees as a population exhibited some sort of psychopathology. Even as they saw children who had experienced trauma as ever less fixable, psychologists also described the relationship between trauma and adoption as "ever more fixed."[8] At the end of the twentieth century, adoption researchers framed adoption itself as a risk factor for personality disorders like reactive attachment disorder. Many believed that such issues were unavoidable for adoptees.[9] Reflecting these beliefs, some psychiatrists and psychologists advocated a new diagnostic category of adopted child syndrome, which alleged that adoptees experienced an extreme form of primal rejection that resulted in significant trauma. The symptoms of this mental disorder included stealing, substance abuse, lying, running away, fire setting, and promiscuity.[10]

Psychologists' and psychiatrists' portrayal of adoptees as pathological resonated for many Americans; the move posited adoption per se as an independent risk factor for behavioral problems, separate from certain conditions of family living and other extenuating social factors in adoptees' lives. It configured all adoptees as at risk for emotional disability because of the way they entered families. As such, this profile reflected the fundamental role disability played in the public's fears and ideas about adoption during this period. Even today, as we will see in the epilogue, many Americans believe that large numbers of foster care children and adoptees are risky; they assume these children are more likely to have medical, academic, and behavioral issues despite the public's positive views of adoption itself.[11]

Drugs, Damage, and New Children in Foster Care

Special needs foster children awaiting adoption bore the brunt of Americans' tendency to pathologize adoptees. Americans' deep and growing fears about both the drug and AIDS crises helped shape public and professional concerns about damage and disability among waiting children. They also linked the issue of dependency with damage and disability.

Conservative attacks on the welfare state and the social safety net, and policies that criminalized poverty and increased incarceration, created economic and social instability for marginalized and vulnerable sectors of American society. These policies all had racist consequences and impacted children in devastating ways. They led to the increasing numbers of children, particularly African American children, who needed to be placed in foster care when their birth parents were left in economic distress, were imprisoned for drugs, or were homeless. Children's affiliation with these problems, and their physical and psychological ramifications, made it easy for the public to attribute damage and risk to them.

Even though Nixon spoke of a "war on drugs," Reagan's war on drugs, which started in October 1982, brought illicit drug use to the forefront of American politics and culture. The George H. W. Bush and Clinton administrations sustained and amplified the political racialized panic about drugs.[12] In the late 1980s and into the 1990s, this alarm led to draconian measures against drug users, like minimum sentencing and more funding for drug enforcement. These policies led to a cycle of increased arrests, imprisonment, and mounting foster care needs. Clinton's "tough on crime" policies intensified the drug war further, so that by 1991 the United States incarcerated its citizens at rates unprecedented in world history. This pattern of mass incarceration disproportionately affected African American communities.[13]

Particularly devastating to Black women and their families, the drug crisis and its attendant policies left women to raise their children alone while their partners were in and out of jail. Then, following the Bush-era 1986 Anti-Drug Abuse Acts, mothers were incarcerated at dramatic rates, a 433 percent increase between 1986 and 1991 alone.[14] Under the Omnibus Anti-Drug Abuse Act of 1988, judges could not consider family situations in sentencing decisions, including whether a female defendant was the sole caregiver for her children.[15] In all, more than a quarter of African American children with parents who did not have a college degree saw their parents imprisoned during the 1980s. Some of these children ended up in the foster care system while others were cared for by extended family members.

Following Reagan's racialized targeting of "welfare queens" and his attack upon food stamps, Black mothers became increasingly associated with welfare.[16] Even as it claimed that its socially conservative policies promoted family values, the Reagan administration's cutbacks to welfare payments frustrated child welfare services that tried to preserve families. As a result, states depended more on foster care.[17] In addition, the welfare policies of AFDC included more rules about behavior change and work requirements until Clinton abolished the entitlement altogether in 1997 with the Personal Responsibility and Work Opportunity Act. He replaced it with state block grants called TANF (Temporary Assistance to Needy Families). The Personal Responsibility and Work Opportunity Act required states to sustain foster care and adoption assistance programs to receive TANF funds. It also pressured child welfare workers to monitor families for child neglect, which increased the likelihood of child removal.[18] Along with the Adoption and Safe Families Act, the Personal Responsibility Act caused courts to terminate parental rights at an accelerated pace immediately after 1997.[19]

Women and their children also increasingly became homeless because of new public housing policies that cracked down on drug use. When

Congress revisited the Anti-Drug Abuse Act in 1988, for instance, it provided funds for prevention and treatment programs for women. But Congress also authorized new legislation that allowed public housing authorities to evict any tenant who permitted any drug-related activity to occur on or near the premises. Under this pressure, many mothers felt they had no choice but to place their children in foster care.[20]

Harsh drug policies also blocked the expansion of clean needle access during the HIV/AIDS crisis and contributed to the rapid spread of the virus through the Clinton years. Media reports described mothers, especially African American mothers, who engaged in sex work and injected illicit drugs, passing HIV to their fetuses. Once born, the babies entered the foster care system, often involuntarily. These reports were not entirely reflective of reality; the number of white women who used illicit drugs while pregnant significantly surpassed the number of minority women. Yet the public's impression that poor minority women used drugs more derived from laws mandating public hospitals to test and report on maternal drug use.[21]

Public fears about HIV and its transmission only compounded the idea of foster care children as damaged and fragile and raised quandaries for foster and adoptive parents during a time when knowledge about the disease and its treatment was limited. One *Ladies' Home Journal* article (1988) titled "The Baby Nobody Wanted," for example, featured a child whose mother was a heroin addict and contracted AIDS from dirty needles. The baby was at risk of contracting the disease. Once his foster parents found out about a possible diagnosis of HIV, they returned him to the system. The article details how the child's risk for HIV was kept secret, how the foster parents took daily care precautions due to fears of transmission, and how they could not adopt him because of high medical costs.[22] Indeed, in 1989 the American Academy of Pediatrics Task Force on Pediatric AIDS highlighted the "serious burden" an HIV-infected infant posed to any family. The acute bouts of illness, the frequent medical treatments, the lack of respite care, community fears of transmission, and the child's death made foster care or adoptive placement "exceedingly difficult" for these children.[23]

The field of foster care and adoption responded to the pressing issues of "crack babies" and HIV-infected babies in the foster care system by declaring a need to refocus its programs. By 1988, the Child Welfare League of America (CWLA) not only called for "energizing the special needs adoption system" but specifically suggested that adoption professionals develop best practices for babies and children with "special needs related to drugs and HIV infection."[24] The CWLA acknowledged by 1990 that the project to establish best practices for these children would have to be at the top of their adoption agenda.[25]

Fears of Dependency and Hesitancy to Adopt

The CWLA's call was consistent with wider cultural trends that focused on illicit drug use in inner-city neighborhoods. The inflamed rhetoric of Black "crack whores" and "crack babies" animated this discourse and conjured up the language of defect and the imagery of damage that Americans had long used to justify the marginalization of poor African Americans.[26] This racialized discourse, itself unjust due to its representational distortions and punitive implications, was also reflective of and intersected with American society's tendency to devalue and marginalize people with disabilities of all races. Such public rhetoric persisted, despite intensified disability activism that sought to change the social meaning of disability and gain access to various avenues of civic life.[27]

Conservative claims about Black pathology centered on illegitimacy and a reliance upon welfare. According to this argument, irresponsible women on welfare were allegedly producing a generation doomed to fail, posing a "menace to the future" of America.[28] Press coverage added to the focus on welfare and dependency. Reportage leveraged public fears about both disability and race by representing crack babies as having limited horizons, as having no potential of being "normal," and as having "permanent brain damage."[29] Commentators called crack babies the new "bio-underclass," a term that historically underscored the distinction between the "worthy" and "unworthy" poor that so often applied to policies concerning people with disabilities of all races. The term also reinforced deeply ingrained racial and gender stereotypes about women and men of color. Conservative columnist Charles Krauthammer, for example, warned that an "exploding" crack baby crisis where a "generation of physically damaged cocaine babies whose biological inferiority is stamped at birth" was emerging, "whose future is closed from day one. Theirs will be a life of certain suffering, of probable deviance, of permanent inferiority."[30] A well-known Native American adoptive parent and author, Michael Dorris, echoed these sentiments about crack babies' damaged futures and applied them to children with fetal alcohol syndrome (FAS). He even represented his son as irredeemable. Writing about babies exposed to crack or alcohol, he wrote: "A drug-impaired baby is destined for, at best, an adult life of sorrow and deprivation, and at worst, for a fate governed by crime, victimization, and premature death."[31] His words point to how the crack baby discourse and the discourse about FAS among Native American women and children mirrored one another. One Native American professional working with children with FAS even remarked that they were never able to become humans, never being able to love or be accepted into society, and never being capable of "living even in *this* world."[32]

Magazine articles also described foster and fost-adopt mothers who raised children with crack addiction, hyperactivity, or AIDS as saintly selfless rescuers and inspirational "supermoms" who used fostering to satisfy maternal drives and enact motherly behaviors. Reminiscent of the late 1950s and 1960s, the article described these women as nursing these children back to health, offering them the "gift of love," and gaining their ultimate fulfillment in doing so. The article explained that these children were the rejected "little sufferers" whom "nobody wanted."[33]

Disability Rag magazine, a disability rights magazine, called out the problematic nature of these depictions in their March/April 1989 column "What?" The column focused on the problematic statements of a pediatric nurse and single adoptive mother of several children with multiple disabilities. She remarked, "I lovingly call these kids my little factory seconds. . . . Each one has a flaw that's visible." *Disability Rag* highlighted her choice of words to show its readers the power of the terms of public discourse about damage and disability. By featuring this story, the magazine emphasized how even this mother portrayed her adopted children with disabilities as defective. By contrast, two other articles featured in media outside of the *Disability Rag* presented this mother, Jude Lincicome, in a more positive light. They depicted her as an advocate of finding adoptive homes for disabled children (some of her testimony uses similar language as the *Disability Rag* piece) and as someone who fought for services and believed in her children's abilities. She even stated how amazing she thought her children were.[34]

As historian Laura Briggs has argued, the particularly strong symbolic power of crack babies and their care rested on the role these babies inhabited as poster children for the War on Drugs. The image of crack babies presented moral failure, criminal behavior, and bad parenting as the problems; it offered a "biologized account of the growing impoverishment of urban communities of color."[35] Just as importantly, it also reified disability as biologized failure, inevitable ruin, burden, tragedy, and a threat to the nation. Images of brain-damaged babies costing the nation millions tapped into long-held moral judgments and fears about disabled people draining the economy and being perpetually dependent. In this way, conservatives played on the public's deep-seated existential anxieties about the all-too-familiar link between disability and dependency, while medical and psychological discourses of the time associated dependency with pathology.[36]

Although policy experts and social scientists of all political stripes decried dependency as bad, conservative policy makers saw social welfare programs as producers of dependency. They therefore called for dismantling the welfare state as *the* way to produce reform and to rehabilitate those on welfare, particularly Black families.[37] But for foster children with disabilities who were exposed to drugs or alcohol, the disability-dependency nexus compounded the dependencies of being a child and being poor. Within the neoconservative political climate and its assault upon the welfare state, these children evoked intense cultural fears in the American public about dependency and actual or assumed Blackness that had deep historical roots.[38] These anxieties now resurfaced through the crack crisis.

The stigma of being a poor foster child with a disability, however, exceeded the expected and acceptable form of child dependency, where a child is presumably able-bodied but socially vulnerable (because of age) and is a legal dependent. By contrast, the layered dependency of being a disabled foster child was socially unexpected because of its complex multidimensional nature. The dependent disabled foster child uniquely required either state funds and services to function in daily life or efforts to take care of her bodily and emotional needs.[39] Importantly, the status of occupying interwoven dependencies had significant implications for these children's familial fitness and citizenship.[40] They delimited which children's bodies Americans believed had worthy and contributive lives. Given the pejorative notion of dependency and its racial, class, and disability axes during this time, many Americans conceptualized these children as inherently a burden, a lack, and risky candidates for family life.[41] Instead of recognizing the "inevitable dependencies" inherent in all social relations, the ideologically charged meanings of these intertwined dependencies butt up against American historical myths about rugged individualism, personal responsibility, and independence (now framed as a matter of personality). The latter ideals not only applied to political citizenship but also translated into the norms of familial citizenship.[42]

Moreover, particularly when there was a political assault on public, and therefore private, dependency, the federal government harnessed these myths to rationalize economic retrenchment and family values. The government engendered antipathy toward crack mothers and mothers addicted to alcohol towards these same ends.[43]

Scientific ideas about the physical consequences of crack in infants helped substantiate and intensify already panicked ideas about dependency. Stories in major newspapers and scientific articles about crack babies centered around the medical complications allegedly caused by their mothers' addiction during pregnancy and babies' suffering during withdrawal. According to these reports, crack babies faced early birth and an array of neurological, respiratory, cardiac, and digestive conditions (e.g., paralysis, seizures, abnormalities in the genital and digestive tracts, etc.). They also had an increased risk of learning disabilities and behavioral problems. Crack babies were allegedly at much higher risk for sudden infant death syndrome and accounted for the growing rates of infant mortality in many US cities.[44]

But later medical reports in the 1990s disputed these claims. They showed that babies' medical and neurobehavioral complications could be caused by exposure to a variety of different drugs, not just crack. These challenges to the crack narrative mollified medical practitioners' fears regarding the sole culpability of crack cocaine. They also provided evidence that the medical outcomes of crack babies were along a spectrum, ranging from "severely damaged" to falling within the "normal range of development." But during the 1980s, common medical and popular belief held that there were substantial risks of impairment due solely to crack.[45]

Given the stated medical complications from crack and the public hype, many hospitals, especially those serving Black patients, began to institute screening tests for cocaine in delivery rooms. Those women who tested positive lost their babies immediately, which contributed to what child welfare professionals termed a "boarder baby crisis." The boarder baby crisis involved babies left at hospitals for a variety of reasons. The babies taken from women who tested positive for crack were counted as part of this group.

Sometimes women who tested positive were arrested and sent to jail. Criminalizing them validated the stereotype of the Black "crack mother" as irresponsible and selfish and contributed to the foster care crisis. The public strongly opposed returning the children to these women, even after they had undergone drug rehabilitation. This position meshed with broader conservative trends opposing, and therefore restricting, the welfare state.[46] But these indigent women were actually caught in a bind, having no choice but to bear children because of Medicaid restrictions to abortion but who, because of drug use, were deemed unfit mothers.[47] Feeding the stereotype, the number of these women's arrests was disproportionate to the arrests of pregnant women using other drugs. Because of drug-related arrests, from 1986 to 1989, San Francisco alone saw a 148 percent increase in foster care placements from 1986 to 1989. New York faced a similar rise.[48] In 1989, child welfare services received referrals for an estimated 100,000 crack- or cocaine-exposed infants across the US.[49]

The boarder baby crisis was so substantial that it prompted the Abandoned Infants Assistance Act of 1988 (amended in 1991, PL 102-236). The act gave money to recruit foster families or fund residential programs for these children. The statute's recruitment provision was based upon what professionals believed constituted a viable family. It therefore reflected where they felt these dependent children belonged: either with their birth families or with foster or adoptive parents. Some child welfare professionals argued that the crack epidemic put children at too great a risk for their health and safety to remain in their birth homes. But caseworkers, who were often inadequately trained on matters of addiction, had to decide whether and when parents' drug use put a child at *too great* a risk such that it necessitated foster placement. Moreover, a limited number of places to refer drug-addicted parents for rehabilitation frustrated any well-intentioned plans for birth parents to recover and reclaim their children to reestablish an intact family.[50]

The CWLA took a more equivocal approach about the viability of families and where these children belonged. In 1992, it contended that when a drug-exposed child was legally declared abandoned (when parenting was effectively not functional), child welfare services should move to terminate parental custody and either place the child with relatives (kinship care) or put the child up for adoption. For babies not in these circumstances, the CWLA supported making "reasonable efforts" to preserve the biological family. For its part, the Department of Health and Human Services promoted the idea that when family reunification was impossible for drug-exposed children, child welfare services should terminate parental rights quickly and should begin the adoption process swiftly.[51]

Beyond the field of child welfare, the drug crisis stimulated strong political debate about welfare, family preservation, child neglect, and dependency, and its relation to foster care and adoption. Newt Gingrich's *Contract with America* proposal to put welfare mothers' out-of-wedlock children in orphanages (after denying the 14.3 million on AFDC welfare, 9 million of them children; "We'll help you with foster care, we'll help you with orphanages, we'll help you with adoption"), along with the

Republicans' Personal Responsibility Act, signified the extent to which punitive policies around poverty coupled with angst about dependency and race deeply affected and targeted children, even to the point of institutionalizing them.[52] Though institutionalization ran counter to the prevailing child welfare belief that family-based care served the best interest of children, Gingrich saw Black families as unlikely to rehabilitate and therefore in need of a congregate solution.[53] Conservatives like drug czar William Bennett and Douglas Besharov of the American Enterprise Institute also strongly promoted expediting adoption procedures once drug-exposed children had been removed from parental custody.[54]

Poor disabled children's dependencies, coupled with the highly stigmatizing effects of drug use and HIV/AIDS, ultimately undermined the support for children with disabilities as desirable candidates for adoption. The moral panic surrounding crack during this period played into the social and cultural obstacles keeping many social workers from placing, and many parents from adopting, children from foster care because of worries about damage and disability. When given the choice, families preferred healthy children over drug-exposed or otherwise disabled children. Some looked to international adoption as a result. They considered the high medical costs relative to any available state or federal subsidies and the social stigma that could come from adopting a drug-exposed child. This made the permanent placement of such children very difficult.[55]

The answers that Michigan's Lutheran Child and Family Service gave to the questions of fost-adopt applicants Karen and Guenter Lahr (a white couple), for example, reveal the challenge. The agency did not receive any acceptable responses from African American families to a newspaper posting about a Black boy with mild cerebral palsy that allegedly resulted from "his mother's drug abuse." Although originally placed in foster care at two months old, he wasn't permanently placed with the Lahrs until three and a half years of age. Other children with disabilities of all races faced similar delays and problems with regard to finding a permanent home.[56]

Damage, (Im)perfection, and Reproductive Technologies

At the same time as the drug and AIDS crises, the 1980s and 1990s saw the expanded use of reproductive technologies. These technologies elevated the public's concern about damage, disability, imperfection, and risk in American family making in new ways.

Although some journalists, ethicists, and physicians saw technologies like in vitro fertilization as a threat to the American family and to society in the 1970s (some even spoke of "test-tube babies" as "monstrosities"), other commentators understood that the "dramatic biological revolution" underway was highly significant; it was a revolution that was becoming a common part of the family, medical, and adoption landscape of America.[57] Central features of this new landscape included the growing use of prenatal screening (including the use of amniocentesis earlier in pregnancy), the expanded category of high-risk pregnant women (advanced maternal age), the use of preimplantation genetic diagnosis, and the increased support for terminating a pregnancy for a "defective fetus" (for those conditions that amniocentesis could detect at the time). The latter was an option that women had not had before.

The presence and social potential of reproductive technology reconfigured ways of conceptualizing family, lineage, pregnancy, futures, identity, and kinship while it also retained old ways of favoring biological parenthood and relatedness, the category of the "natural," and the cultural premium of genetic kinship. These were all questions the field of adoption had struggled with for decades, as adoptive applicant criteria, matching practices, medical disclosure, and the debates around open records demonstrate.[58] Recognizing the impact these technologies had on creating new forms of kinship and identity, the CWLA suggested extending services that adoption agencies traditionally gave to prospective adoptive parents to families using assisted reproductive technologies (ART) because "there is a similar family dynamic for the child and the family using these new technologies for family development as there is with adoptive families."[59] But as ARTs became real alternatives to adoption for the first time, more people who would otherwise be adoptive applicants turned first to technology-based conception. Only thereafter did they turn to adoption.[60] For some couples, adoption was not even considered. As Burton Sokoloff a pediatrician involved in adoption affairs, noted in 1987, "Adoption remains an acceptable option that is all too frequently not even considered by the infertile couple."[61] The adoption world took notice, publishing articles in social work journals and offering expanded agency services to couples considering reproductive technologies.[62]

Even though there were some similarities between adoption and ART in terms of family building, there were also striking differences. In no small way, these technologies changed the parental calculus about reproduction; they allowed parents to feel that they had more control over family-making processes and gave the impression that parents could better manage the type of children they would bring into the world. In essence, they tapped parents' ·wariness about risk in family making and mobilized the cultural hierarchy of biological family over alternative forms. The availability of these technologies put questions about desirable children front and center at the same time as questions about damage and disability hovered over the foster care crisis and adoption. As a result, adoption was often reconfigured as a "less desirable, last resort option" for infertile couples.[63] Despite its low success rates, assistive technologies also created a historically distinctive, new sense of obligation by couples to consider initiating, and then continuing, the use of reproductive technologies to treat infertility, and, along with the birth control pill, it gave women the option to delay childbearing—to push back the biological clock, or at least try to.[64]

But there were limits to the promises of these technologies. Even as parents believed they could better control family building, especially the types of children they would produce, the particular use of prenatal testing was, as Ginsburg and Rapp have shown, "antiseptically removed from the world it is designed to predict"; that is, it disassociated the idea of disability from the lived experience of disability. As such, it could lead parents to make decisions based on social or medical misconceptions or conventional tropes about disability, rather than grounding their decisions upon a rich, complex, and nuanced understanding of the lives of people with disabilities.[65] Prenatal testing also assumes that disability primarily occurs before or at birth, as noted by Perri Klass, a Boston physician. Reminiscent of postwar adoption debates, Klass stated that prenatal testing offered no guarantee of a perfect baby. Parents therefore needed to ask themselves, "How great is their need for a perfect child? And, if not a perfect child, how much imperfection can they tolerate—or love?" He cautioned that even with all the new technology, the growth of a fetus and a baby's birth still escaped human's full control.[66]

Klass's words point to the role that a child's imagined future played during this specific historical moment. This imagined future operated not only in shaping physicians' and parents' investment in reproductive technologies, but it also evoked the meaning of risk as a marker of "danger from future damage."[67] As in adoption, reproductive technology generated a web of disability, risk, and futurity. It affirmed Americans' inherent anxiety behind the pressure to produce a family with healthy, idealized, white children as its desirable members. It also deployed the idea that controlling risk could guarantee a "perfect" child.

By asking his audience about the parental limits of imperfection, Klass challenged the blanket notion that "disability destroys the future." He clearly referenced the ideals of perfection that bolstered Americans' investment in reproductive technologies.[68] Despite the "indeterminacy lurking in the certitudes of fetal testing," however, these tools allowed physicians and parents to make decisions based on a process of "naming and ranking defects and the defective." This process delineated the imperfect and perfect fetus and reified impairment as indicative of the whole fetus.[69] Doctors offered testing to pregnant women (most of whom had little knowledge about the conditions that the test detected) as a way to have a normal child and experience normalcy in motherhood.[70] But at the same time, the process of defect sorting shows how fetal testing reflected a deeper level of ambivalence about impairment; it revealed that physicians and parents could indeed accept *some* level of difference. The technology's ability to rank impairments exposed its limits; it revealed medicine's hesitancy around guaranteeing a perfect fetus, even as it allowed the fantasy of that child to remain intact.

Moreover, the federal government at the time provided monies to states for genetic screening and services. In so doing, it communicated a broad social commitment to managing and preventing disability and supported the cultural push to have a normal family.[71] Indeed, the embrace of ART shows that it was not just about fulfilling parents' wishes for a normate family, but how it was also about a wider social investment in those imagined families.[72]

Ideas swirling within the new sphere of reproductive technology about perfect or "damaged" children played themselves out in the field of adoption. Leveraging consumerist notions about children, people feared getting damaged goods through adoption.[73] A child welfare handbook used in the 1980s to recruit families for disabled children stated this set of ideas clearly: "The concentration on the adopted child as a substitute for the unavailable biological child limits the interest of such families in handicapped children."[74] Here, prospective parents' vision of the perfect child they believed they could have biologically had colored their ability to accept a waiting disabled child. This stance excluded children of color and disabled children, as disability scholar Alison Kafer has observed, from the "privileged imaginary"; that is, they were cast "out of reproductive futurism."[75] Indeed, unlike the truncated, dismal futures medical providers described for children exposed to drugs or infected with HIV, physicians provided hopeful prognoses for children produced through ART.

ART thereby resolved prospective parents' conflict between the lack of available healthy white infants for adoption and the cultural mandate to have a healthy child. As Margarete Sandelowski wrote about subjects she interviewed in 1985–1986:

> there is now increasing competition among white couples for a decreasing number of available white infants to adopt and, as mentioned by respondents, an increasing concern about adopting because of fears of AIDS, drug addiction, and the impact of genetic factors on abilities and behavior.[76]

A 1985 Senate Committee hearing on barriers to adoption confirmed the same. Senator Howard Metzenbaum (D-Ohio) cited healthy white infants as clearly in demand, with long waiting lists for them, whereas older, minority, and disabled children—about 14,000 per year in 1985—aged out of the system. Until that time, they lived in foster care homes, "never knowing the psychological and emotional security of a permanent home."[77] By 1988, although at least 34,000 children, most of them special needs, were legally free for adoption, prospective adoptive parents waited years for white healthy infants instead of adopting those children most available.

Because of those long waits, parents often turned to international or independent adoption. Ellen Herman contends that one of the primary reasons international adoption increased during this period related to the "specific kind of racial difference that had bothered Americans and had tortured their history most. Children adopted from overseas were not black."[78] Laura Briggs and Ana Teresa Ortiz concur but suggest that the "moral panics over the scarcity over white children for adoption" and the "medical fragility of crack babies" as they interacted with the rise of international adoption had to do with two competing notions of childhood. The 1991 adoption boom of Romanian children, they argue, was not simply about race but was also a response to a disparate cultural logic operating among adoptive applicants that configured the childhood of American foster children as "pathological and irredeemable." They contend that as part of the urbanized poor, these children are cast as "similar to the chronically ill and disabled" in their social invalidation. Even as they make this comparison, Briggs and Ortiz do not take up disability as an analytic nor do they recognize that many poor children (often of color) in foster care were disabled and older.[79] The two groups were neither mutually exclusive nor actually distinct during this time—they are in fact often co-constituted.[80] Instead, in their description, the disabled merely serve as a referent while the co-constitution of these two groups and normative standards of the social body go unexplored.[81] Still, in contrast to Black foster children's childhood, they explain that Americans saw Romanian children as pliable and retrievable from trauma; only the latter set of children could be transformed into independent, productive citizens.

Fundamentally, this rehabilitative and redemptive transnational narrative hinged on normative notions of US citizenship that were foreclosed to American special needs children, be they minority children, older children, children with disabilities, or some intersection thereof. As a result, parents adopted Romanian children even though family service support or subsidies to raise these children were unavailable. What seems equally important in the turn to Romanian adoption, however, were the images of large amounts of institutionalized children living in terrible conditions, not unlike the exposes televised in the 1970s about American institutions for disabled children. Here the rescue narrative, a common dynamic in international and some forms of domestic adoption, was likely operative. Furthermore, even if Romanian children were at first thought pliable, follow-up study on these adoptions and other international adoptions showed that adoptive parents often sought later to dissolve their adoptions due to disability. Thus, these actions ultimately reinforced the notion that disability and family-building were incompatible (despite the fact that Americans always had disabled children in their families).[82] The director of one California agency, Holy Family Services, for example, reportedly received weekly calls from parents seeking readoption for their children from Romania after discovering they had medical conditions.[83] Well before the Hansen case, seen at the beginning of this book, a Massachusetts couple elicited press attention when they tried to send a three-year-old "severely handicapped" boy whom they had adopted in 1993 back to Lviv, Ukraine, because of excessively high medical bills.[84] Disability may have been a reason not to adopt domestically but it was also a reason not to sustain transnational adoptions.

There are certainly many intersections between disability, transnational adoption, and domestic trends deserving of comprehensive study. But what is most important to this chapter's argument is that adoptive applicants' cycle of waiting and turning to other avenues to start their family decreased the pool of possible parents to adopt children with disabilities and further exacerbated the special needs foster care problem. As a result, many special needs children ended up waiting an average of two years to be placed in adoptive homes.[85]

Questioning the Lives of Children with Disabilities

The medical and cultural themes of biological perfection, disability, and notions of futurity, seen in discussions of ART, also played out in a vigorous cultural debate in the 1980s about whether to withhold treatment from disabled infants. Physicians and ethicists focused on the cases of Baby Doe and Baby Jane Doe as the debate's centerpieces. Adoptive parent applicants and adoption workers could not have been ignorant of the debate's tenor, not only because of the public potency of the issue but also because ethicists and physicians offered adoption as a solution to birth parents' rejection of disabled infants. Prospective adoptive parents were likely also aware of the issues of assisted suicide and euthanasia of adults with disabilities featured in the news, with the stories of Larry McAfee (1988) and Terri Schiavo (1990) as key cases.

Baby Doe and Baby Jane Doe prompted bioethicists Helga Kuhse and Peter Singer to write a book titled *Should the Baby Live? The Problem of Handicapped Infants*. The book discusses euthanasia or infanticide of children with disabilities. They argued that since parents would be the ones taking care of a "severely handicapped infant," they should be key decision-makers about whether that child should live or die. Invoking futurity, the authors claimed that when a family does not wish to care for their disabled child, the state should take over the responsibility of the child only when "life may be in the best interests of the person the infant will become"; that is, when the state deems the child's future life as potentially worthwhile.[86] Kuhse and Singer contended that in the latter cases, the best form of care would be the adoptive family, reasonably adding: "but we would be pleasantly surprised if there were enough families willing to adopt these children."[87]

The Baby Doe case allowed doctors to withhold routine life-saving surgery to fix tracheoesophageal fistula (opening between trachea and esophagus) and esophageal atresia (esophagus ends in a pouch instead of continuing to stomach) from a baby with Down syndrome in 1982. The baby eventually starved to death. But the story was more complicated. A surrogate mother, inseminated for a couple who later separated, gave birth to Baby Doe. The alleged biological father initially accepted the child but later rejected the baby, arguing that Baby Doe was actually not his own (a blood test attested to this fact). Not only did the case involve a multimillion-dollar lawsuit and allegations of fraud and baby selling, but Baby Doe's physical and intellectual disabilities intensified the case's cultural import. Media reports utilized the rhetoric of the day, describing him as inferior, disposable, and as damaged goods. They commodified him as someone who could be discarded or exchanged. As a critique of these depictions, journalist Roger Rosenblatt reminded his readers that "what is being cooked up in each instance is not a cake or a car or a mail-order watch but a person, small-headed or not, and any situation that suggests otherwise is not just dismaying but dangerous."[88]

Despite disparaging media representations, public outcry about the Baby Doe case led the Department of Health and Human Services (HHS) to make "medical discrimination against handicapped infants" unlawful under Section 504 of the Rehabilitation Act of 1973. The regulation made withholding nutritional, surgical, or medical treatment from a disabled infant illegal "when treatment was not contraindicated by the condition." But the final HHS regulations in 1984 invoked medical custom and "reasonable judgment" as the principles upon which physicians should rely, even though many neonatal treatments were relatively new at the time and so medical custom had not been established. Furthermore, the regulations did not clearly delineate the ability to use quality of life judgments to determine medical benefit.[89]

A year later, the Baby Jane Doe case continued the debate about whether disabled infants should be denied treatment and allowed to die. It involved a child with spina bifida whose parents refused (against physicians' recommendations) to place a ventricular shunt because of the multiple disabilities she would have after the surgery. After making its way through several layers of the court system, during which time her parents allowed some surgery, the District Court of Appeals determined that the Rehabilitation Act did *not* give HHS authority to interfere in any medical decision-making regarding the treatment of disabled infants, thus undermining the original HHS regulations.[90] The Supreme Court agreed in 1986, arguing that it was parents, not the hospitals or physicians, who had the right to decline to give consent to the infant's treatment and that only states had the power and right of enforcement in this area. The judges who dissented noted that parents did not make these decisions in a vacuum and that physicians routinely influenced the decisions. Ultimately, the Court struck down the regulations that made withdrawal or withholding treatment unlawful.[91]

Although it did not amend the Rehabilitation Act to reinstate the Baby Doe regulations, Congress turned to child abuse as a way to address whether physicians could withhold medical treatment to an infant on a state level. Concerned primarily with antiabortion politics rather than enforcing Section 504 or a concern for disabled infants, Reagan signed the Child Abuse Amendments of 1984, which made withholding or withdrawing medical treatment and nutrition from a disabled infant an act of child abuse.[92] But like the Baby Doe regulations, the law allowed physicians to withhold medical treatment on the basis of "reasonable medical judgment" when treatment would prolong dying, or when it was deemed medically futile. Medical and disability advocacy groups articulated strong principles for dealing with the medical treatment of disabled infants that same year, erring on the side of providing treatment, community support, and protecting the rights of disabled infants. The Child Abuse Amendments of CAPTA deepened this debate and intensified its already principal focus on child abuse that had started in the 1970s.[93]

As a result of the amended CAPTA, state child protection services (CPS) began to spend more time and resources on potential abuse or neglect in neonatal care. This emphasis closely tied to foster care and adoption services in that when CPS turned its attention to medical neglect, it made that kind of neglect an adjunct to general neglect as a basis for placing a child in foster care. The law also required state-level programs to facilitate adoption opportunities for disabled infants with life-threatening conditions. This is one of the reasons why "chronic care" and "terminally ill" children became new constituents of the foster care and adoption populations during this time.

Even prior to the law, some pediatricians and adoption workers proposed that adoption be a solution to withholding treatment from infants with disabilities. Dr. Reba Michels Hill of St. Luke's Episcopal Hospital in Houston and Jo Ann Caldwell of Homes of St. Marks Adoption Agency, for instance, suggested that adoption be used as "an alternate method for handling cases of malformed or damaged infants who are unacceptable to biologic parents."[94] Hill and Caldwell described Susie Q, who exhibited a variety of impairments at birth. Upholding cultural notions of perfection, her parents asked "if she is not normal, why salvage her?" Susie's parents refused to see or touch her; they refused to visit her in the hospital. They decided to send her to an institution and were adamant that she would not be allowed into their home. The neonatologist requested that they consider relinquishing her for adoption. Even though they "were appalled that anyone would want to adopt an imperfect child," they eventually agreed. Luckily, Susie was adopted three days after discharge from the hospital.

Various parties paid for several subsequent surgeries. According to Hill and Caldwell, Susie developed into a "vivacious 6½ year old, who has cerebral palsy but now walks independently. . . . She is living proof that a child with a handicap can flourish in a loving, concerned family in which her personality and self-worth are nourished by being loved, wanted and accepted."[95]

More optimistic than Kuhse and Singer, Hill and Caldwell continued arguing for adoption as an alternative to medical neglect and rejection by birth parents. But they neither challenged parental rejection of a child based on disability nor substantially discussed supports that parents might need to navigate childcare for these children. However, they did try to find a solution to the problem of unwanted children through adoption.[96] They explained that for those biological parents who could neither cope with nor nurture a child with physical, mental, or neurological disabilities, adoption was a better alternative than death by starvation, permanent institutionalization, or physical abuse. The children had a right to this option, rather than death. But, they claimed, because "the attitude that adoptive parents only want a perfect child has been so ingrained," doctors were unaware that there were adoptive parents who could love and accept an "imperfect" child.[97] Some physicians could not imagine that possibility. Some parents who adopted severely disabled or seriously ill children reported that their doctors had told them: "I have no time for this child. He's better off in an institution—or dead—anyway. Why do you care what happens to him? He isn't *really* yours."[98]

Imperfect Children and Adoption Disruption

As we saw in the 1960s and 1970s, and during this period as well, there were certainly parents who could love and accept an " 'imperfect' child" and could sustain their adoptions. But others struggled with addressing the daily emotional or physical needs of their children with disabilities. Parents who confronted challenges defied the figure of the selfless adoptive parent whose love could conquer all. Indeed, harsh realities sometimes clashed with the ideal. One parent, speaking about her child who was neglected and abused, revealed that adoptive parenting a child who suffered this trauma was often complicated by the child's "profound inability to trust" that infused a family's life. "It was a painful learning experience for us as parents to come to terms with the reality that there are some aspects of their personality development and their very beings that no amount of our love, nurturance and family stability can overcome."[99] Still other parents who adopted children with disabilities despaired; they found that there were insurmountable challenges and that they could not sustain the placement. Many families faced "stigma and isolation" due to their family's difference (called "courtesy stigma" by psychologists; see epilogue).[100] This shunning by the community, family, and friends revealed the societal consequences of not having a "perfect" family and the emotional implications it had for families.[101] One handbook on adoptive parenting of children with disabilities stated that any family that has a disabled child has to "learn to deal with relatives, neighbors and strangers who are likely to have a strong reaction to the child's handicap." But, the handbook warned, in adoption, the family who has intentionally chosen to parent such a child experiences added hostility; "they may become a target for the community's hostility," particularly if the child exhibited antisocial or disruptive behavior. The handbook pointed out that there are some parents who would not have the "internal strengths to accept such a child" if their friends and relatives disapprove.[102]

These situations could end in what adoption professionals and researchers called adoption disruption. Although the term "disruption" did not have a uniform definition, it usually meant when a family terminated an adoption before it was legalized. This concern was not new; it animated many of the decisions regarding adoption practice during the twentieth century. But in this period, agencies and researchers used the term as a move away from the earlier label of "failed adoption," which placed blame on both child and parents for being unable to sustain the adoption despite all efforts to do so.[103] Ironically, adoption professionals and researchers reinscribed such blame when they invoked a disruption risk in relation to children with disabilities.

In contrast to disruption, dissolution meant the removal of a child *after* an adoption was legally finalized. The Hansen case we saw at the beginning of this book was a controversial transnational example of dissolution. Because agencies frequently did not follow outcomes after an adoption was finalized, researchers suspected that the number of dissolutions was vastly underreported, although they characterized disruption as having higher rates than dissolution.[104] Another term, set-asides, were legalized adoptions that the courts dissolved; they usually resulted from an agency misinforming or defrauding parents.[105]

Adoption disruption happened to many children in residential care or in mental health or juvenile detention facilities. Adoption professionals considered these cases "out-of-home-care disruptions" because parents had placed these children in other residential settings. When adoptive parents retained legal custody of these children, states did not generally report it in adoption statistics because they did not commonly require treatment program staff or foster care providers to inform adoption agencies of extended out-of-home services.[106]

As the population of children waiting for adoption drastically changed from healthy infants to special needs children, agencies, researchers, and state governments reported what they saw as a remarkable rise in the rates of disrupted adoptive home placements, up from 3 percent in the 1970s.[107] These growing rates, reported as ranging between 10 percent and 20 percent, shook "the faith and foundation of child service providers" such that by 1990, child welfare experts considered the problem substantial.[108]

Disruption was serious, painful, and highly stressful for all parties involved.[109] But inasmuch as researchers produced a plethora of studies that included stories of disruption to understand what was going on in order to prevent disruption, their clear emphasis upon it over success reinforced the dominant belief (certainly among social workers but also in the public sphere) that foster care children with disabilities were risky and damaged; researchers' messaging implied that they were, in fact, not the most desirable children to adopt. Numerous studies, for instance, looked at the various child populations inhabiting the disrupted category, the coping strategies of families who adopted them, the successes and failures of these adoptions, and the impact of supports.[110]

In stark contrast to the perfection discourse underlying reproductive technologies, the actual occurrence of disruption, and the social science of disruption that studied it, highlighted the imperfection of children with disabilities (particularly those with emotional disability) and the turbulence that these children may bring to family life. With its growing incidence, researchers, social workers, and even parents expected that disruption for special needs adoptions would prevail.[111] But, as Mr. and Mrs. Avegno, who adopted six children with disabilities, claimed: "Special needs is difficult; the children are extremely challenging. . . . We have tamed disruption and, painful though it is, we have learned to live with it."[112] Challenging the common claims of the day, the Avegnos contended that the idea of disruption was too available for parents; parents harbored the notion that if a special needs adoption didn't conform to their expectations, then "we can terminate it." Using consumerist language, they remarked: "In our world of disposable beer cans and disposable diapers, our children are disposable too. Like no-fault insurance and no-fault divorce, no-fault adoption offers us a tidy solution to a tragic and complex problem."[113] Here, the Avegnos' comments, and their play on the word "no-fault," reveal the reductive thinking that implicitly operated when parents commodified children; parents treated these disabled children as products whose value depended upon parents' expectations. Underneath the idea that damaged children were returnable and that disruption was an easy, legitimate, and viable alternative for challenging adoptions, however, laid many "complex problem[s]" rooted in a cultural intolerance for imperfection, in intransigent social issues, and in unsatisfying political answers, all of which could lead to tragic consequences for children and families. Despite the Avegnos' indictment of parents who commodified children, for a good many deciding to disrupt or dissolve an adoption was extremely difficult; many cases occurred only after painstaking efforts to get children and families the help they needed.

Adoption disruption in the 1980s and 1990s became a new locus of the discourse of risk in adoption circles. Social workers used risk to focus primarily, but not exclusively, on disabled children as the *cause* of disruption. Risk, yet again, reinforced the idea of disability as lack, burden, and tragedy. It configured children with disabilities as those who were "high risk."[114] This framing of risk, which circulated among agencies and among parents who experienced disruption, could not have helped agencies recruit families for children with disabilities. Though they did not agree upon which impairments led most to disruption, adoption researchers believed that "the placements of children with extensive physical, medical, intellectual, social, and/or emotional handicaps are judged to be vulnerable to disruption or discontinuation."[115] Even with these warnings, some parents still decided that "the chance to help a child would be worth the risk." But even experts who noted high success rates of disabled children's adoption inevitably entangled children with disabilities with risk.[116] One might expect this attitude from public agency workers who were not generally trained in special needs adoption practices, but even Spaulding for Children, a specialized agency considered quite progressive in its approach and advocacy, accepted the link: "One fact is clear. When placing older and handicapped children, the rate of disruption increases dramatically."[117] Inasmuch as agencies like Spaulding tried to focus on a child's individual attributes to find families to place her, some researchers who categorized disruption by "handicap" did just the opposite. In their quest to find singular explanations to adoption outcomes, they reified a reductionist approach to impairment by stratifying children according to their impairment in their analyses. As a result, they tended to flatten or disregard individualized characteristics (likes, dislikes, talents) of the child.[118] Instead, researchers' focus on handicap often treated the impairment itself, and not the meaning and treatment of it in society, as deterministic of a disruptive or successful adoptive outcome. As such, expert discussions mostly focused on which impairments (such as emotional or intellectual disabilities) caused the most disruption, over analyses of family dynamics. They sometimes also framed successful placements as taking place *in spite* of disability.[119] Consistent with child welfare workers' treatment of risk in this period, researchers of adoption disruption once again allowed a slippage to occur between children being "at risk" to being inherently "risky." As we will read in the epilogue, this trend continues in the twenty-first century.

Most child welfare professionals considered disruptions a necessary risk of adoptive placement, but some scholars acknowledged that risk operated differently for various segments of adoptees.[120] "In the final analysis," adoption researchers Ann Coyne and Mary Ellen Brown wrote, "the adoption of any child, but most particularly an older or handicapped child, is an act of courage that carries risk as well as opportunity to love."[121] Social workers had to assess disruption risk as one of many factors when they made a placement. In fact, most adoptions resulted in "lifelong gratitude that families and children assumed the necessary risk."[122] Children who unfortunately experienced disruption were usually either returned to their old foster families or to new ones, or they found new adoptive homes. In any case, disruption was not a desirable outcome for any of the parties involved: child, adoptive parents, or social workers.

Though many caseworkers and researchers believed that a child's disability was the major reason behind a disruption and that certain children were inherently riskier than others, several social conditions also contributed to disruption. Many of these children were older, had waited longer for placement, and had numerous, previous foster care placements or previous disruptions. At a time when infants continued to be the preferred type of child to adopt, being an older child remained a huge disadvantage to placement. But older children also had higher chances of acquiring an emotional or behavioral disability because of foster drift or because they had been shuffled back and forth between their biological parent and foster care. As one researcher explained: "It is truly a system in which those who have suffered most are the most likely to continue to suffer."[123]

Beyond age as a complicating factor, researchers and parents cited trauma, abuse, and neglect as reasons for disruption.[124] Yet children with past histories of abuse who had experienced disruption were often "re-adopted." Readoption was a new phenomenon that emerged in the 1980s. It meant the agency placed the child in a different adoptive home.[125] At the same time, many adoption advocates began to argue that adoption was perhaps not a viable family alternative for children who had suffered trauma or had severe behavioral or emotional problems; that *not* every child was adoptable.[126] Even as they considered social conditions as major factors in disruption, advocates also contended that this particular type of child was not fit for adoption. They still framed the child's risks on an individual level, rather than addressing contextual issues.

Another factor causing disruption was the gap between what kind of child parents wanted to adopt and the child they actually adopted. This chasm exposed the negative aspects of social workers' use of stretching as a casework strategy to recruit families. As one report stated: "Typically they had sought to adopt a younger child without any disabling conditions but eventually agreed to adopt an older child or one with serious emotional problems."[127] Although not every parent who adopted a special needs child was infertile, researchers found that parents who sought adoption to resolve their infertility often had an idealized notion of what kind of child they would raise. They expected their adopted child to exhibit high performance, more warmth, and stronger closeness than their child actually could give in the way they envisioned. These parents tended to have a lower tolerance for difference, which could consequently lead to disruption.[128] When parents struggled to raise a child, their struggles challenged not only how they had envisioned their child's future, but it also raised self-doubt about their own capacities as parents.[129]

Experts disagreed on whether income level or race mattered to the success or disruption of a placement, but one key study on race, class, and intact adoption showed that minority families tended to adopt fewer children with physical, intellectual, emotional, or psychiatric disabilities or those who were sexually abused. The researchers surmised that, due to the disproportionate (to their numbers in the general population) number of minority children in the foster care system, minority parents could more easily adopt a younger, less disabled child and they chose to do so. According to the researchers, this was one reason they had fewer disruptions. But parental attitudes distinct from white parents also made a difference. Emphasizing the contextual nature of disability (in this specific case, behavioral disabilities), the same researchers stated that "behaviors that are problems in some contexts—for instance, in conservative, middle-class [white] communities—may be less of a problem in other settings, for instance in some minority and lower-income communities."[130]

The issue of parents' expectations made it ever more important for social workers to match parents' strengths and resources with children's needs.[131] The example of a disabled single mother (with a "mild neurological condition") who adopted Amos, an eleven-year-old who had spent four years in foster care and was "aphasic, encopretic and effectively mute," is a case in point. To a degree, Amos's case challenged the idea that certain children were inherently risky. Amos's adoptive mother was a special education teacher and speech therapist. She had not parented before but had had prior contact with Amos's foster mother and understood his background. Researchers found that Amos's adoptive mother had abilities that were a "beautiful match" with the child's needs; the case aligned with the social work ideal during this period that no child was unadoptable.[132] Given this goal, the social worker's task was to find the right family to care for and address the child's special needs. This role was usually gendered, with the mother traditionally the one expected to fulfill the child's needs. As such, if a child and mother did not mesh, the mother endured the blame and guilt.[133] In Amos's case, when the agency matched the mother's professional expertise with the child's particular medical condition, as in the 1950s and 1960s, they expected that she serve as the source of care and as the sphere for his rehabilitation.[134] At the same time, Amos's case also reflects a set of changing gendered dynamics during this period, when experts and American society could envision that women's professional skills could be legitimately incorporated into mothering.

Still, child risk and parental characteristics cannot fully explain the causes of an occurrence as complex as disruption. Parents' clear need for additional support and resources, for example, contradicted American society's propensity to privatize family responsibility in a neoliberal age. Adoption professionals, doctors, legislators, and permanency planning advocates could seek adoption as the solution to unwanted children, like those with disabilities; such permanency certainly seems better than congregate care, foster care, or infanticide. But without adequate support systems in place, adoption ostensibly became a sort of dis-located solution—one that easily recreated the "problem" of disability for new adoptive parents by transferring the same lack of needed services and supports for biological parents ("I don't think I can adequately care for this child") to adoptive ones.

Disruption forced the question of how structural supports enable or constrain the limits of parenthood; that is, what Americans believed were the acceptable and unacceptable reasons to allow or disallow a child into one's family and what level of caregiving Americans felt should be needed to sustain belonging. When a family accessed adequate supports, it substantially decreased the chances of disruption. Proactive agencies therefore offered more consistent communication and psychotherapy to help families through crises and lower the risk of disruption.[135]

Researchers also acknowledged that appropriate community resources, like a child's access to suitable public or private education, often served as a "turning point away from a disruption."[136] These structural supports forced social workers to think about family as an entity that extended beyond the personal. In no small measure, they allowed parents to create and sustain a family. As Lynn G. Gabbard, an adoptive parent, testified to Congress in 1993: "Too often, adoptive and foster families are viewed as part of the problem and not part of the solution when mental health issues arise. As it continues to be the expectation, both the love and nurturance of a stable family can overcome all obstacles and repair all damage."[137] Yet adoption experts Madelyn Freundlich and Lisa Peterson acknowledged that there were limits to the discourse of love. They maintained that agencies needed to "explain [to adoptive parents] that love may not always be enough."[138] Gabbard agreed, arguing that parents desperately needed stronger support services and more supportive environments. She called on schools to develop "mentally healthy environments capable of accepting children who may never be capable of conformity," and for medical providers, coaches, and community members to understand that these families were not perfect "and do not need to be and that they cannot repair the injuries and damages that their children have sustained."[139] Care in this sense was both a personal *and* a public/social endeavor.

In contrast to researchers, parents focused on the intense emotions involved in caring for a child with severe behavioral or other disabilities and in their experiences with disruption. They either recounted the episodes that led to disruption or shared the impact of their decision. Even for those whose adoption did not ultimately disrupt, adoptive parents charted their expectations, frustrations, feelings of isolation, intense grief, loss, and distress through interviews, memoirs, and other writings.[140] For example, Michael Dorris, whose adoption did not disrupt but who mirrored the intense feelings of parents whose did, had been told by the agency that Adam, his son, was small for his age. His agency relayed that his son

Adam had been diagnosed as "mentally retarded." But Dorris held fast to the belief that good parenting would overcome any delays. When he discovered that his son had fetal alcohol syndrome, and that his impairments would not improve, he began to focus on Adam's limitations. He and his wife blamed Adam's birth mother for producing a child they saw as damaged and as having a limited future. They began a quest to combat maternal alcoholism within the Native American population to prevent similar births from happening.[141]

Some parent stories, relayed to scholars, acknowledged that extended family members and social workers had "warned" them of serious challenges if they were to pursue a special needs adoption; others reported either that their preplacement expectations had not been met, that the child never attached to the parents, or that they felt wholly unable to cope.[142] They reported a variety of challenges to raising a disabled child, from time commitment and financial strain to a breakdown of marital or family relationships and social stigma.[143] Parents felt tapped by frequent appointments to address educational, physical, emotional, or medical problems. This feeling could lead them to terminate an adoption. They also described feeling overwhelmed, helpless, and without the tools to handle their child's behaviors, which could include failing to attach, soiling clothes, stealing, suicidal threats, sexual promiscuity, criminal behaviors, drug abuse, eating disorders, and physical injury. Parents who felt that they had exhausted all options usually disrupted their adoption. As adoption experts Susan Partridge, Helaine Hornby, and Thomas McDonald wrote: "Consider, for example, how important it is to be able at least to feed and watch a child grow, and how distressful a child's suicidal desires are to the parents' attempts to nurture the child. These and other needs, problems and struggles are the legacies of the unique histories brought to adoption by special-needs children."[144]

Sometimes parents, despite best efforts, were unsuccessful in accessing community supports, and this was often no through fault of their own. Available resources for families reflected the hierarchy of care that mirrored the social hierarchy of kinship in America; that is, even though adoptive families were given equivalent legal rights as birth families, the services accessible to adoptive families were often less adequate than those for birth families. This disparity led to lower levels of service for special needs children.[145]

Adoptive families also had more limited access to services than foster families. Ann Kimble Loux, for example, wrote about her own struggle to adopt her two daughters from foster care (although her adoption was finalized) in 1997. According to Loux, adoptive parents with abused or neglected children needed continued professional, financial, and emotional support, not unlike those services offered to foster parents.[146] But many agencies did not proactively provide these services to adoptive parents; they often failed to support postplacement services like respite and temporary out-of-home care or other family preservation services. This led to higher chances of disruption. With this lack of resources, parents were left feeling desperate and rejected by the agencies with whom they had worked. Speaking about her own situation with a disabled Native American son, Marie Adams writes: "I was also frustrated when I came to realize that adoption of Native children, who, we once had been told, were in desperate need of good homes, was now no longer viewed as desirable." Adams presumably meant that doctors and social workers no longer considered Native American children with FAS adoptable as they became more aware of fetal alcohol syndrome and its symptoms.[147] To Shane Salter, a former foster care child who testified before the Senate Subcommittee on Children, Family, Drugs and Alcoholism in 1993, the lack of support services caused his disruption: "problems that I believe could have been resolved escalated to a point of no return."[148]

In addition, certain casework practices put children at risk for disruption. When casework prepared the child for her move from foster care to the adoptive family, the risk for disruption decreased. But when there were several caseworkers involved in the multiple aspects of this work, disruption tended to increase.[149]

Many parents claimed to have never received the full information on their child's disability nor the child's exposure to prior trauma. This often factored into why certain adoptions disrupted and others did not.[150] When social workers in Arizona in 1985 listed the child's problems or parents' expectations as the reasons for disruption, for instance, parents highlighted the lack of disclosure. They noted that either agencies did not fully inform them about the extent of a child's disabilities prior to placement or that they were ill-informed about adoption subsidies.[151] In California in 1988, more than one-third of adoptive families claimed that their agency did not tell them about their child's history of physical abuse. More than half said their agency failed to disclose their child's history of sexual abuse.[152]

There were several reasons why families felt they were not told pertinent information about a child. Sometimes, parents *did* receive psychological or educational reports, dental histories, neurological reports, birth histories, physical therapy, or early childhood reports, but they did not understand the information fully or still expected a less difficult child.[153] Other times, social workers failed to gather this information from the birth parents, particularly if it pertained to sensitive topics. High worker turnover (particularly in public agencies) also led to problems with information transfer between social workers.

But not having information about a child's disability history affected a family's ability to provide adequate treatment. It impacted their ability to emotionally and financially prepare for the child and their capacity to deal with issues that came up.[154] This knowledge also influenced the potential for an adoption to disrupt, especially for families who had "stretched" their preferences. In cases of stretching, parents claimed that knowing the information would have definitely affected their decision and may have led them not to adopt. This is a scenario that caseworkers often deeply feared.[155]

Experts therefore recommended that social workers engage in much more careful information gathering. They urged social workers to more effectively communicate and prepare prospective families. Indeed, the way social workers gave detailed background information about the child influenced a family's adoption future. Parents who felt that caseworkers unrealistically presented a child's record in too positive a light were more likely to disrupt, whereas those who reported having received realistic information seemed to be stable.[156]

When an agency failed to disclose a child's disability or medical history, it had serious consequences. In the 1980s and 1990s, it led to wrongful adoption lawsuits in which litigants sued agencies for their failure to disclose the presence or likelihood of a child's disability. If they had known, the parents argued, they would not have adopted the children. These cases mirrored wrongful birth lawsuits emerging at the same time that posited a similar line of argument about prenatal testing and physician liability.[157] Even though the wrongful adoption lawsuits focused on misinformation or agency fraud, they also revealed the persistent notion that disability and family building were incommensurable. These cases called into question whether there were children who simply could not be expected to function in *any* home and contributed to the idea that the adoption of certain children, particularly those with serious disabilities, was "unthinkable."[158] As parents and experts argued, a lack of family support services and guaranteed medical insurance that refused to acknowledge the needs of the caregiver and cared for influenced and exacerbated this notion of incommensurability.[159]

Agency practices changed in light of these lawsuits. Legal experts rec-ommended that agencies clearly describe the "risks and uncertainties as-sociated with adoption."[160] These risks were essentially about disability; agencies had to state to adopters that any child could have diagnosed or undiagnosed physical, intellectual, behavioral, or developmental condi-tions and they only had the information that the birth parents disclosed. They had to inform applicants that they could not guarantee the present or future health or development of a child.[161]

In sum, the heightened litigation of disruption and wrongful adoption cases contributed to the public and professional conversations about chil-dren with disabilities as damaged goods and as risky. This observation is not to discredit the painful experiences of families with regard to disruption and wrongful adoption, but rather to point out that *as a social problem*, as these cases emerged during this period, social workers and prospective parents became increasingly exposed to messaging that the adoption of dis-abled children was risky, problematic, and perhaps unavoidably so.

Conclusion

Unlike many "healthy" children, the adoption of children with disabilities in the 1980s and 1990s was not a foregone conclusion. Disabled children's uneven access to family lay not only in the sheer numbers of children needing placement or in the tenacity of institutional barriers. It also lay in the ideological environment that culturally supported and even exac-erbated the reasons and motivations behind parental hesitancy. In many ways, the experiences of disabled waiting children reflected the larger paradox of disability experiences at this time, with legislative and even cultural gains that were accompanied by continued social exclusion for people with disabilities.

For disabled waiting children, the stigma of damage, the crack and AIDS baby crises, the emergence of reproductive technologies, and the withdrawal of treatment for disabled infants all served to counter the so-cial work ideal that "all children are adoptable." Adoption disruption and wrongful adoption were, in part, a function of this ideological environ-ment. A lack of sufficient supports and a lack of full agency disclosure also reflected this environment. All of these forces positioned disability as a problem to be solved or to be rid of. They reinstantiated the notion that disabled children were risky.

At the same time, child welfare professionals deemed these children as at risk because of the social and structural reasons behind their placement. Indeed, adoption professionals' diagnoses of disabled children as both "risky" and "at risk" coexisted during this period. Sometimes they conflated these ideas. Meanwhile, Americans upheld the image of the "perfect" and "normal" child, which heightened expectations of potential parents in their family-making pursuits. Questions about the attractiveness, value, and worthiness of disabled waiting children, then, shaped the worries, concerns, and decisions of parent applicants. These questions helped keep waiting disabled children from being seen as desirable for family as a matter of course. Ultimately, this set of social and cultural dynamics, along with structural and procedural barriers, help explain why there were never enough parents to adopt disabled children. Thus, by the end of the twentieth century, disabled children were only partially included in adoptive family making.

A Usable Past:
Thinking about Contemporary
Practice in Light of History

This book is dedicated to the late disability historian Paul Longmore, who described the pertinence of disability history as a search for a usable past to create more accessible futures for people with disabilities.[1] Longmore's vision resonates with a 2009 conference panel by historians of childhood that examined whether historians can or should inform children's policy.[2] Like Longmore, these scholars argued that one role of historians is to "provide context, illuminate issues, or even offer caveats about the utility of popular prescriptions based on past experience."[3] Historians can unravel social, political, cultural, or economic phenomena to enhance our understanding of the present; in particular, they can help policymakers understand how the past has structured policy decisions but "without being presentist."[4]

Acknowledging continuities and discontinuities from adoption's past, for instance, can help make sense of contemporary debates about children's rights and needs and which policies would improve their lives.[5] Through such an analysis, one clearly observes the contingent nature of concepts like childhood, family, disability, and risk. As we learned from the trajectory traced in this book, these concepts are shaped by historical processes, social and cultural contexts, and economic and demographic forces. Thus, thinking about contemporary issues in light of the past helps us understand where we are in the ongoing trajectory of the adoption of children with disabilities. We also can discern how much of the language and practices that were established in the twentieth century structure our present moment, and what possibilities (or combination thereof) could champion children's best interests in adoption.

What Matters for Access to Family?

Informed by the past, and with Longmore's charge in mind, this epilogue reviews what (continually) matters for disabled children's access to, and thriving in, adoptive families in a landscape after the Adoption and Safe Families Act (ASFA). Although many of the themes I delineate apply to both private and public adoptions, my discussion concentrates on adoption from the foster care system for three reasons: ASFA itself spurred an increase in adoptions from foster care (one million children adopted in twenty years, although this rate seems to have declined), the scholarly and policy literature subsequently overwhelmingly focused on this sector, and adoption from foster care is now a significant twenty-first-century American social problem.[6] My discussion here cannot encapsulate all of the trends, programs, or issues that have surfaced since ASFA. That requires another book-length history. Rather, I posit what issues and frameworks I believe still matter for improving that access. In so doing, I articulate the conceptual and social implications of my work. I hope policy scholars and child welfare practitioners more knowledgeable than me can use this analysis to construct ever more adoption possibilities for children with disabilities.

Striving to provide better access to adoptive families should not undermine the great need to keep biological families with children with disabilities thriving and intact.[7] Preventing family separation while protecting children should be a central goal of all child welfare policy. Targeting the structural barriers to prevent separation and providing medical, childcare, and financial supports is unequivocally vital. In those instances where foster care or adoption is necessary for disabled children, however, we should make concerted efforts to meet children's needs. In the event of adoption, we should optimally assist those families, providing the same supports as biological ones to ensure permanency and prevent disruption.[8]

In trying to imagine robust options for disabled children's adoption, we must analyze why the inclusion is still incomplete and why hierarchies among children still remain. We must question why ideologies and practices with exclusionary outcomes still occur, even amid broad adoptability definitions and wider programmatic and policy efforts. As much of this book has shown, we must recognize that decisions about disabled people—even ones about intimate matters—are political decisions commonly shaped by ableist notions of family. Exposing those notions and reconceptualizing family in new ways is necessary for improving access for disabled children.[9] But we must also understand how and why this dynamic has occurred to think of scenarios and solutions that focus less on disability as a personal or parental problem and more on structural limitations and broad sociocultural trends. Such a focus allows us to extend the notion of care beyond neoliberal configurations of the private sphere and shift the language of risk from individuals to one that centers on social and political responsibility.

The Landscape after ASFA

Since the passage of ASFA, the same themes that surfaced throughout the twentieth century are reoccurring now but under new conditions. As a result of twentieth-century transformations in the family, in the notion of risk, in recruitment strategies and financial programs, and in critiques of disability stigma, disabled children's inclusion in adoption has expanded significantly, but, as at the end of the twentieth century, is still incomplete. Perhaps the best proof of this claim is that children with disabilities still remain one of the least desirable child populations to adopt, particularly from the foster care system.[10]

According to the most recent data gathered from the Adoption and Foster Care Analysis and Reporting System (AFCARS) for 2018, there are 437,000 children in foster care (with almost 700,000 served in some capacity that same year); almost half of those children have chronic medical issues.[11] Approximately half of the children in the child welfare system under five years of age have developmental delays. Upward of 80 percent of all children in foster care have physical or emotional disabilities. Many children have multiple disabilities.[12] Overall, researchers have reported that a disproportionate number of children with disabilities are represented in the child welfare system, many of them placed in group homes or residential treatment programs, which often compounds their embodied vulnerability.[13] Some states have adopted the model of therapeutic foster homes, where foster parents are trained in therapeutic care, as an effective alternative to communal care (especially for children with emotional disabilities). But therapeutic homes are sparse due, in part, to state funding arrangements that still tend to favor institutionalization.[14] Despite significant improvements to family access over the twentieth and twenty-first centuries, disability (especially as it intersects with age) remains a major barrier to adoption.[15]

In 2021, about 125,000 children in foster care are eligible and waiting for adoption, a rise of about 23 percent from 2012.[16] Many children wait more than two years to be adopted; children with disabilities wait even longer.[17] One reason for this long wait is that although four in ten Americans consider adoption as a way to form a family, few actually go through with it. Most adoptions today are either fost-adopt or relative adoptions.[18] In the years after ASFA, kinship care has become the preferred form of foster placement, but when caregiving relatives are not formally licensed with the state (as is common) they do not receive foster care payments.[19] It is hard to know how many informal relative adoptions actually take place. American taxpayers spend about $8.7 billion a year on foster care programs (15 percent of the overall budget dedicated to children and families) but the system itself is continually in crisis.[20]

Many legal changes have occurred since ASFA. In 1998, as part of the Clinton administration's Adoption 2002 Initiative, the federal government released funds to reward states that had increased the number of children adopted from foster care, giving qualifying states bonuses of up to $4,000 per adopted child, and $6,000 for each child with special needs. It also awarded Adoption Opportunities grants to states with innovative proposals to remove barriers to adoption for children with special needs.[21] But the bonuses did not apply to kinship care or guardianships, nor did the initiative account for the stability of placements, only a rise in them. States used the funds for postadoption services, adoption awareness programs, subsidy increases, provider trainings, legal services, and adopter recruitment, but not to increase the number of caseworkers to lower caseloads.[22]

Additional laws during the twenty years after ASFA continued to try to address and correct the inadequacies in support services and promote adoptions from foster care.[23] In 2018 the Family First Prevention Services Act marked the largest change to the structure of financing child welfare since the Adoption Assistance Act of 1980. The act amends the Title IV-E entitlement to provide more federal funds for family preservation and limits funds allocated to congregate care in order to emphasize family foster homes for foster youth.[24] Residential treatment group homes that remain approved must follow a trauma-informed treatment model with licensed staff, children must be monitored to make sure the placement is suitable, and states must undergo concurrent planning for permanent placement.[25] The law also slowed down the process of unlinking income from adoption assistance that was mandated with the Fostering Connections to Success and Increasing Adoptions Act in 2008. Now, states can opt into using Title IV-E funds to pay for foster care prevention services, which could help prevent children from being placed into the child welfare system in the first place and work to keep biological families intact. Quite significantly, the act also eliminated ASFA's term limit on providing family preservation services and its mandate to terminate biological parental custody for any child who had been in foster care for fifteen months out of the last twenty-two. At the time of ASFA's passage and afterward, child welfare advocates, scholars, and social work researchers, as discussed in chapter 5, fiercely criticized this limit because it did not allow enough time for reasonable reunification efforts to work and it prejudiced families of color.[26] Although ASFA increased the number of adoptions and sped up the time to adoption—increasing adoptions between 1995 and 2005 from 28,000 per year to more than 50,000 and decreasing the time spent in foster care by 30 percent—researchers found it did not improve the well-being of adopted children overall.[27] It is too early to know whether removing this family preservation time limit will result in higher rates of foster drift or whether it will increase the incidence of children's movements in and out of foster care again, as the 1960s through the 1990s, or in higher family reunification rates and a decrease in adoptions.

The former seems more likely. Much like the crack epidemic in the 1980s, the recent opioid crisis in America and its policing have driven even more children into the foster care system amid a dearth of foster families. Yet, instead of the assumed Black racial profile of crack addicts in the 1980s, the profile of the opioid addicts today is white. Still, involuntary relinquishment related to neglect and abuse remains a significant reason for foster care placement, with 36 percent of foster children entering the system because of biological parental drug use.[28] Children with disabilities today remain particularly at risk for neglect and abuse; they are in fact three times more likely to be maltreated than children without disabilities.[29] These adverse childhood experiences can lead to new or additional emotional, cognitive, and physical impairments, including numerous types of developmental disabilities.[30] The effects of these childhood experiences can also strain adoptive families, thereby destabilizing adoptive placements.[31] If history is any guide, the foster crisis will continue to get worse unless concomitant structural changes involving health care, drug policy, income inequality, and incarceration follow, and services to vulnerable biological families are offered. These moves seem highly unlikely in the current political environment.

Stigma, Attitudes, and Concepts Matter

Despite a definitive social shift in the past century in society's openness to adoption as an alternative family formation and in its broader recognition of disability rights, long-standing notions that pathologize adoption and disability persist among adoption professionals and the public. Some social workers continue to question whether all children are adoptable, for example, despite social work principles that espouse this notion of adoptability. A study by Rosemary J. Avery found that 40 percent of social workers believe that children with severe behavioral issues were not adoptable because they require high levels of care. Social workers fear that these children's issues may be too much for adoptive parents to cope with. Many believe that a child's physical, psychiatric, and behavioral disabilities are critical barriers to placement. Prospective parents also fear the lack of support during the postadoptive period.[32] Medical experts often concur with these decisions and have advised against adoptive placement for children with behavioral challenges. Such fallacious attitudes, according to the study, "aris[e] from various misplaced beliefs such as that the child is too emotionally troubled, too old, too damaged by the system, that the level of care needed to support the child is too intensive, and that no family would want to adopt a child with such severe special needs."[33] This may sound familiar.

As this history has shown, such attitudes do children with disabilities a major disservice; if a child's caseworker is not convinced of a child's adoptability, she will not dedicate the effort to recruit adoptive parents. Even when the social work notion of adoptability is broad—certainly compared to a hundred years ago—attitudes can still hinder access to family.[34] Indeed, adoption professionals recognized in the 1960s and 1970s that caseworkers' beliefs in the adoptability of every child was the starting point to any successful effort to place children with disabilities.[35] This remains the case; as adoptive mother Patricia Harris remarked, "The stigma that sees foster kids as unlovable and unadoptable should be changed."[36]

Adoptive parents of a disabled child acknowledge the intense stigma that still surrounds disability. No matter which types of impairments a child might have, researchers have found that caregiver commitments remain the same.[37] Social attitudes about disability in adoption, as in other spheres, are inflected by such factors as the presumed etiology of disability, race, gender, and disability (in)visibility. An adoptive mother in one study noted that although she doesn't publicize that her daughter with fetal alcohol spectrum disorder is adopted, her doctor and counselor advised her to do so as a countermove to providers and citizens who blamed her for her daughter's impairment. Ascribing culpability reveals that value judgments that are still entangled with disability, risk, and guilt. "They said whenever you're talking to someone advocating for her you need to be upfront and say, 'This is my adopted daughter,' so that you'll just release all the antagonism that's going to be thrown at you."[38] At first glance, this advice seems highly problematic since it shifts blame and guilt from adoptive to biological mother, rather than fundamentally calling out others' ignorance and prejudice no matter the mother's status. But this mother thought the doctor's suggested strategy was protective; he pointed to the necessity that she may have to employ to avoid having her own legal custody status challenged on the basis of child neglect and endangerment. For this reason, the mother admits: "I've got a letter on me from the pediatrician . . . that states her diagnosis," and the business card of a lawyer in the event someone questions her custody.[39]

Assumptions like these about disability etiology invoke the same damage rhetoric we found in the 1980s and 1990s about children in foster care. They reflect and perpetuate disability stigma. But they also point to the actual problem of neglect and abandonment that affects disabled children more than their peers. Instead, as adoptive father Ralph Savarese asks, shouldn't we move our attention to systems-level culpability by questioning whether foster care *itself* is intrinsically damaging, rather than the children in it or the children who come from/out of it?[40]

Negative views about disability and disabled people continue to pervade American society and its policies. Despite disability activism and empowerment, many Americans still see disability as a tragedy and a burden. Although the Americans with Disabilities Act Amendment (2008) and the UN Convention for the Rights of People with Disabilities (2006; which the US hasn't ratified as of 2020), Americans still assume disabled people are dependent, incapable, and incompetent; in many spheres people with disabilities are still deprived of full social and political citizenship. Like child abandonment and neglect, hate crimes, violence, and social exclusion all disproportionately affect people with disabilities. Discrimination in sectors like education, housing, employment, medicine, and family is still widely prevalent. As in the case of Tiffany Callo, disabled parents' ability to parent is continually challenged, with many losing custody of their children for no reason other than their disability. In fact, at least 19 percent of children in foster care enter the system because their biological parent has a disability. Although some states have passed legislation to protect these parents from losing their custody rights, others have not yet succeeded.[41]

Parents of color with disabilities are particularly affected by child welfare practices that allow the state to use disability as a reason to terminate rights.[42] But there are counternarratives that resist these trends. As opposed to the legal focus on how disabled parents are compromised as parents, Heather Watkins, a Black disabled mother, has emphasized how disability generates parental adaptability and accountability:

> Disability permeates every aspect of my lived experience and has factored in key quality of life decision-making. . . . My parenting has benefited as I've had to consider how I would respond to challenges knowing that my child would be a direct recipient of how I internalized my disability.[43]

Adoption is also a site of social stigma. Although Americans express positive views of adoption today, many still harbor biases about it. Stigma about adoption—tied as it is to disability—is so prevalent in American culture, like movies, books, and television, that it is often glossed over or dismissed.[44] Psychologist Abbie Goldberg summarizes the components of adoption stigma: "Beyond the stereotypes that children who are adopted are damaged in some way, there are many other dominant stereotypes and myths about adoption," such as: adoptive parents cannot love an adopted child as much as a biological one; open adoption causes problems for children; bonding between a child and her adoptive parents is inherently harder to achieve than when there are genetic ties; and birth parents can reclaim their child at any time.[45] Ideas about (ab)normality, authenticity, legitimate motherhood, and the nature of genuine love suffuse these myths. As the use of genetic and reproductive technologies intensified, the mandate of biogenetic ties has become ever more forceful.[46] No longer a retort between siblings, for instance, children are increasingly using the phrase "you're adopted" pejoratively with their peers.[47]

The rhetoric of "realness" (as in, "is she your *real* child?"), which reflects the power of biological kinship as the most authentic form of family in America, enables Americans to see adoption as a "last alternative" or as a nonchoice because they view it as a risky venture (although how embryo adoption rates in this calculus are unclear).[48] According to Goldberg, adoptive parents of all types perceive adoption stigma, but some adoptive parents internalize these stereotypes more than others, particularly heterosexual couples with in-racial adoptions. Others feel they must defend their families and push against the idea that pursuing adoption is second rate to biological parenthood.[49]

Addressing and alleviating disability stigmas and adoption stigmas are important steps toward improving access to family for children with disabilities. Addressing both forms of prejudice will likely help validate the multiple types of families that exist in America, make adoption more attractive to prospective parents, and, in the end, lower the gap between available children and parent applicants. As we have seen throughout the twentieth century, as notions of adoptability, family, and disability widen, so too do more expansive opportunities for the permanent placement for children with disabilities.

Personal Stories Matter

Personal stories matter in the quest to make family more accessible to and for children with disabilities through adoption. Families' and adoptees' lived experience, and their self-representation, add texture to policy debates and research, reveal expertise in navigating needed supports, services, and family dynamics, and show the incredible heterogeneity of adoptive families.[50] As I noted in the introduction, finding twentieth-century personal stories unmediated by social workers' perspectives is difficult. Since the 2000s, however, several adoptive parents have published memoirs about raising children with disabilities. Some disabled adoptees have addressed their disability and adoptee identities in blogs.[51] These memoirs and writings are much more critical of the prejudice against their children (or themselves) than those published in years prior. Although parent memoirs chart the struggles involved in adopting and parenting children with disabilities, twenty-first-century authors as a whole do not posit disability as burden, as those from the 1990s did; they use memoir as a "medium for counter-discourse that challenges stereotypes and misconceptions."[52] Such memoirs are a small body of work, and the authors possess more varied perspectives than those of the past.

Perhaps the best-known memoir about adoption and disability is Denise Jacobson's *The Question of David*, published in 1999, one of the first
memoirs by a disabled mother of a disabled child. This book captures the
need for help, the misgivings family members express about Denise and
her husband Neil's decision to adopt, the ups and downs of parenting David, and the support of disability community activists.[53]

Denise, Neil, and David all have cerebral palsy. In fact, the family came
together through this bio-familiarity. David became available for private
adoption to Denise and Neil after another couple set to take him started
having doubts about adopting a baby with a disability. Denise could not understand how the couple could want a baby so badly but did not want David
because he might have a disability (at the time undiagnosed). She writes:

> I had already concluded, too, that if he had a disability at all, it would have
> been relatively insignificant (to Neil and me, at least). If I was wrong and his
> disability turned out to be more involved, well. . . . I'd deal with that too, even
> though I always told Neil I wouldn't have another wheelchair in the house. . . .
> But there are never any guarantees.[54]

Denise's understanding of the contingency, of corporeal vulnerability,
and of a rejection of conditional parenthood is a direct result of Denise's
own disability experience.[55] Throughout the book, Denise candidly writes
about how that experience informs her parenting style, her worries and
fears, her recognition of disability prejudice (she calls it "cripophia"), her
need for parenting assistance and its chronic inadequacy, and barriers for
people with disabilities to adoptive parenthood.[56] Denise recounts the
adoption process, with all the insensitive and discriminatory things people
tell her, the typical historical assumptions about her that experts and family still make ("damaged goods"; "tragedy"; "a potential hazard in raising
a child"; "aren't fit to be parents"), the childhood memories it invokes,
and the fortitude it gives her to resist negative views about herself, Neil,
and David.[57]

At one point in the narrative, Denise raises the issue of labeling a baby's
disability as either mild, moderate, or severe—a mode of risk coding, as
we saw in chapter 3, that became prominent in adoption discourse in the
mid to late twentieth century and beyond. Denise calls this hierarchy out;
she argues that categorizing people with disabilities according to medical
and societal beliefs leads to a "dim view of children and adults with CP and
other developmental disabilities and our potential."[58] To Denise, it was

understandable for prospective adoptive parents without her medical savvy to be scared off when an expert labeled a relinquished child "severely disabled." Without the knowledge of lived experience, they would not necessarily know how to critically assess expert claims.[59] But Denise is also realistic and practical; she describes the extensive paperwork needed to get David the services he needs, the strategies she creates and learns to care for him, and the threat she feels of losing David because of her disability.

Reasonable People: A Memoir about Autism and Adoption follows a similar disability perspective to that of Jacobson's book. The book, about a boy named DJ, is written by his father, Ralph Savarese, a poet and professor. Savarese's astute academic commentary about disability, family, class, social responsibility, and accountability offers a unique layer of analysis in the memoir that merges the personal with the structural. Savarese provides a stinging critique of an American culture that romanticizes children while it also enables extreme child poverty, trauma, and violence. He is highly critical of foster care as a deeply flawed, underfunded institution, one that completely failed his son. Given the shortage of foster homes and the population of foster kids, Savarese wishes for a "common commitment to the well-being of children, not some fatuous cultural sentimentalization of them." This is the only way he sees an opening for the system to transform.[60] At the same time, Savarese is troubled that economic retrenchment and the decline of the welfare state have only intensified the "fetish of blood relations," which, in turn, has produced a narrower sense of the "human family to which we might feel obligated" and a zero-sum sense of "competitive happiness," where one group's well-being must come at the expense of another's.[61] DJ concurs: "Politicians present kids as very important but only pointing out that millions of kids look poor might not get them homes. Thinking group homes respect kids, they hurt them. . . . Kids love very much being safe. They get put in dangerous situations."[62]

Savarese also disputes feminist critiques of ASFA that state that the law is fundamentally an attack on single mothers. He contends that commitments to motherhood should not ignore the urgent and desperate needs of children like his own.[63] Additionally, Savarese takes issue with his social circle's comments about the decision to adopt DJ. Friends remarked on how saintlike he and his wife were to go through with DJ's adoption. Savarese calls out these claims:

> Selected not as a last resort, adoption—particularly of a disabled child—
> seemed to constitute a challenge, even a threat, to the comfortable assumptions

of our friends and relatives. Nearly everybody wanted to identify the adoption as, on the one hand, an act of altruism and, on the other, foolhardy, even self-destructive.[64]

Still, Savarese writes candidly about his own doubts about whether he and his wife have the skills necessary to parent DJ (his wife is a specialist in autism).[65]

The memoir is a tome on disability as deeply relational. In fact, Savarese powerfully captures the questions this book poses in his own retelling; questions about the implications of disability and difference for building and sustaining families. Like the history I present here, *Reasonable People* raises Americans' reticence about disabled children as worthy and fit candidates for family, and grapples with the workings of love (DJ: "I'm nervous love is hard. It breathes hard; Mom: Not always. Sometimes love quietly approaches to calm and soothe you just when you need it").

Beyond social analysis, this deeply honest, self-reflective memoir is fundamentally a story about DJ, a nonverbal child with autism, becoming the "author of his own story." DJ writes the last chapter, which is a radical departure from other memoirs by adoptive parents about their disabled children.[66] The memoir also maps DJ's path from not being able to communicate to gaining an aptitude for expressing his experiences, feelings, and insights. Ironically, as DJ gains language, his fears about being returned to foster care create extreme anxiety. As his adoptive parents ease DJ's fears and establish constancy, their own parental journey takes shape. *Reasonable People* is not an overcoming narrative, however, but rather one about disregard and underestimation, belonging, pain, and empowered difference as inextricably linked; it is about the road from "lost normalcy" to disability pride.[67]

DJ is now an advocate who educates others on neurodiversity and is an author/poet in his own right. His autobiographical documentary film, *Deej* (2017), a Peabody awardee, speaks to DJ's fight for "autistic human rights and universal inclusion." Much like this epilogue's contention about access to family, one of the film's key statements is "Inclusion shouldn't be a lottery."[68] *Deej* traces DJ's transition from eighth grade to Oberlin College, all the while forcing viewers to rethink society's devaluing ideas about disability and autism.[69] The film also asks viewers to reconsider whose stories matter and which voices count as authentic.[70]

The documentary *My Flesh and Blood* (2003) highlights the stories of Susan Tom and five of her eleven disabled adopted children. The film shows how disability experiences are not monolithic; they are shaped through a mixture of social, physical, psychological, and structural issues. Viewers see these children as social actors, with opinions, interpretations, and stories of their own.[71] The film chronicles this adoptive family's life over a year, in which each child's personality is highlighted alongside sibling dynamics, individual identity struggles, Tom's own personal travails (including her mother, who is distant and judgmental), and the need for more mental health support, adoption assistance, and respite care. It explores many of the children's physical and emotional needs, how they take care of one another, how each is vulnerable, and how some periodically cause tensions and problems. In so doing, the impairments themselves increasingly disappear from viewers' minds as they continue to watch the film; an erasure no doubt the director intends to create so as to demonstrate the ways in which this adoptive family is just like many others.[72] This latter message is reminiscent of the photo-listing strategy we saw used in the 1970s, which focused on the specific personalities of waiting children so that prospective parents could see them as more than their impairment and just like others.[73]

Less well-known memoirs include a set of (presumably) able-bodied female authors who describe their journeys with adoption and disability. *Not Always Happy: An Unusual Parenting Journey* (2017), by Kari Wagner-Peck, is a memoir about parenting Thorin, a child with Down syndrome. Unlike many narratives about disability, this one refuses to engage with tropes of heroism, pity, or tragedy.[74] Yet Wagner-Peck shows how those tropes are still operative among her peers. When she began to consider adopting Thorin, people focused solely on his disabling traits as a signifier of an inevitable unrewarding life; disability, in their construction, stood in for Thorin himself.[75] None of Wagner-Peck's peers "said anything close to 'Hey awesome, you found a kid!' It was more like 'Why do you want to do that to yourself?'; 'That sounds hard'; or even 'Don't do that, please.'"[76] The author asks why it is necessary to defend one's decision to adopt a child with a disability: "Why couldn't we love him freely without question?"[77] In her pursuit of a fost-adoption, Wagner-Peck explicitly recognizes the role that ableism and racism play in determining which babies are available and which babies are most wanted. Wagner-Peck contends that damage imagery and the discourse of risk are foregrounded rhetorics in fost-adopt training and discussions, making her wonder, with sarcasm, if the children themselves could sue for defamation of character.[78] Wanting to explore the attitudes about adoption and Down syndrome, Wagner-Peck established a blog called the *A Typical Son* to give a "nonlinear telling" about state adoptions, her experience of being a new parent, and the typical and complex ways Thorin developed and behaved.[79]

Three other of these less-known memoirs merge the authors' religious beliefs and a discussion of disability, foster care, and adoption. *Loving the Unadoptable* offers a brief reflection on the fost-adoption of Cory who, in his teenage years, is diagnosed with bipolar disorder and goes in and out of hospital and residential care.[80] A play on the label of the disabled child as unadoptable, the title of the book poses a challenge to that position. Patricia Harris, Cory's mother, merges religion and activism in her call to create a Christian Residential Treatment Facility that merges prayer with medication, well-trained staff, mental health services, and empowerment. Harris believes that this combination can help Christian adopted children with mental illness like her son achieve a "normal life."[81] Harris's book is a mixture of commentary about her experience parenting Cory, advice for parents in a similar situation, and reflections about the role of her faith in motivating her to love in a way that is "patient, kind, longsuffering, and accepts Cory for who he is. This is unconditional love."[82] Harris's description of love harks back to the adoption overcoming narrative we saw in the 1960s. Like much religious commentary about disability, Harris believes God brought Cory to her for a reason. Harris hopes for a supportive community and changed attitudes that will resonate with the values of her religious community.

Born Broken: An Adoptive Journey (2017), by Kristin Berry, was published with the permission of Berry's son Alexander, diagnosed with fetal alcohol spectrum disorder (FASD). The memoir describes similar themes of prejudice, frustration with societal views of disability and transracial adoption, medical misconceptions, confusion and delayed diagnosis, social isolation, critical allies, and family love. Berry, a foster and adoptive mother of several children, depicts how Alexander's distress affects her other children.[83] Berry describes her complex emotions regarding Alexander's quick marked shifts from being happy, calm, and gracious to frenzied outbursts, anxiety, and dangerous behavior.[84] She shares the anger she felt toward the hypocrisy of church members who "claimed to love God [but] couldn't see my son for more than his outbursts."[85] Although she remains devout and prays to find guidance and healing for "our own brokenness" (that of her family) throughout the narrative, she increasingly realizes Alexander needs therapy and residential care.[86] Like some of the other memoirs, Berry's explores her emotional journey as an adoptive parent with a parallel journey of the child's "coming of age," through education, communication, residential care, and disability pride. Part rescue and resentment, Berry points to the fragility of both her son and herself, the balancing act of parenting her other children, and her recognition that love may not be enough.[87]

Finally, *Forfeiting All Sanity* (2010), by Jennifer Poss Taylor, highlights the central role religious faith plays in parenting an adoptive child. Unlike the aforementioned memoirs, however, Poss Taylor's book describes a litany of pathologies about her daughter, Ashley; she does not resist the biases of disability but rather reproduces them. As such, the reader never gets a sense of Ashley's personality; she is reduced to a set of behavioral challenges. Poss Taylor has certainly had to confront serious challenges, and her frustration is palpable. She seeks expert advice and turns to her religious community.

Access to therapeutic expertise, however, is only made possible by having access to health care. Even with private insurance, Poss Taylor admits, most families cannot afford all the needed medical care. Recognizing the value of respite care as well, she shares her desire to open a home for children and families with special needs that is staffed with trained, nurturing professionals so that parents could have the space and time to take care of daily demands and rest. These two programs/services are key to the author's family.

Poss Taylor's narrative seems much like Michael Dorris's *The Broken Cord* (1989) in that it portrays disability as "confining" rather than "defining."[88] She sees her memoir as a medium to advocate making drinking by pregnant women illegal; she views it as a "selfish decision" to torture an innocent child who will "never experience normalcy again."[89] The narrative is infused with the language of risk, damage, and resentment. Poss Taylor herself admits to the latter in a confessional chapter. She acknowledges her resentment toward her daughter, her tendency to blame Ashley for her struggles, and her need to cease "hiding behind the diagnosis."[90] In the final chapter, in a question-and-answer format, the author asks Ashley her opinions about FASD and about the memoir. These few simple lines are the only ones where we hear Ashley's voice; she states that FASD makes her feel worried that she will drink when she grows up, she wants to be an artist when she grows up, and she appreciates her brother and sister.

With their array of perspectives, these memoirs shaped by ASFA reflect the diverse experiences of adoptive parents and their children with disabilities. As adoptees after ASFA age, it is possible we will see more memoirs that explore growing up and living as an adoptee with a disability. Much as childhood studies scholars have argued elsewhere, these narratives could move our attention from stories *about* children's needs and parents' protection, to subjective accounts of being adopted and disabled.[91] By writing or recording their own stories, disabled adoptees could define their own best interests and those of their peers. They could resist, accept, or reformulate American notions of belonging and worth. These works may enable policymakers, social workers, scholars, and the public to fully consider adoptees' ideas for targeted programs to ensure that they thrive.

Community Matters

What these memoirs demonstrate is that navigating disability and adoption necessitates interdependence and solidarity with other people. A sense of community matters for humans to connect and flourish. Families who adopt children with disabilities emphasize this need.

As we saw in the middle of the twentieth century, adoptive parents of hard-to-place children politically organized for permanency planning and sought community support among those parents who sought similar paths to family building, all in order to effect change for themselves and for other prospective adoptive families and children.

New needs for help and advice arise across the adoption life course. As children grow, some of these developing needs can be attained through social work services, but others can only be gathered from others who have experienced these needs directly. Adoptive families with disabled children today find nurturing in support group networks with families who have similar experiences.[92] Community reduces isolation and enables families to share tips, insights, and strategies. As one adoptive mother in a study of fetal alcohol spectrum disorder remarked: "I feel so much better talking to other parents [who have children with FASD] knowing it's not just my child. It's not just us."[93] Similarly, a community of adoptees with disabilities could help form friendships, provide guidance, and create new forms of knowledge about the uniqueness and value of such experiences.

Advocacy Matters

If we think about children's access to family as a basic right, then obligations and responsibilities to ensure that right should not be completely dependent upon the nuclear family but should also be a concern and obligation of the community.[94] Child welfare professionals made this argument almost a century ago in the Children's Charter of 1930, which articulated a loving and secure home (or its substitute where necessary) as a fundamental right and, for disabled children, the right to become an asset to society.[95] The charter recognized that if costs relating to the latter could not be fulfilled privately, then they should be borne publicly. It did not explicitly state a provision relating to the question of access to family, but such a right is certainly not anathema to child welfare sentiments expressed since. The pertinent issue is that to uphold children's rights, including the right for disabled children to have access to family, it takes political and social will on the federal, state, and local levels, and it demands that we reconceptualize the scope of care.

Like those in the latter part of the twentieth century, adoptive parents of disabled children report needing to know their rights and to keep on top of things, like up-to-date records, and to monitor the appropriateness and adequacy of their child's support services. This legacy continues. Parents report the need to be constant advocates for their disabled children. One adoptive mother stated of her thirteen-year-old son: "You have to fight for your child. You cannot sit back and let the teachers tell you, 'Well this is what we're going to do.' You have to be willing to fight constantly to get your child what he needs to get them to listen to you. Because a lot of times they won't listen to you."[96] Showing a penchant for resourcefulness, many parents read research about their child's impairment to most effectively advocate for her and to educate others when necessary. Other parents use advocacy services to help their child.[97] Like those in years past, adoptive parents today describe advocating for one's child as a reflection of their unconditional love for, and acceptance of, her.[98]

Parent, adoptee, and disability self- and community advocacy matters to enact political and structural change. In twentieth-century adoption, reformers, activists in the permanency planning movement, and advocates for deinstitutionalization changed standards of adoptability, foster care, adoptive practices, and norms for upholding the dignity and treatment of people with disabilities. These advocates improved opportunities for children with disabilities to live within adoptive families and within their communities. Parents of children with special needs and forward-thinking adoption professionals helped create and sustain specialized services for children for whom families were hard to find. By challenging adoption agencies and social worker attitudes, and by engaging legislators as allies, advocates opened opportunities to family that had been closed just decades before.

Practices Matter

Such advocacy must be followed by clear, systematic, and extensive practical steps to make a tangible difference for access to family. Social work practices, including postplacement services, matter for the sustainability of disabled children's adoptive placements, private or public. Only a few years after ASFA, social workers pointed out that states and agencies could significantly facilitate the adoptive placement and security of disabled children by providing better services.[99] Social workers recognize the need for intensive adoptive parent training, higher adoption subsidies, more accurate photo listings, more effective recruitment and postplacement services, and more interagency cooperation to enable optimal access to family for children with disabilities.[100] But social workers' workload is already overwhelming and most cases are enormously complex. They must try to recruit parents, coordinate due process hearings, arrange visitations, access service providers, find appropriate educational settings for children, manage the personalities and emotions of all those involved, and more. Finding foster parents, much less adoptive parents, for waiting children is difficult, especially because of the complex care that is often needed for disabled children.[101] Even with ASFA's mandate to perform concurrent planning of family reunification and adoptive placement, the latter is frequently not pursued for children with disabilities. When it is, placement planning tends to be different from how it is for children without disabilities, especially for older children.[102] Disabled children are less likely to be reunified with their biological parents and tend to change placements more often. Social workers more often place disabled children in settings like non-kin home foster care, group homes, and institutions compared to children without disabilities.[103] The pressures of the foster care system tend to create a generally high rate of turnover of caseworkers. But disabled children in foster care tend to have even more caseworkers because of the added demands on social workers to address their needs, creating a discontinuity in placement planning that then contributes to longer wait times in foster care until a permanent placement. Furthermore, in some cases, available recruitment tools are not even utilized for these children, and public and private agencies still do not adequately recruit disabled parent applicants to adopt and raise children with disabilities.

Understandably, specialized agencies, certainly those modeled after Spaulding for Children, tend to have the most success in placing waiting children with disabilities. When social workers do refer these children's cases to specialized agencies, multiple foster and adoptive placements tend to be avoided.[104] As in the late twentieth century, specialized social work training programs that adapt recruitment and services necessary for children with disabilities continue to engender success.

A plethora of training programs after ASFA now focus on children with disabilities and their permanent placement. Yet there are limits to training programs; they ultimately cannot fully prepare social workers for the "overwhelming tasks and skills needed to interface with children with disabilities . . . family members, and other service providers."[105] Training programs are similarly designed for prospective adoptive parents with the belief that more informed adoptive parents can help create sustainable families. Social workers who believe that disabled children are adoptable and that their adoptions can be "successful" also believe that prospective parents should be adequately informed about a child's past experiences in her biological family and in foster care, her personality, and her challenges so that parents can have adaptable expectations and encourage her to excel in the ways she is able while advocating for their child's needs and rights.[106]

To enable access to family, training programs and other services need to embody terms, concepts, and goals that promote a flexible idea about family. Definitions inform practices and should be critically reassessed. Redefining placement success, for instance, can be a first step toward changing attitudes and building practices that enable better access. Policy scholar Rosemary Avery argues that the bar for success—"strong attachments, harmonious relationships, and warm reciprocal affection"—may be too high for some families with adopted children with special needs to fulfill. This observation is reminiscent of social workers' revision of the standard of mutual affection for adoptive families that we saw at midcentury. Avery adds: "But that does not mean that adoption is not possible or has failed. Situations where adoptive parents can model stability, consistency, and reliability, and advocate to ensure that the child's needs are met, should be regarded as a highly successful adoption."[107]

Adoption leaders were right when they strongly recommended postplacement services for adoptive families in the late 1970s. Their insights are still salient today. Robust postplacement services, including respite care, can help adoptive parents and children navigate and meet their disability needs and adoption goals. More recently, researchers have noted that there is a high demand for postadoption services by adoptive families, but they fail to access or underutilize these services. Often they do not even know about these services, or they do not have enough information to access and utilize them successfully.[108] Families who adopt children with disabilities (whether there is a diagnosis before finalization or a child develops a disability postadoption) have the largest needs for tutoring, medical treatment, crisis intervention, and counseling. Easily accessing these supports significantly helps adoptive families thrive.

In this sense, subsidies remain very important to enable ongoing support for a prospective disabled adoptee. Medicaid is a lifeline for many adoptive families to be able to access medical services, but not all adoptive families qualify. In the midst of economic retrenchment, parents worry that cuts to services and subsidies could jeopardize their ability to care for their adopted children.[109] As the gains from the Adoption Assistance Act of 1980 showed, higher subsidies that keep up with medical costs and cost of living could alleviate the higher cost of caring for children with disabilities in families and lead to both greater access and placement stability.[110]

Informal and formal respite care helps adoptive families who need it to attend to home obligations, self-care, or other commitments. Adoption leaders argued for respite care decades ago, understanding that it increases family stability. Yet it remains one of the greatest unmet service needs of families who have adopted disabled children from foster care.[111] Policies and programs that are serious about permanent placement of children with disabilities need to include respite care funding and provision as an integral part of expanded postplacement services.

All these services help families a great deal, but even with their use, families experience additional stresses in that they have to repeatedly educate others about their child and her impairment to access care across the life course, especially when there is high provider turnover. This is especially true for children with invisible disabilities and rare diseases for whom social service provider knowledge is generally inadequate or goes unrecognized.[112] A lack of adoption-specific competence in disability services also contributes to family stress.[113] Moreover, restricted geographical access to services in some states leads to longer wait lists and ultimately further reduces the likelihood of sustaining stable adoptive families. Parents who have to travel hours to get the services they need for their child feel frustrated, unsupported, and emotionally taxed. By contrast, families thrive when they access effective preadoptive services, whole-family support, and networks with adoptive parents who are experienced in navigating adoptive and disability services. Thus, social work practices matter to recruit parents, to offer advice on the right resources for optimal care, and to furnish families with comprehensive supports to ensure sustainability.

Coordination Matters

Adoptive parents simultaneously navigate multiple complicated legal, medical, and service systems to take care of their disabled children. The fragmentation of these systems, and even the inconsistent definitions of "disability" and "special needs," creates additional struggles for parents seeking help.[114] That is why coordinated child welfare and disability policies matter for children's permanency in an adoptive family.[115] Making child welfare and disability systems more strongly coordinated is a massive endeavor, but families' experiences and frustrations within and between these two complicated systems merge together and become inseparable. Solutions must therefore serve—to adapt a long-standing historical phrase—the best interests of the whole child.

However, comprehensive reforms are extremely hard to make. For one thing, the child welfare "system" consists of several agencies that deal with multiple matters (e.g., mental health counseling, public assistance, substance abuse treatment, Medicaid), making coordination quite difficult. For another, disability services at the federal, state, and local levels are delivered separately from child welfare services, frustrating any moves for coordinated care. Third, because foster care is administered by states, any federal moves toward comprehensive reform results in a cascade of additional state actions and decisions that, in turn, create a plethora of nonstandard practices across states.[116] States invest differently in (or divest from) child welfare services, have different definitions of maltreatment, and have different laws that implement federal regulations. Variations in court processes also contribute to a complicated system. Some states contract private agencies to deliver their fost-adopt services, blurring the public-private divide. As a result of all these structural barriers, social workers and foster and adoptive parents need incredible endurance to navigate the system's bureaucratic web to advocate for disabled children in both foster care and adoptive families.

Health care provision is a significant area that needs to be coordinated with child welfare and disability policy. Fortunately, the Affordable Care

Act (ACA; 2010) expanded health care access and coverage for millions of Americans and, in some states, expanded Medicaid access. Through expansion, the ACA has reportedly helped stabilize vulnerable biological families and the health of their child(ren) with a disability. We should remember that ASFA guaranteed health care for adopted special needs children, but the ACA also enabled low-income parents to adopt a child with medical needs. The ACA amended the financial incentives to adopt by increasing the maximum tax credit for adoption and the employer-based adoption assistance tax exclusion threshold.[117] Any moves to overturn the ACA or significantly weaken it could upend these provisions. If the ACA is kept relatively intact, universal health care could build upon and expand the benefits of the law to potentially alleviate access and utilization disparities for adopted children with disabilities and relieve some of the financial barriers to adoptive placement.

A national coordinated approach to child welfare in the US would continue to revamp the foster care system in a systematic way to address inconsistencies and problems across and within states, create additional mechanisms to facilitate cross-agency and cross-service delivery systems, and promote the integrity of all types of families (biological, foster, and adoptive). This is no small feat. The federal government has recommended enhanced coordination of public health, community, and child welfare programs toward this end, but much more work remains to be done.[118]

This approach would ideally be multipronged, with funding to support adoptive families and vulnerable biological families as well; it would provide treatment and prevention services to parents to keep children safe and consistent screenings for children entering the foster care system to understand their physical, cognitive, and mental health needs. It would buttress trained human resources to lower social worker caseloads, reduce wait lists and wait times to receive needed services, enact any necessary legal/court reforms, tackle the need for foster aging-out supports, and better assist prospective adoptive parents in their quest to start and preserve a family from the public or private agency system.[119]

A comprehensive approach would also align and coordinate child welfare and disability policy goals, mechanisms, and procedures as a way to "imagine and materialize the widest array of bodies and minds" for family formation and flourishing.[120] Changes to disability policy to support foster and adoptive families could start with education. Practices relating to the Individuals with Disabilities Education Act (IDEA), for example, are not foster-informed and so they account neither for children's school moves as foster drift occurs nor for foster parent's lack of authority over the educational decisions relating to their foster children. A lack of sufficiently funded mental health services and crisis support underserves children with disabilities writ large, but these services are especially important for adoptive families to remain intact.[121]

Historically, rights-based legislation and deinstitutionalization have had positive impacts upon adoptive families with a disabled child. But implementing these policies in an underfunded environment without adequate mechanisms for enforcement remains a major problem. Unlike other civil rights legislation, integrating people with disabilities in society costs money. Disability policies that include sufficient federal and state funding for discrimination prevention and training, support staff for implementation and assurance of the law, and proactive enforcement mechanisms (including in education)—to name a few—are necessary to make steps toward disability justice for all children, adoptive or otherwise.

It goes without saying that such social and service supports do not have to be limited to adoptive families; they should also extend to *all kinds of families to which children with disabilities belong*. A comprehensive coordinated approach would need to streamline relevant disability and health care policies to make sure children with disabilities have adequate educational opportunities, medical care, respite care, and community supports in an integrated fashion. The conceptual model of wraparound services may be instructive here. Wraparound services are currently a therapeutic model of foster care. Similar to the concept of a medical home but more extensive and directed at service provision, this approach places the family and child at the center of a set of health, mental health, educational, and social welfare services coordinated by a caseworker.[122] The wraparound model could be expanded, adapted, and developed as a systematic approach to improving child welfare.

Research Matters

The sheer number of reports and research articles about the landscape after ASFA is overwhelming, but there are many areas where research into adoptive children with disabilities is still needed, like their experiences within the child welfare system and with placement stability and instability, and thus their ongoing access to family.[123] State child welfare systems do not collect standardized information on children with disabilities, and child welfare workers are inadequately trained, so they underidentify disabled children and therefore fail to connect them to disability-specific services.[124] This needs to change. Policies need to be evidence based, but to be so inquiries that seek data about these children—their biological and adoptive parents, outcomes, services utilized, aging-out experiences, and adoption facilitators and barriers—are necessary.[125] Social scientists (mainly in psychology, social work, and sociology) and medical researchers mainly address these areas; historians and humanities scholars have yet to engage deeply with the landscape after ASFA, and they should. As a result, extant knowledge tends to be historically superficial; research fails to frame or analyze developments in child welfare and adoption within broad American social and political contexts. Extensive, multidisciplinary research on a diverse set of topics pertinent to children with disabilities matters.

As a field, adoption research has drawn its working assumptions, definitions, and agendas from wider intellectual trends in psychology, social work, and medicine; trends that must continually be critically reassessed by those within and outside of these fields. Developmental psychopathology, for instance, has shifted away from employing fixed notions of risk and pathology to a model that views "the transaction between risk and protective factors in an individual's developmental trajectory."[126] Similarly, critical and community psychologists have reconceptualized marginalization to highlight its relational character, as arising from the interactions and daily routines of disabled and nondisabled people; disability, in this view, is an embodied relationship.[127] What new insights about adoption and disability can be borne out of these intellectual shifts?

Despite these disciplinary shifts, the research about adoption and disability after ASFA is generally bifurcated: researchers report either beneficial outcomes among families who adopt a disabled child, or higher rates of adoption disruption and dissolution for children with a variety of disabilities. These conflicting findings seem to reflect the different child populations researchers have studied, the kind of research questions they ask, and social, economic and political changes over time that support or frustrate adoption permanency. The findings about adoption disruption or dissolution for adoptive families with disabled children suggest that rates may not necessarily be directly due to medical or behavioral challenges but rather to a complicated mix of structural and financial forces and the attendant time demands that undermine the placement. Lower parental commitment to placement sustainability and unrealistic expectations (based on insufficient information about a child's history, not understanding the parenting implications of that history, failing to adapt to their child's changing behaviors or needs, or lacking adequate skills to manage those needs) also seem to play a part in adoption disruption, particularly for families who adopt children with behavioral or mental disabilities.[128] Conversely, researchers who have detailed positive outcomes link these experiences to the ability of families to gain access to pre- and postplacement planning and services. Adoptions with parents who understand what to expect of their adoptive child—and who can access appropriate services—thrive.

The discourse of risk, however, permeates this research.[129] Social work researchers, for instance, describe "preadoptive risks" as either environmental (e.g., outside factors such as age at time of adoption) or biobehavioral (e.g., disability status or drug exposure). They continue to conceptualize risk in a way that combines ecological and embodied notions of risk that we found in the late twentieth century.[130] Reminiscent of the postwar period, public perceptions about the alleged greater risks of adoption, as compared to bio-genetic kinship, continue to relate to fears of disability risk, particularly an adopted child's "unknown or problematic background."[131] Researchers even study adoption itself as a risk factor in creating child development issues.[132]

Even though the vast majority of adoptions include parents who are satisfied with their child(ren) and who report a well-functioning family dynamic, much of adoption research tends to focus on the negative and pathological aspects of the adoption experience, and thus reinforces the societal stigma of adoption.[133] This research has largely focused on the individual behavioral outcomes of children, rather than their interaction with larger medical and social systems like mental health, schools, and communities. Further, it tends to base its results on clinical populations or use the comparison group of nonadopted children in intact families to study issues of psychological adjustment. A good proportion of this research explicitly focuses upon risks.[134] A "litany of distresses faced by many children who have been adopted" pervades scholarly and public inquiries into this form of family.[135] For their part, mental health experts have assumed that adoptees come from "less optimal hereditary backgrounds," which leads to research that pathologizes adoptees, disregards social and cultural context, and tends toward reductionist, rather than complex, interactionist explanations.[136] On the other hand, studies that compare adoptees to children in foster care or in institutional care show that adoptees do much better than their counterparts.

Much of the research on adoptees, however, falls into the "adjust-ment" category and starts with the premise of loss. This work mainly sits squarely within a deficit model. Scholars apply this model particularly to studies about disabled adopted children and their families; in this way, they do not differ much from the medical and rehabilitation approaches scholars have traditionally used to conduct disability research.[137] Studies and policy papers still emphasize individual risk factors to adoption dis-solution relating to preadoption history, rather than take an ecological approach that probes a wide range of reasons.[138]

To be sure, data about the prevalence of problems and barriers in adop-tion is needed to inform ways to improve systems, supports, and experi-ences. But since, as Katarina Wegar notes, "identities, attitudes, and be-havior patterns of stigmatized individuals cannot be understood apart from the social context that shapes them," much more work needs to be done by historians, social scientists, and clinical researchers alike (preferably as a collaborative team) to understand the mutually constitutive factors of bodies, social oppression, and specific contexts, including how these fac-tors are continually contested and revised in adoption.[139] With these ques-tions in mind, we need to learn and gather data about advantageous ex-periences; facilitators of placement; adoptive parents' actions to empower their disabled children, themselves, and their families; and adolescent and adult adoptee self-empowerment. The data on self-empowerment can show how, as historians of childhood have argued, adoptees are social ac-tors and change agents in their own right.[140]

Conceptual knowledge and information about practical strategies used in adoptive families with disabled children, for example, can provide action-able ideas for policymakers and service providers. These experts can apply their knowledge to formulate ways both to adapt or reform child welfare practices and to formulate family-focused interventions and childcare poli-cies that support, rather than undermine, American families of all types. As in trends in other fields, social work, psychology, policy, and disability re-searchers could engage adoptive families with disabled children and disabled adoptees themselves to help identify research priorities and research ques-tions; adoptive families can play central roles in designing and implementing research about and for them. Certainly, research and policy agendas would benefit greatly from the experiential expertise of adoptive families and of adoptees with disabilities, as the aforementioned memoirs demonstrate.[141]

To parse these questions, a more complex multi- and interdisciplinary approach to research on adoptive families with disabled children, foster children with disabilities, and disabled adoptees is necessary.[142] This approach could, for example, start with the notion of disability as dis/ability; that is, as theorist Anna Waldschmidt suggests, an "always 'embodied' type of difference relating to the realms of health, functioning, achievement and beauty (and their negative poles)."[143] By taking this approach, adoption research about disabled children and their adoptive families could provide not only new knowledge about dynamics within those particular families, but also "essential knowledge about the legacies, trajectories, turning points, and transformations of contemporary society and culture," including further insights about normality, childhood, parenthood, and family.[144] Research that explores the strategies adoptive families with disabled children create and utilize to optimize their family members' lives could reveal unique perspectives about the meaning and practice of care that are relevant for *all* families, biological and adoptive, with or without able-bodied or disabled family members.[145]

Disability studies, family studies, and childhood studies scholars could utilize these insights to further theorize notions of family, caregiving, fragility, vulnerability, and intimacies; they could chart new directions in these respective fields that interrelate with and buttress one another. Precisely because this type of research starts with the social location of family, such research can unveil a deeper understanding of disability and the constellation of disability experiences as inherently relational and intersectional, and of the family as both an inclusionary and exclusionary, material and social, institution.[146] This book is one such work on adoption and disability toward that end, but the fields of adoption and disability history need many more inquiries to gain a fuller picture. It is only through a set of multiple historical studies, broad and deep, that we can map additional avenues for increasing disabled children's access to family. In sum, all types of research that can capture broad and micro-trends about foster and adoptive children with disabilities and their families, could move analyses away from predominantly pathologizing these children and their families or treating them as an aberration, to situating them with the broad range of family life that exists, and as such, capturing the rich complexity of their contexts and their lives.

Inclusion Matters

Today, all children are considered adoptable, no matter their disability status. But many barriers remain to their sustained adoption. The current status of adoptability's definition ostensibly removes ideological and definitional barriers but, as this history has shown, stronger community supports, more extensive social services for adopted children with disabilities, and financial assistance for adoptive families with these children must also ensue. Indeed, this history has shown the ways in which ideologies and attitudes inform child hierarchies in adoption practices but also how demographic demands change those practices. These dynamics will likely remain at play and need to be contextually understood if they are to effect improvements to family access. The social meaning of disability must be markedly transformed to elicit new practices that will continue to preserve biological families and facilitate more special needs adoptions so that children in need can enter a permanent family. Poverty prevention, adequate social welfare, and general family supports should enable even more biological families who *want to and feel they can* take care of their disabled children to do so, so that voluntary and involuntary relinquishment is minimized.

This book asks readers to think deeply about the multiple forces that shaped, and continue to shape, practices to place disabled children in adoptive families and that have impacted parental willingness to accept those children into their family. Both in the past and in the present, these complex dynamics continue to play key roles in determining which children have the opportunity to be nurtured in a permanent family. One of this book's broad lingering questions, however, is: can a sweeping conceptual transformation about disability and people with disabilities take place in a society where there has been (and still is) a tenacious idea about the (un)desirability of certain disabled children in the most intimate of settings, like family?[147] Or alternatively: how are social and familial citizenship connected?[148] The historical trajectory I trace suggests that without the full inclusion of disability and disabled children in the sphere of family, the social, political, economic, and cultural inclusion of people with disabilities in American society will very likely remain limited.

Acknowledgments

This book has been a long time in the making, with many people who have deeply informed its content and offered their support toward its completion. I owe special thanks to Paul Longmore (now deceased), Sander Gilman, Sue Levine, and E. Wayne Carp, who mentored me during this project's various stages. I remember emailing Paul from the archives about what I was finding and him encouraging me to dig deeper and keep going, even when historical inquiries into disability and family were off most historians' radars. Paul saw my potential as a disability historian before I did. I wish he could have seen this book once published, but I have no doubt that if he were still here, he would offer some quip, and lots of critique, that reflected how much he truly cared. I miss him every day. Sander has provided me with unwavering support and guidance throughout my professional career. He expressed his excitement for this project since its infancy and believed in its value when others questioned it, including myself. He saw, early on, the policy potential of this book and provided me and this project with steadfast endorsement and incisive suggestions. Sue generously offered her office during a fellowship year and read several early chapter drafts, providing keen feedback about constantly keeping in mind "who was doing what" and the wider context of child welfare and social work. E. Wayne Carp (who always reminds me to use the "E") has read drafts with a keen eye and checked every footnote. I do not know a more meticulous scholar. Over drinks, Korean food, and email, he has offered his expertise in adoption history and in American history to me. This work is so much better for it.

I owe a great debt to the archivists and librarians who enabled this research, particularly David Klassen and Linnea Anderson of the Social Welfare History Archives. Linnea even helped me from afar. It has been a pleasure working with such professionals who know their collections so well.

Karen Darling of University of Chicago Press shepherded this book from its inception to its completion. She has been more than patient with me and with this project and has offered such priceless feedback along the way. I feel so lucky to have found such an incredible editor. I am grateful to the reviewers for their exceptional comments on my manuscript; their reports truly improved this work. I am grateful to Tristan Bates and Michael Koplow for helping me with the final publication process and to Cheryl Green for providing the visual descriptions of the book's images. Audra Wolfe of the Outside Reader helped me reconceptualize this book and focus it. She significantly helped my writing, such that I will never write in passive voice again. Her patience with me over a decade of collaboration has been impressive. She is tough, ethical, and committed. Her brilliant editorial skills have drastically improved this manuscript. It would literally not be the same book without her incisive input. Similarly, Amberle Sherman's suggestions in the later stage of my writing allowed me to progress with confidence and get across the finish line.

I am very thankful for the financial support I received from the National Endowment for the Humanities Summer Stipend program, the University of Illinois-Chicago (UIC) Institute for the Humanities Faculty Fellowship, and UIC's Faculty Support grant program. My colleagues during my Institute for the Humanities fellowship year gave me the intellectual sustenance I needed and the humanities environment I craved. Jeff Sklansky and Javier Villa-Flores were/are exceptionally important colleagues from that time. Linda Vavra has always welcomed my engagement with the Institute and for that, I am grateful. I have benefited as well from the Mid-Career Writing Program at UIC, and especially from Sydney Halpern's professional and intellectual guidance and chapter review through that program and beyond. Without the sabbaticals granted to me by my university, I could have never finished this book.

My colleagues in the Departments of Medical Education, Disability and Human Development, and History at the University of Illinois at Chicago have offered their encouragement and feedback on chapters and conference papers throughout the past decade. Aly Patsavas offered incredibly valuable ideas during our monthly writing lunches. Sarah Parker has modeled leadership, scholarship, keen PowerPoint skills, and loyal friendship. Our weekly lunches provided the gossip and support I needed to keep things in perspective. Carrie Sandahl has provided important scholarly and personal insights about this book and has shown me through her example, advocacy, and sensitive care that this history matters. Carol Gill read chapter drafts, offered her pertinent expertise in psychology and disability, and has provided professional and personal mentorship throughout my career. Her friendship with Paul led me to my current position. Lenny Davis has provided guidance and support throughout this project and my career; he has seen and supported my development as a scholar from my graduate school days in New York City to my time at UIC. Tamar Heller and Alan Schwartz have been patient, receptive, understanding, and affirming chairs. Toby Tate provided me with invaluable career advice during this past decade. Michele Mariscalco has been an amazing, fun, and no-nonsense mentor who respects and honors my diverse interests and is also a supportive friend. Jay Mueller, Michael Blackie, Laura Hirshfield, Kristi Kirshner, Laura Schaaf, Janet Settle, Joanna Michel, Abbas Hyderi, Ray Curry, Christine Park, and so many others have been incredibly smart, decent, and compassionate colleagues to me. Suzanne Poirier has provided her steadfast mentorship to me over the years and has validated my work and my struggles with positivity and grace. Claire Decoteau has been a wonderful coorganizer of our Health and Society series and is such an impressive thinker and friend. My undergraduate assistants over the years, Kim Hu, Bhargavi Dhanireddy, and Lily Zheng, helped with literature searches, book and article procurement, citation management, and other important aspects of research and writing. I am incredibly grateful to them for their hard work, quick turnaround, and responsible follow-through. Similarly, my colleagues in the History Department—Jennie Brier, Robert Johnston, Kevin Schultz, Chris Boyer, and others—have reminded me that my work makes a significant contribution to the wider field of history.

My colleagues and students in Disability History and Disability Studies invigorate me every day. They offer the world new ways of thinking about disability and show that our history is full of texture. I draw from so many of their insights in this book. Particular thanks go to Julie Livingston, Sue Schweik, Licia Carlson, Rosemarie Garland-Thomson, Catherine Kudlick, Lenny Davis, Susan Burch, Kim Nielsen, Audra Jennings, Ann Fox, Katarina Kolarova, Michael Rembis, Rebecca Garden, and Lex Owen. I have benefited so much from their intellectual generosity and their innovative thinking about the experience(s) of disability. They, and so many others in this field, have demonstrated how generative a community of scholars can be.

Colleagues in Adoption Studies like Catherine Rymph, Emily Hip-chen, Margaret Homans, Karen Balcom, and Marina Fedosik have made room for disability as a valid area to explore within the field. I am indebted to the work of Molly Ladd Taylor and Ellen Herman, which has been essential to the way I conceptualize and narrate the intersection of disability, adoption, and child welfare.

I learned a great deal from the scholars in my fellow history of medicine writing group, Sarah Rodriguez and Sydney Halpern. Reading and discussing their work, and engaging with mine, pushed my thinking in productive ways. It also provided me with the companionship and expertise of fellow historians from the Chicagoland area when I desperately needed it. Historians of medicine, like Nadav Davidovitch, Ellen Amster, Beth Linker, Randall Packard, Rhona Seidelman, Jeremy Greene, Keith Wailoo, Matthew Gambino, Lara Freidenfelds, Leslie Reagan, Janet Golden, Mical Raz, and many others, are models for me in terms of intellectual and personal integrity.

More recently, fellow advisory panelists from the Patient Centered Outcomes Research Institute and colleagues from PaCE (Patient and Clinician Engagement) have welcomed me into their worlds and honored my voice and expertise in our joint mission of making patients' lives care better. Similarly, my colleagues and peers in CFReSHC (Cystic Fibrosis Reproductive and Sexual Health Collaborative) have given me a new space within which to use my disability expertise and to make an intellectual and personal difference. My Health Humanities Portrait colleagues have given life and substance to my proposed educational intervention that centers patients' sociopolitical context to understand the illness and disability experience. I am invigorated by their commitment to health humanities education and am very honored to have worked with them.

Friends outside of work near and far have given me perspective and rest from what has been an all-consuming process. They housed me while I was doing research for this book and made the inherently isolating process of research less so. For that I am thankful. Eugene Sheppard deserves a special mention here. He is my intellectual rock of twenty years, a treasure, and a mensch. I truly adore and cherish him. Similarly, Zvi Ben-Dor has been not only a historian that I respect greatly, but also a true long-lasting friend.

My health care providers have looked after various aspects of my health and made sure I was taking care of myself despite how grueling and intense this job can be. Patricia Walker is particularly worthy of mention here. Since graduate school, she has believed in me when others doubted. She is truly a one-of-a-kind physician, friend, and my hero. My mom, dad, sisters, brothers-in-law, sisters-in law, and father-in-law have provided their unwavering support and love. I don't know where I would be without them; they have never questioned my commitment to my work nor underestimated my ability, the latter being a historically ableist disability trope. Nati made sure my house, my son, and my health remained intact and for that I owe her my deepest gratitude. I hope this book will make them all proud.

Finally, I am beyond blessed for my husband, Elias, our son, Joseph, and our dog, Oreo. Joseph has grown up with this book. He came into our lives during the research phase of this project and he reminds me every day what is ultimately important in life. His love of life, of people, and of learning makes me so proud and happy. He is growing up to be a wonderful, sensitive, and kind person. Elias has offered laughter, sustenance, friendship, and steady guidance. He has taken on the bulk of the childcare and cooking when I needed to spend time quietly reading, writing, and thinking about this project. I am looking forward to returning to a more balanced life with him, Joseph, and Oreo now that this book is making its way out into the world.

Suitability of the Child for Adoption

Questionnaire to Mental Hygiene Professionals

From Hyman Lippman, "Suitability of the Child for Adoption," *American Journal of Orthopsychiatry* (April 1937). 270–273

$n = 30$

Question 1. Do you consider a child unsuitable for adoption if there is a history of psychosis in his immediate family?

Did not recommend

- 11: Did "not recommend a child for adoption if there is a history in the family of psychosis which cannot be explained on an organic basis. They consider schizophrenia and manic depressive psychosis hereditary."
  - 1 "refers to the scarcity of information generally obtained regarding the father's background. With one known case of psychosis in the family of the mother he would want to be certain there was no psychosis in the father's family before recommending the child as suitable."

Did not state whether they would recommend the child or not

- 1: "Feels there is less risk involved if there are two cases of psychosis in the family of one of the parents than if there is one instance in each family of both parents."
- 5: "Attach special significance to the child's having lived in the same home as the psychotic individual. As a result of this exposure they consider such a child unsuitable for adoption. Duration of exposure not referred to."

Recommended

- 7: "Recommend such a child if there is only one instance of psychosis in the family."
- 9: "State that there is no satisfactory evidence to indicate that psychosis is hereditary. They therefore recommend the child for adoption despite the existence of psychosis in the family if the child is in other respects suitable."
- 2: "Consider a child suitable for adoption despite a family history of psychosis, if the prospective adoptive parents are willing to accept the risk."

Question 2: Do you feel that it is necessary to observe the child some time before you are satisfied that he is a safe risk?

- "Because of the vagueness of this question the information was not obtained. . . . Despite the vagueness of the question, eight (8) answer that here is little to be gained from such observation, since one would have to wait long after the age when the child is no longer placeable before being reasonably certain that he might not develop a psychosis."

Question 3. Do you think he is unsuitable for adoption if there is feeblemindedness in the immediate family, assuming that the child has been tested more than once and the psychologist is satisfied that the child has at least average intelligence?

Recommended

- 14: "Recommend for adoption a child who comes under the above classification."
  - 3 "recommend waiting until the child is three to five years of age, in such cases where there is more than one instance of feeblemindedness in the family."
  - 2 "state that if the child had a superior rating they would recommend him for adoption even though there was more than one instance of feeblemindedness in the family."
  - 12 "recommend the child for adoption if there is only one instance of feeblemindedness in the immediate family. If more than one, the child is considered unsuitable."

Did not state whether they would recommend the child or not

- 8: "Emphasize the unreliability of psychological tests during the early years."

- 1: "Waits at least three years before advising adoption even if there is only one instance of feeblemindedness in the immediate family."
- 1: "Leaves the decision to the prospective adoptive parents"
- 1: "Feels there is less risk involved when there are two instances of feeblemindedness in the family of one of the parents than when there is one instance of feeblemindedness in the family of both parents."
- 1: "Stresses the fact that the danger does not lie entirely in the eventuality of the child's becoming feebleminded. The tragedy may be equally great if a child who originally tested superior later showed a slowing down, perhaps ending as a child of low average intelligence in a superior family."
- 1: States that "the mental level of the parents is important in helping us to evaluate our study of the child — our experience would lead me to feel (though this is purely a personal hunch) that if the parents are distinctly below normal, I would look for a probable slowing up of the mental growth in the child. Contrariwise, if the parents are above average and the infant shows only average development, I would feel few qualms about placing the child in an above average home."

Question 4A. Do you consider serious delinquency or bizarre behavior in the immediate family such as transvestism or homosexuality sufficient cause to make the child unsuitable for adoption? Do you consider in the same category the child who is a product of an incestuous relationship?

Recommended

- 14: "Feel that such a child is suitable for adoption."
  - 5 "consider as unsuitable a child who has lived in an atmosphere of delinquency. Under such conditions they prefer a longer period of observation before recommending such a child for adoption."

Did not recommend

- 12: "Refuse to recommend a child coming from an environment of delinquency if this delinquency appeared to express a fundamental character in the family that was quite general."
  - 1: "Makes an exception of the child living under such conditions who presents an unusually good adjustment in his general behavior. Under such conditions he would discount the family background."

Did not state whether they would recommend the child or not

- 3: "Refer to the factor of neurosis complicating the delinquency, emphasizing the fact that they would consider in a different light the delinquency that was deeply ingrained in the pattern of behavior."

In commenting on the product of an incestuous relationship:

Did not recommend

- 3: "Answer that they unqualifiedly reject the child."
- 7: "Feel that the child should not be considered unsuitable because of the incestuous origin per se."

Did not state whether they would recommend the child or not

- 6: "Say that they are on a sharper lookout for serious character pathology if the child is a result of an incestuous union."
- 1: "Refers to the fact that the results of a pregnancy of a sister by a brother would be less significant than that between a son and the mother or a daughter and father."

Question 4B. Are there any other conditions in the immediate family which in your opinion make a child unsuitable for adoption?

"Other conditions mentioned are those of hereditary origin, such as hereditary degenerative diseases of the nervous system, congenital blindness and deafness, Huntington's chorea, and so forth. Epilepsy was frequently referred to. There was an occasional reference to hemophilia and pathology of the endocrine glands."

Question 5. How much of the family history and background of the child do you think should be told to the prospective adoptive parents?

- 1: Nothing

- 13: As little as possible, particularly material of a negative nature.
- 1: That which the child will need to know later on.
- 3: As much as is felt can be accepted.
- 9: Everything the adoptive parents wish to know. All their questions should be answered, withholding only names and addresses of parents.

Chronology of Relevant Federal Bills and Their Provisions (1970–1980)

1973: Vocational Rehabilitation Act (P.L. 93-112)

- Section 504: promotes civil rights for persons with disabilities.
- Prohibits discrimination against persons with disabilities by federally funded programs, organizations, schools and employers.

1975: Developmentally Disabled Assistance and Bill of Rights Act (P.L. 94-103) (also known as DD Act)

- To receive a grant, each state has to establish advocacy and protection programs charged with ensuring the well-being and safety of people with developmental disabilities.
- Bill of Rights of DD Act: "Individuals with developmental disabilities have a right to treatment, services and habilitation for such disabilities . . . . designed to maximize the potential of the individual and should be provided in the setting that is least restrictive of the individual's personal liberty."[1]

1975: Education for All Act (P.L. 94-142)

- Children with disabilities have right to public school education in an integrated environment.
- Eliminated education as a reason to institutionalize children.[2]

1978: Developmental Disabilities Assistance and Bill of Rights Act (P.L. 95-602)

- Otherwise known as the Rehabilitation, Comprehensive Services, and Developmental Disabilities Amendments of 1978. Amended the Rehabilitation Act of 1973 to address the needs of persons with developmental disabilities.
- Defined developmental disability as: "a severe chronic disability of a person attributable to a mental or physical impairment, is manifested before age 22 years, is likely to continue, results in functional limitations in 3 or more major life activities, and reflects need for lifelong services."[3]
- Worked to provide comprehensive services to people with developmental disabilities whose needs were not met by the Education for All Act, the Vocational Rehabilitation Act of 1973, or other health and welfare services.
- Provided aid to states to develop coordinated care and services for people with developmental disabilities. Provided planning, monitoring, and evaluation of services.
- Assisted states and other agencies to establish model programs, develop innovative housing services and arrangements, and train professionals to provide services to people with developmental disabilities.
- Offered demonstration grants to universities to provide new ways of delivering services to people with developmental disabilities. Sponsored interdisciplinary training programs that offer specialized services for people with developmental disabilities.
- · Gave grants to states to ensure the legal and human rights for this population.

1978: Child Abuse Prevention and Treatment and Adoption Reform Act of 1978 (Adoption Opportunities Act, P.L. 95-266; amendment of CAPTA as Title II). Reauthorized in 1991

- Special needs adoption advocates' advocacy helped get this act passed.
- Intended to "promote the health development of children who would benefit from adoption by facilitating their placement in adoptive homes."
- Intended to improve upon Child Abuse Prevention and Treatment Act (CAPTA, 1974).
- Established model adoption legislation available to states to remove obstacles to adoption.
- Developed an information exchange system that matched families to foster children legally free for adoption.
- Funded regional adoption resource centers to enable permanent placement of special needs children.
- Expanded interstate adoption exchanges.
- Funded public service announcements about special needs adoption.

- Implemented social worker training programs to help agencies prepare prospective adoptive parents to adopt foster care children.
- Established programs to recruit adoptive families from minority groups.
- Enacted as a response to outcomes research in the 1970s that showed that families who adopted abused children struggled to raise them, causing some families and professionals to think that it might be better for these children to remain with their birth families.[4]
- Offered two demonstration programs: (1) postadoption legal services for families with special needs children; (2) placement of minority children.
- First federal role in adoptive placement of special needs children.

1980: Adoption Assistance and Child Welfare Act (P.L. 96-272)

- Most expansive federal policy on special needs adoptions.
- Amended Title IV of Social Security Act.
- Made preserving birth family and permanent placement the goals of child welfare.
- Adoption should be considered only when family preservation and reunification fails.
- Intentions: to reduce the number of children going into foster care, prevent foster drift, and control costs of foster care.
- First instance of federal role in monitoring the financing of foster care services and in the delivery of state child welfare foster care and adoption services.
- To receive federal funding, a state had to develop a plan for foster care and adoption assistance, track every child, and create individualized case plans in "least restrictive setting" for each child to lessen foster drift.
- To receive additional funds, a state had to create a system that prevented family breakup, tried to reunify birth families, and, as a last resort, place children in adoptive homes. It also had to review cases every six months and consider permanent placement for children in long-term foster care.
- Courts had to determine future status within eighteen months after initial foster care placement.
- First federal financial incentives for states to develop an alternative to foster care through federal subsidies.
- Established Title IV-E: Federal Payments for Foster Care and Adoption Assistance.
- Guaranteed subsidies to families who adopted special needs children eligible for SSI (Social Security Income) or ADC (Aid to Dependent Children). States had to create an adoption assistance program to continue in ADC.

- Allowed children on ADC to continue to receive these payments and receive Medicaid, without consideration of income level of adoptive family.
- States should define special needs broadly to receive subsidies; children had to have a "special condition" that required assistance to be placed.
- States should first try to find an adoptive home that did not need subsidy (except for fost-adoption).
- Provided federal money to states for administrative costs of pursuing special needs adoptions.
- Paid a percentage of adoption subsidy cost.
- Reduced federal support for foster care costs to deincentivize agencies from using foster homes, leading to foster drift.

Handicapping Conditions of Children Listed on Adoption Exchanges in 1985

Type of handicap	percentage of handicapped children with condition
Emotional disturbance/behavioral problem	51
Mental retardation	38
Specific learning disability	22
Correctable problem	22
Hearing, speech, or sight impairment	12
Allergies/asthma	16
Diabetes	11
Cerebral palsy	8
Multiple handicaps	6
2% of the handicapped children had the following conditions:	Mild physical problems, colon problems (distended bowel), orthopedic problems, spina bifida, endocrine problems, epilepsy/seizure disorder, cleft palate/harelip, quadriplegia/paraplegia, fetal alcohol syndrome, ear problem (chronic infections)
1% of the handicapped children had the following conditions:	Heart problems, sickle cell anemia, cancer, neurological condition, nonambulatory, cystic fibrosis, spasticity, urticaria pigmentosa, deformity (no upper ear), stomach problems, Hydrocephalus, adenoidal hypertrophy, albinism
Among the conditions that less than 1% of the children had were:	paralysis, lung and kidney problems, muscular dystrophy, blood disorders, autism

Data from Penelope Maza, "Trends in National Data on the Adoption of Children with Handicaps," in *Formed Families: Adoption of Children with Handicaps*, ed. Laraine Masters Glidden (New York: Routledge, 1990), 134–135.

List of Archives

American Academy of Pediatrics. Itasca, Illinois
National Archives. College Park, Maryland
National Library of Medicine. Bethesda, Maryland
SWHA (Social Welfare History Archives). Minneapolis, Minnesota.

Notes

A Note on Language

1. Erving Goffman, *Stigma: Notes on the Management of Spoiled Identity* (Englewood Cliffs: Prentice Hall, 1963).

Introduction

1. David Batty, "US Mother Sparks Outrage after Sending Adopted Child Back to Russia Alone," *Guardian*, April 10, 2010, https://www.theguardian.com /world/2010/apr/10/torry-hansen-artyom-savelyev-adoption.

2. Masha Lipman, "What's Behind the Russian Adoption Ban?," *New Yorker*, December 21, 2012.

3. US-Russian adoptions began in 1991, with Americans only being allowed to adopt disabled children. Lily Rothman, "How Russian Adoptions Became a Controversial Topic," *Time*, August 1, 2017, https://time.com/4868968/donald-trump -russia-adoption-history/.

4. Damien Cave, "At a Family's Home in Tennessee, Reminders of a Boy Returned to Russia," *New York Times*, April 11, 2010, A16.

5. Evan Donaldson Adoption Institute, "Keeping the Promise: The Critical Need for Post-adoption Services to Enable Children and Families to Succeed, Policy and Practice Perspective," October 2010, 4.

6. An extensive examination of transnational adoption and disability is beyond the scope of this study, although it is a much needed area of historical research.

7. P. O. Holliday, "A Judge Considers Adoption," *CWLA Bulletin* 17, no. 3 (March 1938): 1.

8. Alison Kafer, *Feminist, Queer, Crip* (Bloomington: Indiana University Press, 2013), 2 (Kindle); Rosemarie Garland-Thomson, "Eugenic World Building and Disability: The Strange World of Kazuo Ishiguro's *Never Let Me Go*," *Journal of*

Medical Humanities 38 (2017): 142; Rosemarie Garland-Thomson, "The Case for Conserving Disability," *Journal of Bioethical Inquiry* 9, no. 3 (2012): 351.

9. I borrow this phrase and definition from Julie Livingston, *Debility and the Moral Imagination in Botswana* (Bloomington: Indiana University Press, 2005), 7. See also Douglas C. Baynton, "Disability in History," *Disabilities Studies Quarterly* 28, no. 3 (Summer 2008), DOI: http://dx.doi.org/10.18061/dsq.v28i3.108; Liat Ben-Moshe and Sandy Magana, "An Introduction to Race, Gender, and Disability: Intersectionality, Disability Studies, and Families of Color," *Women, Gender and Families of Color* 2, no. 2 (Fall 2014): 106; Rosemarie Garland-Thomson, "Misfits: A Feminist Materialist Disability Concept," *Hypatia* 26, no. 3 (Summer 2011): 591–592; Ellen Herman, *Kinship by Design: A History of Adoption in the Modern United States* (Chicago: University of Chicago Press, 2008), 7.

10. Barbara Yngvesson, *Belonging in an Adopted World: Race, Identity, and Transnational Adoption* (Chicago: University of Chicago Press, 2010); Judith Schachter, review of *Blue-Ribbon Babies and Labors of Love: Race, Class and Gender in US Adoption Practice*, by Christine Ward Gailey, and *Belonging in an Adopted World: Race, Identity and Transnational Adoption*, by Barbara Yngvesson, *Journal of Sociology* 117, no. 1 (July 2011): 341; Erving Goffman, *Stigma: Notes on the Management of Spoiled Identity* (Englewood Cliffs, NJ: Prentice-Hall, 1963); Garland-Thomson, "Misfits," 592. For insistence on normality in American culture, see Robert McRuer, *Crip Theory: Cultural Signs of Queerness and Disability* (New York: New York University Press, 2006). For stratified reproduction, see Faye Ginsburg and Rayna Rapp, "Introduction: Conceiving the New World Order," in *Conceiving the New World Order: The Global Politics of Reproduction*, ed. Faye Ginsburg and Rayna Rapp (Berkeley: University of California Press, 1995), 3.

11. By the 1980s, social workers often used *handicapped* and *disabled* interchangeably. Michael Omi and Howard Winant, *Racial Formation in the United States: From the 1960s to the 1990s*, 2nd ed. (New York: Routledge, 1994), 4, 56.

12. Garland-Thomson, "Case for Conserving Disability," 340; Garland-Thomson, "Misfits," 594, 602; Rayna Rapp and Faye Ginsburg, "Enlarging Reproduction, Screening Disability," in *Reproductive Disruptions: Gender, Technology, and Biopolitics in the New Millennium*, ed. Marcia C. Inhorn (New York: Berghahn, 2008), 100.

13. Carol Singley, "Childhood Studies and Literary Adoption," in *Children's Table: Childhood Studies and the Humanities*, ed. Anna M. Duane (Athens: University of Georgia Press, 2013), 185.

14. Christine Ward Gailey, *Blue Ribbon Babies and Labors of Love: Race, Class and Gender in US Adoption Practice* (Austin: University of Texas Press, 2010).

15. Gailey; Kim Park Nelson, "The Disability of Adoption: Adoptees in Disabling Societies," *Adoption Quarterly* 21, no. 4 (2018): 288–306.

16. Donald N. Levine, Ellwood B. Carter, and Eleanor Miller Gorman, "Simmel's Influence on American Sociology," *American Journal of Sociology* 81,

no. 4 (January 1976): 813–845; Sue Schweik, *Ugly Laws: Disability in Public* (New York: New York University Press, 2009), 166–167; Garland-Thomson, "Case for Conserving Disability," 340.

17. Herman, *Kinship by Design,* 7; Barbara Melosh, *Strangers and Kin: The American Way of Adoption* (Cambridge, MA: Harvard University Press, 2002), 2.

18. Jessaca Leinaweaver, "Little Strangers: International Adoption and American Kinship: A Review Essay," *Comparative Studies in Society and History* 54, no. 1 (2012): 206, 208, 209. See also Heather Jacobson, *Culture Keeping: White Mothers, International Adoption, and the Negotiation of Family Difference* (Nashville: Vanderbilt University Press, 2008).

19. Herman, *Kinship by Design,* 7; E. Wayne Carp, Introduction, *Adoption in America: Historical Perspectives*, ed. E. Wayne Carp (Ann Arbor: University of Michigan Press, 2004), 2.

20. Ellen Herman, "Child Adoption in a Therapeutic Culture," *Society* 39, no. 2 (January 2002): 11–18; Herman, *Kinship by Design*, 190.

21. Melosh, 4.

22. See Douglas C. Baynton, *Defectives in the Land: Disability and Immigration in the Age of Eugenics* (Chicago: University of Chicago Press, 2016); Douglas C. Baynton, "Disability and the Justification of Inequality in American History," in *The New Disability History: American Perspectives*, ed. Paul Longmore and Lauri Umansky (New York: New York University Press, 2001), 33–57; Schweik, *Ugly Laws*.

23. Eli Clare, *Brilliant Imperfection: Grappling with Cure* (Durham: Duke University Press, 2017).

24. Garland-Thomson, "Eugenic World Building," 135.

25. Laura Briggs, *Somebody's Children: The Politics of Transracial and Transnational Adoption* (Durham: Duke University Press, 2012), Loc. 834 (Kindle); Melosh, 5.

26. Rapp and Ginsburg, "Enlarging Reproduction," 99, 106.

27. Deborah Lupton, *The Imperative of Health: Public Health and the Regulated Body* (London: SAGE, 1995), 77. On disability and existential anxiety, see Paul Longmore and Lauri Umansky, introduction, "Disability History: From the Margins to the Mainstream," in *The New Disability History: American Perspectives*, ed. Paul Longmore and Lauri Umansky (New York: New York University Press, 2001), 6; Gay Becker and Robert D. Nachtigall, " 'Born to Be a Mother': The Cultural Construction of Risk in Infertility Treatment in the US," *Social Science and Medicine* 39, no. 4 (1994): 507; M. Margaret Clark, "The Cultural Patterning of Risk-Seeking Behavior: Implications for Armed Conflict," in *Peace and War: Cross-Cultural Perspectives*, ed. Mary LeCron Foster and Robert A. Rubinstein (New Brunswick, NJ: Transaction, 1986), 79–81. Clark describes risk taking as a conscious evaluation of what can be gained by doing something against the harm that can be done by inaction. Tobin Siebers, *Disability Theory* (Ann Arbor:

University of Michigan Press, 2008), 6, 9. It is for this reason that disability scholar Adrienne Asch has argued for a shift from using the term *risk* when speaking of disability to terms like *likelihood* or *possibility* to wrest meaning making from health professionals to parents. Adrienne Asch, "Why I Haven't Changed My Mind about Prenatal Diagnosis," in *Prenatal Diagnosis and Disability Rights*, ed. Erik Parens and Adrienne Asch (Washington, DC: Georgetown University Press, 2000), 252.

28. Schweik, *Ugly Laws*, 61.

29. Melosh, 39.

30. Melosh, 38.

31. Lupton, *Imperative of Health*, 80. For risk as lived experience and state of being, see 85. See also Dorothy Nelkin, "Communicating Technological Risk: The Social Construction of Risk Perception," *Annual Review of Public Health* 10 (1989): 96.

32. Shelley Tremain, as quoted in Alexa Schriempf, "(Re)fusing the Amputated Body: An Interactionist Bridge for Feminism and Disability," *Hypatia* 16, no. 4 (Fall 2001): 70; Schweik, *Ugly Laws*, 61; Deborah Lupton, "Introduction: Risk and Sociocultural Theory, in *Risk and Sociocultural Theory: New Directions and Perspectives*, ed. Deborah Lupton (Cambridge: Cambridge University Press, 1999)," 6.

33. Longmore and Umansky, introduction, 6–7. For Douglas on the Other blurring boundaries and overtaking the self, see Deborah Lupton, *Risk: Key Ideas*, 2nd ed. (London: Routledge, 2013), 124; Garland-Thomson, "Case for Conserving Disability," 340; Mary Douglas, "Risk as Forensic Resource," *Daedalus* 119, no. 4 (Fall 1990): 1–16; Michael V. Hayes, "On the Epistemology of Risk: Language, Logic and Social Science," *Social Science and Medicine* 35, no. 4 (1992): 401–407; Kim E. Nielsen, *A Disability History of the United States* (Boston: Beacon, 2012), xii.

34. Siebers, *Disability Theory*, 6, 9; Asch, "Why I Haven't Changed My Mind," 252; Anna Waldschmidt, "Who Is Normal? Who Is Deviant? Normality and Risk in Genetic Diagnosis and Counseling," in *Foucault and the Government of Disability*, ed. Shelley Tremain (Ann Arbor: University of Michigan Press, 2005), 197; Dorothy Nelkin and Sander Gilman, "Placing Blame for Devastating Disease," *Social Research* 55, no. 3 (Autumn 1988): 361–378; Nikolas Rose, "Genetic Risk and the Birth of the Somatic Individual," *Economy and Society* 29, no. 4 (2000): 485–513; Mary Douglas, *Risk and Blame: Essays in Cultural Theory* (New York: Routledge, 1992); Alan Peterson and Deborah Lupton, *The New Public Health: Discourses, Knowledges, Strategies* (London: SAGE, 1996); Ulrich Beck, *Risk Society: Towards a New Modernity* (London: SAGE, 1992); Ulrich Beck, Anthony Giddens, and Scott Lash, *Reflexive Modernization: Politics, Tradition and Aesthetics in the Modern Social Order* (Stanford: Stanford University Press, 1994); Mary Douglas, *Risk Acceptability According to the Social Sciences* (New York: Russell Sage Foundation, 1985); Mary Douglas and Aaron Wildavsky, *Risk and Culture: An Essay on the Selection of Technological and Environmental Dangers* (Berkeley: University

of California Press, 1982); John Tulloch and Deborah Lupton, *Risk and Every-day Life* (Thousand Oaks, CA: SAGE, 2003); Lupton, *Risk*; Deborah Lupton, ed., *Risk and Sociocultural Theory* (Cambridge: Cambridge University Press, 1999); Jonathan Levy, *Freaks of Fortune: The Emerging World of Capital and Risk in America* (Cambridge, MA: Harvard University Press, 2012).

35. David M. Austin, "The Flexner Myth and the History of Social Work," *Social Service Review* 57 (1983): 373.

36. As philosopher François Ewald has argued, the language of risk and the solutions proposed to control it reflect ideology. François Ewald, "Insurance and Risk," in *The Foucault Effect: Studies in Governmentality*, ed. G. Burchell, C. Gordon, and P. Miller (Chicago: University of Chicago Press, 1991), 199, 207, 208.

37. Ellen Herman, "Rules for Realness: Child Adoption in a Therapeutic Culture," in *Therapeutic Culture: Triumph and Defeat*, ed. Jonathan B. Imber (New Brunswick, NJ: Transaction, 2004), 190.

38. Lupton, "Introduction: Risk and Sociocultural Theory," 2, 6; Omi and Winant, 4.

39. Douglas, "Risk as Forensic Resource," 3–4, 5, 7, 9–10; Lupton, *Imperative of Health*, 77, 90; Hayes, 401–407.

40. Sandra M. Sufian, "As Long as Parents Can Accept Them: Medical Disclosure, Risk, and Disability in Twentieth-Century American Adoption Practice," *Bulletin of the History of Medicine* 91, no. 1 (2017): 94–124.

41. Lupton, *Imperative of Health*, 90.

42. Lupton, *Imperative of Health*, 85.

43. Lupton, *Imperative of Health*, 79–80; Mildred Blaxter, *Health* (Cambridge: Polity, 2010), 152–156; Dorothy Nelkin, "Introduction: Analyzing Risk," in *The Language of Risk: Conflicting Perspectives on Occupational Health*, ed. Dorothy Nelkin (Beverly Hills, CA: SAGE, 1985), 20–21.

44. Risk was also related to the pathological framing of adoption itself— whether closed or open adoption (depending upon the time period)—and its effects upon the development of an adoptee. E. Wayne Carp, *Family Matters: Secrecy and Disclosure in the History of Adoption* (Cambridge, MA: Harvard University Press, 1998), 216–217; Katarina Wegar, *Adoption, Identity and Kinship: The Debate over Sealed Birth Records* (New Haven: Yale University Press, 1997).

45. Michelle Kahan, " 'Put Up' on Platforms: A History of Twentieth Century Adoption Policy in the United States," *Journal of Sociology and Social Welfare* 33, no. 3 (September 2006): 51–52.

46. Carp, Introduction, *Adoption in America*, 4–5.

47. Julie Berebitsky, "Rescue a Child and Save the Nation: The Social Construction of Adoption in the Delineator, 1907–1911," in Carp, *Adoption in America*, 124–139.

48. Herman, *Kinship by Design*, 7.

49. Carp, Introduction, *Adoption in America*, 9.

50. Carp, Introduction, *Adoption in America*, 7, 8.

51. Carp, Introduction, *Adoption in America*, 11.

52. Catherine McKenzie, "A Boom in Adoptions," *New York Times Magazine*, November 10, 1940, 1–7.

53. Rebecca Jo Plant, *Mom: The Transformation of Motherhood in Modern America* (Chicago: University of Chicago Press, 2010), Loc. 1451 (Kindle).

54. Kahan, 60; Carp, Introduction, *Adoption in America*, 12–13; Melosh, 107, 111.

55. Sufian, "As Long as Parents," 94–124.

56. Carp, Introduction, *Adoption in America*, 13.

57. Carp, Introduction, *Adoption in America*, 16.

58. Dorothy Barclay, "Adoption Problems," *New York Times*, April 2, 1950, 173.

59. Carp, Introduction, *Adoption in America*, 16.

60. Carp, Introduction, *Adoption in America*, 17–18.

61. Karen Andrea Balcom, "The Logic of Exchange: The Child Welfare League of America, the Adoption Resource Exchange Movement and the Indian Adoption Project, 1958–1967," *Adoption and Culture* 1, no. 1 (2008): 45–49.

62. Carp, Introduction, *Adoption in America*, 15–16.

63. Kahan, 52, 67; Herman, *Kinship by Design*, 252.

64. This reduced number of adoptions, however, is only an approximation because after 1975 the federal government no longer required states to track private adoptions, making adoption statistics incomplete. For its part, the Department of Health and Human Services continued to report on adoptions from foster care, but comprehensive numbers of private and public agency adoptions were lacking. The National Council for Adoption began keeping track of domestic adoption in 1985 but from the mid-1970s to that time, accurate statistics are scarce. Jo Jones and Paul Placek, *Adoption by the Numbers: A Comprehensive Report of US Adoption Statistics* (National Council for Adoption, 2017), i, https://indd.adobe.com /view/4ae7a823-4140-4f27-961a-cd9f16a5f362. See also Jane Jeong Trenka, Julia Chinyere Oparah, and Sun Yung Shin, eds., *Outsiders Within: Writing on Transracial Adoption* (Cambridge: South End, 2006); Briggs, *Somebody's Children*, especially ch. 3; and Laura Briggs, "Mother, Child, Race, Nation: The Visual Iconography of Rescue and the Politics of Transnational and Transracial Adoption," *Gender and History* 15, no. 2 (2003): 179–200.

65. David M. Brodzinsky and Ellen Pinderhughes, "Parenting and Child Developing in Adoptive Families," in *Handbook of Parenting: Children and Parenting*, ed. Marc H. Bornstein (Mahwah, NJ: Erlbaum, 2002), 279–312.

66. Scholars have analyzed the significant impact ASFA has had on children and families, particularly those of color. Dorothy Roberts, *Shattered Bonds: The Color of Child Welfare* (New York: Basic Civitas, 2002).

67. R. L. Jenkins, "Adoption Practices and the Physician," *Journal of the American Medical Association* 103, no. 6 (August 11, 1937): 403.

68. Carp, *Family Matters*, 88.

69. Garland-Thomson, "Misfits," 593, 600, 604; Melosh, 52.

70. Kahan, 52; Carp, Introduction, *Adoption in America*, 2; E. Wayne Carp, *Jean Paton and the Struggle to Reform American Adoption* (Ann Arbor: University of Michigan Press, 2014).

71. Carolyn Steedman, *Strange Dislocations: Childhood and the Idea of Human Interiority, 1780–1930* (London: Virago, 1995), 5; Mona Gleason, "In Search of History's Child," *Jeunesse: Young People, Texts, Cultures* 1, no. 2 (Winter 2009): 128, 130; Patrick Ryan, "How New Is the 'New' Social Study of Childhood? The Myth of a Paradigm Shift," *Journal of Interdisciplinary History* 38, no. 14 (Spring 2008): 567.

72. Kafer, *Feminist, Queer, Crip*, 33.

73. Betty Jean Lifton, *Twice Born: Memoirs of an Adopted Daughter* (New York: McGraw-Hill, 1975); Sarah Saffian, *Ithaka: A Daughter's Memoir of Being Found* (New York: Basic Books, 1998); Marianne Novy, *Seven Adopted American Women's Memoirs of Adoption, Reunion and Its Aftermath* (2010), http://www.mit.edu/~shaslang/ASAC2010/papers/NovySAAWM.pdf; Margaret Homans, *Imprint of Another Life: Adoption Narratives and Human Possibility* (Ann Arbor: University of Michigan Press, 2013); "Memoir/Biography," *Adoptee Reading*, http://adopteereading.com/memoir/; Lijie Zhang and Ming Canaday, "I Was Adopted, My Friend Was Not," *RainbowKids*, April 2019, https://www.rainbowkids.com/adoption-stories/i-was-adopted-my-friend-was-not-1966; Mia Mingus, "Finding Each Other: Building Legacies of Belonging," *Leaving Evidence*, April 10, 2018, https://leavingevidence.wordpress.com/2018/04/10/finding-each-other-building-legacies-of-belonging/; Mia Mingus, "November 6," *Leaving Evidence*, November 6, 2016, https://leavingevidence.wordpress.com/2016/11/06/november-6th/; Mia Mingus, "Moving Toward the Ugly: A Politic beyond Desirability," *Leaving Evidence*, August 22, 2011, https://leavingevidence.wordpress.com/2011/08/22/moving-toward-the-ugly-a-politic-beyond-desirability/.

74. The question of the social workers' racial and (able) bodied identities is a complex and hidden aspect of this history. While these are layers that may be more sufficiently addressed in localized histories where agency records may reveal the nature and impact of those identities, given my sources, I could not responsibly assess these questions without making potentially inaccurate assumptions about these historical actors. I could also neither precisely nor consistently determine the "white" and "nonwhite" classifications of children as they intersected with the ever-shifting understandings of disability across the course of the entire twentieth century. I have engaged these topics at points throughout this manuscript where I found it prudent and supported by my data.

Chapter One

1. Honoré Willsie, "The Adopted Mother," *Century*, September 1922, 657.

2. Florence Clothier, "Placing the Child for Adoption," *Mental Hygiene* 26 (1942): 257. While acknowledging the presence of risk in adoption, adoptive

parents like Lee and Evelyn Brooks put it in comparative perspective. In their popular book *Adventuring in Adoption* (1939), the Brookses recognized that adoption was no riskier than other life adventures and that some people magnified its hazards. Lee Brooks and Evelyn Brooks, *Adventuring in Adoption* (Chapel Hill: University of North Carolina Press, 1939), 5.

3. Clothier, "Placing the Child," 258–259; Ellen Herman, *Kinship by Design: A History of Adoption in the Modern United States* (Chicago: University of Chicago Press, 2008), 31, 39, 45.

4. R. L. Jenkins, "Adoption Practices and the Physician," *Journal of the American Medical Association* 103, no. 6 (August 11, 1934): 403.

5. E. Wayne Carp and Anna Leon-Guerrero, "When in Doubt Count: World War II as a Watershed in the History of Adoption," in *Adoption in America: Historical Perspectives*, ed. E. Wayne Carp (Ann Arbor: University of Michigan Press, 2002), 190.

6. Herman, *Kinship by Design*, 40, 46, 65–66.

7. Bureau of Children, Commonwealth of Pennsylvania Department of Welfare, "The Significance of Children's Records," Bulletin No. 32 (February 1928): 6–7, CWLA Collection, Box 56 Folder: Admin Recording 1928, SWHA; Brian Paul Gill, "The Jurisprudence of Good Parenting: The Selection of Adoptive Parents, 1894–1964," Ph.D. diss., University of California–Berkeley, 1997, 176.

8. Brian Paul Gill, "Adoption Agencies and the Search for the Ideal Family, 1918–1965," in *Adoption in America: Historical Perspectives*, ed. E. Wayne Carp (Ann Arbor: University of Michigan Press, 2004), 161–162. Whether or not such "failure" routinely happened is hard to prove because agencies discouraged their workers from placing children labeled disabled in the first place, so recorded examples of "failures" would have been hard to come by.

9. James W. Trent, *Inventing the Feeble Mind: A History of Mental Retardation in the United States* (Berkeley: University of California Press, 1994), 188.

10. Paul A. Lombardo, "From Better Babies to the Bunglers: Eugenics on Tobacco Road," 62, 66, in *A Century of Eugenics in America: From the Indiana Experiment to the Human Genome Era, ed. Paul A. Lombardo* (Bloomington: Indiana University Press, 2011), 62, 66; Molly Ladd-Taylor, "Eugenics and Social Welfare in New Deal Minnesota," in *A Century of Eugenics in America: From the Indiana Experiment to the Human Genome Era, ed. Paul A. Lombardo* (Bloomington: Indiana University Press, 2011), 131, 136; Mark Haller, *Eugenics: Hereditarian Attitudes in American Thought* (New Brunswick: Rutgers University Press, 1984), 3; Frank Dikotter, "Race Culture: Recent Perspectives on the History of Eugenics," *American Historical Review* 103, no. 2 (April 1998): 467–468; Trent, 136. For more contemporary instantiations, see Karen-Sue Taussig, Rayna Rapp, and Deborah Heath, "Flexible Eugenics: Technologies of the Self in the Age of Genetics," in *Genetic Nature/Culture: Anthropology and Science beyond the Two-Culture Divide*, ed. Alan Goodman, Deborah Heath, and Susan M. Lindee

(Berkeley: University of California Press, 2003), 58–76. Thank you to Aly Patsavas for this insight.

11. Clothier, "Placing the Child," 257.

12. Sandra M. Sufian, "As Long as Parents Can Accept Them: Medical Disclosure, Risk, and Disability in Twentieth-Century American Adoption Practice," *Bulletin of the History of Medicine* 91, no. 1 (Spring 2017): 98.

13. Gill, "Jurisprudence," 139–140; Ida R. Parker, "The Interdependence of the Doctor and Social Worker in Legal Adoption," *New England Journal of Medicine* 220, no. 17 (April 26, 1929): 883; "Outline of Tentative Standards for Adoption," CWLA Collection, Box 33, Folder 33, Surveys, MN 1919, 1929, SWHA. For normal and normality, see Ian Hacking, *The Taming of Chance* (Cambridge: Cambridge University Press, 1990), 160, 163, 166, 168–169; Georges Canguilhem, *The Normal and the Pathological* (New York: Zone, 1989), 51, 107, 118, 144, 240.

14. Thank you to E. Wayne Carp for this insight. Winthrop Jordan, *White over Black: American Attitudes toward the Negro, 1550–1812*, 2nd ed. (Chapel Hill: University of North Carolina Press, 2012), 24, 44–45; G. M. McKinley, "Genetics in Child Adoption Practice," *CWLA Bulletin* 19, no. 3 (March 1940): 3, CWLA Collection, Box 9, Folder: CWLA Bulletin 1939–1941, SWHA; Douglas A. Thom, "Aid of Science in Child Adoption," *CWLA Bulletin* 16, no. 2 (February 1937): 2, CWLA Collection, Box 89, Folder: Bulletins 1934–1938, 1930, SWHA; Herman, *Kinship by Design*, 13.

15. Lombardo, "From Better Babies to the Bunglers," 62.

16. Lombardo, "From Better Babies to the Bunglers," 66; Ladd-Taylor, "Eugenics and Social Welfare," 131, 136. For more contemporary instantiations, see Taussig, Rapp, and Heath.

17. Dikotter, 467–468.

18. Trent, 1994, 136.

19. Herman, *Kinship by Design*, 14, 16; Lennard Davis, *Enforcing Normalcy* (Verso: New York, 1995); Michael Rembis, "Challenging the Impairment/Disability Divide: Disability History and the Social Model of Disability," in *Routledge Handbook of Disability Studies*, ed. Nick Watson and Simo Vehmas (New York: Routledge, 2019), 378.

20. William Slingerland, *Child-Placing in Families: A Manual for Students and Social Workers* (New York: Russell Sage Foundation, 1919); John Tulloch and Deborah Lupton, *Risk and Everyday Life* (London: SAGE, 2003), Loc. 23, 97, 102, 108, 140 (Kindle); Scott Lash, "Risk Culture," in *The Risk Society and Beyond*, ed. Barbara Adam, Ulrich Beck, and Joost Van Loon (London: SAGE, 2000), 55–57; Mary Douglas and Aaron Wildavsky, *Risk and Culture: An Essay on the Selection of Technological and Environmental Dangers* (Berkeley: University of California Press, 1982), Loc. 67 (Kindle).

21. David M. Austin, "The Flexner Myth and the History of Social Work," *Social Service Review* (September 1983): 368.

22. Parker, 884; E. Wayne Carp, *Family Matters: Secrecy and Disclosure in the History of Adoption* (Cambridge, MA: Harvard University Press, 1998), 11, 19; "Timeline of Adoption History," *Adoption History Project*, https://pages.uoregon.edu/adoption/timeline.html.

23. Austin, "The Flexner Myth," 358, 365, 366.

24. Nancy Fraser and Linda Gordon, "A Genealogy of Dependency: Tracing a Keyword of the US Welfare State," *Signs* 19, no. 2 (Winter 1994): 319–321.

25. Slingerland, 185; Carp, *Family Matters*, 8; Catherine E. Rymph, *Raising Government Children: A History of Foster Care and the American Welfare State* (Chapel Hill: University of North Carolina Press, 2017), Loc. 1482 (Kindle); Emma Lundberg, "Child Welfare Services," *Social Work Yearbook* (1939): 2, CWLA Collection, Box 44, Folder 44:5, SWHA.

26. E. Wayne Carp, "Orphanages vs. Adoption: The Triumph of Biological Kinship, 1800–1933," in *With Us Always: A History of Private Charity and Public Welfare*, ed. Donald T. Critchlow and Charles H. Parker (Lanham, MD: Rowman & Littlefield, 1998), 124–144, table 1; Carp, *Family Matters*, 16; Parker, 884.

27. Slingerland, 62–63; Molly Ladd-Taylor, *Fixing the Poor: Eugenic Sterilization and Child Welfare in the Twentieth Century* (Baltimore: Johns Hopkins University Press, 2017), 45.

28. Slingerland, 63, 67.

29. Kriste Lindenmeyer, *A Right to Childhood: The US Children's Bureau and Child Welfare, 1912–1946* (Urbana: University of Illinois Press, 1997), 139, 161; Michael Rembis, *Defining Deviance: Sex, Science, and Delinquent Girls, 1890–1960* (Urbana: University of Illinois Press, 2011), 46–48; Molly Ladd-Taylor, "'Ravished by Some Moron': The Eugenic Origins of the Minnesota Psychopathic Personality Act of 1939," *Journal of Policy History* 31, no. 2 (2019): 195.

30. Sarah F. Rose, *No Right to Be Idle: The Invention of Disability, 1840s–1930s* (Chapel Hill: University of North Carolina Press, 2017), 2, 162.

31. Janet Golden, *Babies Made Us Modern: How Infants Brought America into the Twentieth Century* (Cambridge: Cambridge University Press, 2018), 145.

32. Alice Boardman Smuts, *Science in the Service of Children: 1893–1935* (New Haven: Yale University Press, 2006), 86–91.

33. Cynthia A. Connolly and Janet Golden, "'Save 100,000 Babies': The 1918 Children's Year and Its Legacy," *American Journal of Public Health* 108, no. 7 (July 2018): 905. The 1919 conference ultimately led to the passage of the Sheppard-Towner Act (1921). Golden, 58; Kriste Lindenmeyer, "Saving Mothers and Babies: The Sheppard-Towner Act in Ohio, 1921–1929," *Ohio History* 99 (1990): 110.

34. Wendy Kline, *Building a Better Race: Gender, Sexuality, and Eugenics from the Turn of the Century to the Baby Boom* (Berkeley: University of California Press, 2001), Loc. 53 (Kindle); Regina G. Kunzel, *Fallen Women, Problem Girls: Unmarried Mothers and the Professionalization of Social Work, 1890–1945* (New Haven: Yale University Press, 1993); Barbara Meil Hobson, *Uneasy Virtue:*

The Politics of Prostitution and the American Reform Tradition (New York: Basic Books, 1987), ch. 8.

35. Kunzel, *Fallen Women*, 71–72; Lundberg, 7. For the postwar period, see Rickie Solinger, *Wake Up Little Susie: Single Pregnancy and Race before Roe v. Wade* (New York: Routledge, 2000).

36. Rymph, *Raising Government Children*, Loc. 1035.

37. Kline, Loc. 1134; Kunzel, *Fallen Women*, 5, 50–51, 126, 130; Lundberg.

38. Edwin D. Solenberger, chairman of the executive committee, CWLA, et al., "Adoptions," CWLA Collection, (November 5–6, 1937), 2, Box 15, Folder 15-5, SWHA; Parker, 883; E. Wayne Carp, "Professional Social Workers, Adoption and the Problem of Illegitimacy, 1915–1945," *Journal of Policy History* 6, no. 3 (1994): 162, 167–168; "New Era in Charity," *Minnesota Children's Home Finder* 19, no. 2 (May 1919): 9, Children's Home Society Collection, Box 40, Folder 40:5, Home Finder 1919, SWHA; letter from Mrs. Wilson and Mrs. Medlock to Mr. Sam Grunfest (October 20, 1939): 2, Florence Crittenton Home of Little Rock, Arkansas, Florence Crittenton Collection, Box 16, Folder 4, Little Rock, AK 1926–1943, SWHA; "An Outline of Basic Needs in a Medical Program for Child Placing Agencies and Institutions," Appendix B: "Standards Applicable to Members of the League," 2, CWLA Collection, Box 12, Folder 12-10, Standards General 1936, SWHA; E. Wayne Carp, "The Sentimentalization of Adoption: A Critical Note on Viviana Zelizer's 'Pricing the Priceless Child,'" *Adoption and Culture* 5 (2017): 12.

39. Robert W. Kelso, "The Responsibility of the State," in *Standards of Child Welfare: A Report of the Children's Bureau Conferences* (1919) (New York: Arno, 1974), 308.

40. Alberta S. B. Guibord and Ida R. Parker, "What Becomes of the Unmarried Mother?: A Study of 82 Cases" (1922), 23, CWLA Collection, Box 44, Folder 44-6, SWHA; Rebecca Jo Plant, *Mom: The Transformation of Motherhood in Modern America* (Chicago: University of Chicago Press, 2010), Loc. 111–118, 187–195 (Kindle).

41. CWLA, "Basic Child Care Principles" (1929), 1, CWLA Collection, Box 39, Folder 39-7, Publications, Public Relations 1929, 1940–1960, SWHA.

42. Carp, "Professional Social Workers," 167–168. Many agencies allowed mothers to board their children while making their final decision about relinquishment, although they often asked the mother to pay for it. Ora Pendleton, "Agency Responsibility in Adoption," *Family* (April 1938): 3, CWLA Collection, Box 15, Folder 15-5, SWHA; Clarence Preston, "Highlights of Thirty Years' Service with the Florence Crittenton League, October 1911–October 1941," 6, Florence Crittenton Collection, Box 21, Folder 4, Member Homes, NYC 1926–1946, SWHA. Eugenicists supported the same position, emphasizing motherhood and family preservation as the center of their work in the 1930s. Kline, Loc. 91; Herman, *Kinship by Design*, 35; Lindenmeyer, *Right to Childhood*, 160. For definition of placing-out, see Edmond J. Butler, "Standards of Child Placing and Supervision," in *Standards of*

Child Welfare: Reports from the Children's Bureau Conferences (1919) (New York: Arno, 1974), 353. For infant mortality rates, see Golden, 35; Lundberg, 7.

43. Kunzel, *Fallen Women* 128; Eleanor Gallagher, *The Adopted Child* (New York: Reynal and Hitchcock, 1936), 179; Lundberg, 7–8.

44. Gill, "Jurisprudence," 134; Julia Grant, *Raising Baby by the Book: The Education of American Mothers* (New Haven: Yale University Press, 1998), 116; Gallagher, 179, 189–191.

45. Guibord and Parker, 23.

46. CWLA, "Study of Adoption in New York City" (1938), 6.

47. Preston, "Highlights of Thirty Years' Service," 6.

48. Henrietta Gordon, "Current Trends in Adoption," delivered at New Jersey State Conference, November 27, 1944, *Child Welfare League of America Bulletin*, February 1945, 3, CWLA Collection, Box 15, Folder 5, Adoption: General 1928–1948, SWHA; Preston, 6.

49. Carp, "Professional Social Workers," 172; Charlotte Lowe, "The Intelligence and Social Background of the Unmarried Mother," *Mental Hygiene* 11 (October 1927): 783–784; Florence Crittenton Home of North Dakota, Twenty-second Annual Report, 1930, Florence Crittenton Collection, Box 21, Folder 9, Member Homes Fargo, ND 1924–1929, 1948–1949, SWHA; Gill, "Jurisprudence," 133; Guibord and Parker, 23.

50. "Retarded Intelligence, Feeble-mindedness and Delinquency," *Minnesota Children's Home Finder*, 20, no. 1 (February 1920): 12, Children's Home Society of Minnesota Collection, Box 40, Folder 40-6, 1920 Home Finder, SWHA.

51. For more on the roots of preserving the mother-child tie, see Slingerland, 83. Guibord and Parker's study showed, however, that about half of feebleminded and the borderline mothers in 1922 kept their children. Guibord and Parker, 25.

52. Rymph, *Raising Government Children*, 1409, 1413, 1416; Carp, "Sentimentalization," 15; Carp, "Professional Social Workers," 170; CWLA, "Children in Your America," November 1941, 1, CWLA Collection, Box 59, File 39-7.

53. Solenberger et al., 1, 2; Mona Gardner, "Traffic in Babies," *Collier's*, September 16, 1939, 14; Kline, Loc. 888; "Study of Adoption in New York City," 9; "Social Workers Look at Adoption," *Child* 10, no. 7 (1946): 110.

54. Gardner, 14.

55. Carl A. Heisterman, "A Summary of Legislation on Adoption," *Social Service Review* 9 (1935): 284; Arnold Gesell, "Clinical Phases of Child Adoption," chap. 36 in *The Mental Growth of the Preschool Child: A Psychological Outline of Normal Development from Birth to the Sixth Year, Including a System of Developmental Diagnosis* (New York: Macmillan, 1928), 425; Madelyn DeWoody, "Adoption and Disclosure of Medical and Society History: A Review of the Law," *Child Welfare* 72, no. 3 (1993): 195–218, esp. 196. For more on disability risk and medical disclosure, see Sufian, "As Long as Parents."

56. Gesell, "Clinical Phases," 425 (italics mine).

57. Toward the end of this period, a few agencies began to recognize the calamitous fates of children who were rejected for adoption and began to ask parents to assume disability risks. But for most of this period, the presence or absence of disability risk undoubtedly helped to determine family belonging. Lundberg, 10; Heisterman, 284; "Study of Virginia Children's Home Society" (1926), 50, CWLA Collection, Box 134, Folder: Virginia Children's Home Society 1926–1960, SWHA; Gesell, "Clinical Phases," 425; Arnold Gesell, "Reducing the Risks of Child Adoption," *CWLA Bulletin* 6, no. 5 (May 15, 1927): 2; Sandy Sufian, "Compounded Anxieties: Adoptive Family Building and the Role of Disability in Adoption IQ Studies," *Journal of the History of Childhood and Youth* 7, no. 3 (2014): 406.

58. Gardner, 43.

59. Gladys Denny Shultz, "Who Wants Me?," *Better Homes and Gardens* (October 1939): 71.

60. C. C. Carstens, "Safeguards in Adoption," *CWLA Bulletin* 15, no. 4 (April 1936): 4, CWLA Collection, Box 89, Folder: Bulletins 1934–1938, 1930, SWHA; Trent, 137; Herman, *Kinship by Design*, 39–45. For contemporary experts' critique of sentimental motherhood, see Plant, Loc. 1389–1404.

61. Consistent with their stance to privilege biology, adoption practitioners believed that adoption by relatives was natural and much less risky. Ellen Herman, "Families Made by Science: Arnold Gesell and the Technologies of Modern Child Adoption," *Isis* 92, no. 4 (2001): 684n1.

62. Gallagher, 34.

63. Unsigned review of *The Adopted Child*, by Eleanor Gallagher, *CWLA Bulletin* 15, no. 7 (September 1936): 7.

64. Solenberger et al., 2, 3; Gesell, "Reducing the Risks," 1–3.

65. Carol Prentice, *An Adopted Child Looks at Adoption* (New York: D. Appleton-Century, 1940), 152.

66. CWLA, "Minimum Safeguards in Adoption" (1937), CWLA Collection, Box 15, Folder 5, Adoption General 1927–1948, SWHA.

67. My use of *flexible* here coincides with the imperative for perfectibility in Taussig's flexible eugenics concept, but otherwise differs. Taussig, Rapp, and Heath, 60–66.

68. Herman, *Kinship by Design*, 1, 2, 6, 13; Parker, 883. For similar goal for orphanages, see "An Outline of Tentative Standards for Child Caring Institutions," 1, CWLA Collection, Box 33, Folder 5, Surveys, Minnesota, 1919, 1929, SWHA.

69. Child welfare officials, through the 1930s, often resisted the eugenic assessment that all dependent children were a "dysgenic menace." Patrick Ryan, "'Six Blacks from Home': Childhood, Motherhood, and Eugenics in America," *Journal of Policy History* 19, no. 3 (2007): 255, 263; Ladd-Taylor, *Fixing the Poor*, 21; Anna M. Duane, ed., *The Children's Table: Childhood Studies and the Humanities* (Athens: University of Georgia Press, 2013), 3 (Kindle). For the history of the field of social work, see Austin, "The Flexner Myth," 357–377; Golden, 50; Lennard Davis,

"Introduction: Disability, Normality and Power," *Disability Studies Reader*, 4th ed. (New York: Routledge, 2013), 3.

70. Hacking, 160, 163, 166, 168–169; Canguilhem, 51, 107, 118, 144, 240.

71. Ladd-Taylor, *Fixing the Poor*, 79.

72. For compulsory able-bodiedness, see Robert McRuer, "Compulsory Able-bodiedness and Queer/Disabled Existence," in *Disability Studies Reader*, 4th ed., ed. Lennard Davis (New York: Routledge, 2013), 369–370.

73. Herman, *Kinship by Design*, 60; Kelso, 308; Gill, "Adoption Agencies," 167–168.

74. Before that determination, however, diagnostic testing cast children as potentially dangerous in seemingly objective ways. See Elizabeth M. Armstrong, *Conceiving Risk, Bearing Responsibility: Fetal Alcohol Syndrome and the Diagnosis of Disorder* (Baltimore: Johns Hopkins University Press, 2003), 8, 9; Deborah Lupton, *The Imperative of Health: Public Health and the Regulated Body* (London: SAGE, 1995), 105.

75. Carp, "Professional Social Workers," 172; Gill, "Adoption Agencies," 167.

76. Butler, 354, as quoted in Gill, "Adoption Agencies," 168–169, 174.

77. Thank you to Aly Patsavas for this insight.

78. Florence Clothier, "Some Aspects of the Problem of Adoption," *American Journal of Orthopsychiatry* 9, no. 3 (1939): 604–605.

79. Daniel J. Kevles, *In the Name of Eugenics: Genetics and the Uses of Human Heredity* (Cambridge: Harvard University Press, 1995), 85; Rosemarie Garland-Thomson, "Eugenics," in eds. Rachel Adams, Benjamin Reiss, and David Serlin, *Keywords for Disability Studies* (New York: New York University Press, 2015), 75; "Study of the Virginia Children's Home Society," 32; Sara Vogt, "Bodies of Surveillance: Disability, Femininity, and the Keepers of the Gene Pool, 1910–1925," Ph.D. diss., University of Illinois–Chicago, 2013.

80. Clothier, "Placing the Child," 257; Barbara Melosh, *Strangers and Kin: The American Way of Adoption* (Cambridge: Harvard University Press, 2002), 74; Gill, "Jurisprudence," 140.

81. Kline, Loc. 1349, 1443, 1686, 1691, 1699.

82. Sufian, "Compounded Anxieties," 400; Herman, *Kinship by Design*, 123–125; Gill, "Adoption Agencies," 163–165; Carp and Leon-Guerrero, 197; Guibord and Parker, 41.

83. Gill, "Jurisprudence," 140.

84. Herman, *Kinship by Design*, 50.

85. As quoted in Gill, "Jurisprudence," 191.

86. Ellen Herman, "The Paradoxical Rationalization of Modern Adoption," *Journal of Social History* 36 (2002): 351; Melosh, 69, 74; Julie Berebitsky, *Like Our Very Own: Adoption and the Changing Culture of Motherhood, 1851–1950* (Lawrence: University Press of Kansas, 2000), 138; Herman, Kinship by Design, 123; Herman, "Families Made by Science," 690; Gill, "Adoption Agencies," 164.

87. Gallagher, 110; CWLA, "A Study on the Adoption Situation in New York City," 5; Arnold Gesell, "Psycho-clinical Guidance in Adoption," in Children's Bureau, *Foster-Home Care for Dependent Children* (Washington: US Children's Bureau, 1926), 204; Gill, "Jurisprudence," 149; Prentice, 171; Hyman S. Lippman, "Suitability of the Child for Adoption," *American Journal of Orthopsychiatry* 7 (April 1937): 271; Agnes K. Hanna, "Adoption," adapted from two radio talks given on November 5 and 12, 1935, reprinted in *Social Welfare Bulletin* 7, nos. 9 & 10 (November–December 1936): 2–3, CWLA Collection, Box 56: Adoption, 1925–1966, SWHA.

88. Gallagher, 98.

89. Prentice, 168.

90. Gill, "Adoption Agencies," 166; Sufian, "Compounded Anxieties," 400; Herman, *Kinship by Design*, 122, 123; Herman, "Families Made by Science," 691; Herman, "Child Adoption," 11, 14, 18; Berebitsky, *Like Our Very Own*, 129, 137, 138; Gill, "Adoption Agencies," 161–162.

91. Tanya Titchkosky, "Normal," in eds. Rachel Adams, Benjamin Reiss, and David Serlin, *Keywords for Disability Studies* (New York: New York University Press, 2015), 131–132; Peter Cryle and Elizabeth Stevens, *Normality: A Critical Genealogy* (Chicago: University of Chicago Press, 2017), Loc. 237, 362, 442 (Kindle).

92. For Hall and the three D's (defectiveness, delinquency, and dependency), see Ladd-Taylor, *Fixing the Poor*, 44; Elizabeth Lunbeck, "A New Generation of Women: Progressive Psychiatry and the Hypersexual Female," *Feminist Studies* 13 (Fall 1987): 517; Smuts, 49–52; Dorothy Ross, *G. Stanley Hall: The Psychologist as Prophet* (Chicago: University of Chicago Press, 1972).

93. Kline, Loc. 1235, Loc. 1266; Grant, 120, 152–158; Canguilhem, 286.

94. Gill, "Jurisprudence," 217–218; Golden, 1, 8; Smuts, 149; Plant, Loc. 1398–1400; Jessica Martucci, *Back to the Breast: Natural Motherhood and Breastfeeding in America* (Chicago: University of Chicago Press, 2015), 29–31 (Kindle).

95. Grant, 41, 45–46, 140, 143, 162, 168; Plant, Loc. 209; Cryle and Stephens, Loc. 6541; Gill, "Jurisprudence," 186.

96. Grant, 182, 185.

97. Jesse Taft, "The Need for Psychological Interpretation in the Placement of Dependent Children," *CWLA Bulletin* 6 (April 1922): 3, CWLA Collection, Box 89, Newsletters File: CWLA Bulletins 1921–1939, SWHA.

98. Taft, 7.

99. Taft, 8.

100. Gill, "Jurisprudence," 275.

101. Gill, "Jurisprudence," 275; Davis, "Introduction," 2 (italics mine).

102. Gill, "Jurisprudence," 276 (italics mine).

103. Gill, "Jurisprudence," 170–171; Gesell, "Reducing the Risks," 1; Walter Fernald, "A State Program for the Care of the Mentally Defective," in *Standards of Child Welfare: A Report of the Children's Bureau Conferences* (1919), ed. William L. Chenery and Ella A. Merritt (New York: Arno, 1974), 399; Davis, "Introduction," 7.

104. William Ellis, *The Handicapped Child: Report of the Committee on Physically and Mentally Handicapped, White House Conference on Child Health and Protection* (New York: Century Co., 1933), 330–331.

105. Ladd-Taylor, "Ravished by Some Moron," 195, 206.

106. Adam Cohen, *Imbeciles: The Supreme Court, American Eugenics and the Sterilization of Carrie Buck* (New York: Penguin, 2016), 26; Licia Carlson, "Cognitive Ableism and Disability Studies: Feminist Reflections on the History of Mental Retardation," *Hypatia* 16, no. 4 (Autumn 2001): 125, 126, https://search.proquest.com/docview/61304301.

107. See also Slingerland, 74–75; Haller, 98.

108. Rembis, *Defining Deviance*, 78. For recommended terminology after the White House Conference on Child Health and Protection (1930), see Ellis, *The Handicapped Child* (1933), 333–335.

109. Goddard as quoted in Cohen, 32; Douglas C. Baynton, *Defectives in the Land: Disability and Immigration in the Age of Eugenics* (Chicago: University of Chicago Press, 2016), Loc. 154 (Kindle).

110. S. W. Dickinson, "Borderline Cases," *Minnesota Children's Home Finder* 21, no. 4 (November 1921): 12. SW289, Minnesota Children's Home Society Records, Box 40, Folder 7, SWHA; A 1940–1947 survey: Survey—Children's Service League, Springfield, IL 1948, 13, CWLA Collection, Box 119, Folder: Ill., Springfield, Family Service Center of Sangamon County, 1941, 1970–1985, SWHA; Jeffrey A. Brune and Daniel J. Wilson, *Disability and Passing: Blurring the Lines of Identity* (Philadelphia: Temple University Press, 2013), 1; Carlson, "Cognitive Ableism," 130.

111. Clothier, "Placing the Child," 258–261; Carlson, "Cognitive Ableism," 132.

112. Gallagher, 90.

113. Rembis, *Defining Deviance*, 60.

114. Gallagher, 98, 153–154; Patrick J. Ryan, " 'Six Blacks from Home': Childhood, Motherhood, and Eugenics in America," *Journal of Policy History* 19, no. 3 (2007): 266; Guibord and Parker, 12, 16. See also Rembis, *Defining Deviance*, 44; Carlson, "Cognitive Ableism," 127.

115. Ruth Workum, "The Problem of the Unmarried Mother and her Child," *CWLA Bulletin* no. 11 (May 1924): 7–9, CWLA Collection, Box 89, Newsletters, Folder: CWLA Bulletins 1921–1939, SWHA.

116. Workum, 7, 9.

117. Guibord and Parker, 28.

118. Half of their feebleminded and borderline mothers kept their children, whereas 75 percent of those labeled normal and dull normal kept theirs. Guibord and Parker, 25, 63.

119. S. W. Dickinson, "The Normal Child," *Minnesota Children's Home Finder* 16, no. 2 (1916): 13, Minnesota Children's Home Society Collection, Box 40, Folder 40:2, SWHA.

120. Carp, "Sentimentalization," 14–15; Lundberg, 8, 10; Dickinson, "Borderline Cases," 11.

121. "An Adopted Child," *Minnesota Children's Home Finder* 25, no. 3 (November 1925): 2, Children's Home Society of Minnesota Collection, Box 40, Folder 40:11, Children's Home Society Records Finder, SWHA; Ada Eliot Sheffield, "The Nature of Stigma upon the Unmarried Mother and Her Child," *Proceedings of the National Conference of Social Work* (Chicago: University of Chicago Press, 1920), 119–122; Baynton, *Defectives*, Loc. 314.

122. Ida R. Parker, *Fit and Proper: A Study of Legal Adoption in Massachusetts* (Boston: Church Home Society, 1927), 26.

123. Lupton, *The Imperative of Health,* 78; Tulloch and Lupton, Loc. 57.

124. Gesell, "Reducing the Risks," 2.

125. Slingerland, 87–88.

126. Slingerland, 87–88.

127. Clothier, "Placing the Child," 258–259, CWLA Collection, Box 63, Folder: Foster Care/Mental Health, SWHA.

128. "An Outline of Basic Needs in a Medical Program for Child Placing Agencies and Institutions" (1936), 4, CWLA Collection, Box 12, Folder 12-10, Standards General, 1936, SWHA.

129. Clothier, "Some Aspects," 603–604.

130. Slingerland, 47; Sophie van Senden Theis and Constance Goodrich, *The Child in the Foster Home, Part I: The Placement and Supervision of Children in Free Foster Homes, A Study Based on the Work of the Child-Placing Agency of the New York State Charities Aid Association* (Philadelphia: Wm. F. Fell, 1921), 15.

131. Lucie K. Browning, "The Placement of the Child Needing Adoption: Recent Changes in Practice," *CWLA Bulletin* (September 1944): 6, delivered at CWLA National Conference, Cleveland, May 1944, CWLA Collection, Box 89 Folder: CWLA Bulletins 1944–1948, SWHA.

132. Van Senden Theis and Goodrich, 27–28; Prentice, 158; Charles Dow, *Mrs. Eliot's Adopted Daughter: A Short Story for Adoptive Parents,* 4, Children's Home Society of Minnesota Collection, Box 3, File 3-9: Mrs. Eliot's Adopted Daughter, Miscellaneous Documents 1938–1996, SWHA.

133. This is similar to judging the impaired appearances of immigrants and excluding them. Baynton, *Defectives* Loc. 151.

134. Clothier, "Placing the Child," 259.

135. Dorothy Thompson, "Fit for Adoption," *Ladies' Home Journal,* May 1939, 48.

136. Tobin Siebers, "Disability and the Theory of Complex Embodiment: For Identity Politics in a New Register," in ed. Lennard Davis, *Disability Studies Reader,* 4th ed. (Florence: Taylor and Francis, 2013), 283 (Kindle).

137. Erving Goffman, *Stigma: Notes on the Management of a Spoiled Identity* (Englewood Cliffs, NJ: Prentice-Hall, 1963).

138. Kunzel, *Fallen Women,* 36–48; McKinley, 3.

139. It also recommended relative adoption over nonrelative adoption and laid out the rights of the child, the birth parents, and the adopters. "Principles of Adoption outlined by the Study Group on Adoptions," Cleveland Conference on

Illegitimacy, February 1928, 2, 3, CWLA Collection, Box 15, Folder 15-5, SWHA; C. C. Carstens, "Child Welfare Work Since the White House Conference" (1927), 129, CWLA Collection, Box 44, Folder 5, Child Welfare Articles, SWHA; R. P. Schowalter, MD, "Wassermann Tests for All Children," *CWLA Bulletin* 19, no. 1 (January 1940): 6, CWLA Collection, Box 9, Folder: CWLA Bulletin 1939–1941, SWHA; Kunzel, *Fallen Women,* 41; Gill, "Jurisprudence," 141–143; Rymph, *Raising Government Children,* Loc. 173, 234.

140. Carp, "Professional Social Workers," 163–165.

141. McKinley, 8.

142. Lippman, 270–273.

143. The same respondent who noted that he must know about both sides of the family in terms of psychosis said that in the case of feeblemindedness he would be less concerned because of the tests that existed to rule out feeblemindedness. Lippman, 271.

144. Based on studies of the Judge Baker Foundation, Lippman admitted that a follow-up question regarding the opinions of the group about neurosis in delinquency should have been asked. Lippman noted that he needed to ask more about this issue of exposure and what constituted due exposure to a psychotic parent to disqualify him from adoption. Lippman, 271.

145. Lippman, 273.

146. Because the answers to Lippman's questionnaire were so varied and were not based on any scientific evidence, his staff set out thereafter to study issues of feeblemindedness and psychosis in adoption. "We did not realize how enormous the problem was and have found very little time outside of the everyday clinical work to devote to this research." Lippman, 273.

147. "Study of Adoption in New York City," 6, 13.

148. "Study of Adoption in New York City," 11.

149. Michelle Kahan, " 'Put Up' on Platforms: A History of Twentieth Century Adoption Policy in the United States," *Journal of Sociology and Social Welfare* 33, no. 3 (September 2006): 59.

150. Gill, "Jurisprudence," 187–188, 193, 197–205; Gallagher, 49.

151. Thom; Gill, "Adoption Agencies," 167.

152. Gesell, "Reducing the Risks," 2.

153. Sufian, "Compounded Anxieties," 404.

154. Gesell, "Reducing the Risks," 2.

155. Gesell, "Clinical Phases," 427. Gesell noted that despite establishing clinical safeguards, child adoption should not become entirely scientific so as to lose its elements of sacrifice, faith, and adventure. Laura Curran, "Longing to 'Belong': Foster Children in Mid-century Philadelphia (1946–1963)," *Journal of Social History* 42, no. 2 (2008): 427, for Child Guidance clinics, efforts for family preservation, Aid to Dependent Children and family breakup due to the Depression.

156. Herman, *Kinship by Design,* 66.

157. Sufian, "Compounded Anxieties," 402.

158. Lewis Terman, *The Intelligence of School Children* (New York: Houghton Mifflin, 1919), 5 (italics mine). Thank you to Sue Schweik for the citation. Haller, 100.

159. Willsie, 660; William Sloan and Harvey A. Stevens, *A Century of Concern: A History of the American Association on Mental Deficiency, 1876–1976* (Washington, DC: American Association on Mental Deficiency, 1976), 123.

160. Agnes K. Hanna, "Adoption," adapted from two radio talks given on November 5 and 12, 1935, reprinted in *Social Welfare Bulletin* 7, no. 9 and 10 (November–December 1936): 2, CWLA Collection, Box 56: Folder: Adoption, 1925–1966, SWHA.

161. Jenkins, "Adoption Practices and the Physician," 408; Solinger, *Wake Up Little Susie*, 32–33, 180–182.

162. Usually the Stanford-Binet test for children under four.

163. Jenkins, "Adoption Practices and the Physician," 407.

164. Jenkins, "Adoption Practices and the Physician," 407.

165. Jenkins, "Adoption Practices and the Physician," 407.

166. For other cases, see Melosh, 44–45.

167. Sufian, "Compounded Anxieties," 399.

168. Edith Liggett, "Where to Find a Baby for Adoption," *Woman* (1946): 38, enclosed in letter from Lillian Muhlbach to Miss Martha Wood, San Antonio, July 2, 1946, Box 159, Adoption, January 1, 1947–April 30, 1947, National Archives; Sven Ove Hansson, "Dimensions of Risk," *Risk Analysis* 9, no. 1 (1989): 107–108.

169. Janice Brockley, "Martyred Mothers and Merciful Fathers: Exploring Disability and Motherhood in the Lives of Jerome Greenfield and Raymond Repouille," in *The New Disability History: American Perspectives*, ed. Paul Longmore and Lauri Umansky (New York: New York University Press, 2001), 299–300, 302–303.

170. Sufian, "Compounded Anxieties," 419; Frances Lockridge and Sophie van Senden Theis, "Environment vs. Heredity," *CWLA Bulletin* 26, no. 7 (September 1947): 13, CWLA Collection, Box 89, Folder: CWLA Bulletin 1944–1948, SWHA.

171. Lockridge and van Senden Theis, 14.

172. Gallagher, 102, 112.

173. Some adoption professionals, like Clothier, still espoused hereditarian views in the early 1940s. Florence Clothier, "Placing the Child for Adoption," *Mental Hygiene* 26 (1942): 257–274; Rembis, *Defining Deviance*, 21, 126–127.

174. Thompson, "Fit for Adoption," May 1939, 47.

175. Clothier, "Placing the Child," 260, 261.

176. Gill, "Adoption Agencies," 166.

177. Carp and Leon-Guerrero, 197.

178. Children's Service League, Medical Program, 1–2, CWLA Collection, Box 119, Folder: Ill, Springfield Family Service Center of Sangamon County 1948, SWHA; Gallagher, 97.

179. Gesell, "Clinical Phases," 426.

180. Gesell, "Clinical Phases," 425.

181. Gallagher, 195; Golden, 154.

182. "The Child Neglected for Adoption," *Minnesota Children's Home Finder* (August 1947), SW289, Minnesota Children's Home Society Records, Box 40, Folder 40:13 Children's Home Finder 1947–1948, SWHA.

183. "Child Neglected for Adoption."

184. Mary Frances Smith, "A Study of the Adoption Situation of New York City as it Relates to Protestant Children" (January–April 1938), 4, CWLA Collection, Box 15, Folder 15-5, SWHA.

185. Browning, "The Placement of the Child Needing Adoption," 5.

186. Herman, *Kinship by Design*, 64, 67.

187. Slingerland, 68.

188. Slingerland, 68.

189. Slingerland, 68.

190. Connolly and Golden, 903; Slingerland, 67.

191. William Ellis, "The Handicapped Child," *Annals of the American Academy of Political and Social Science* 212 (November 1940): 138.

192. This stance also preceded this chapter's period. Dickinson, "The Normal Child," 11–12; CWLA, "Standards of Foster Care for Children in Institutions" (February 1937), 5, CWLA Collection, Box 13, Folder 13-1, SWHA.

193. Anne Waldschmidt, "Normalcy, Bio-politics and Disability: Some Remarks on the German Disability Discourse," *Disability Studies Quarterly* 26, no. 2 (Spring 2006), https://dsq-sds.org/article/view/694/871. Softening these parameters was consistent with shifts in eugenic thinking in the 1930s. Haller.

194. Davis, "Introduction," 10, 12 (Kindle).

195. McRuer, "Compulsory Able-bodiedness," 370 (Kindle).

196. Prentice, 54–55.

197. Gallagher, 43.

198. S. W. Dickinson, "The Use of Psychology and Psychiatry in Work among Children," *Minnesota Children's Home Finder* 20, no. 4 (November 1920): 11, Children's Home Society of Minnesota Collection, Box 40, Folder 40-6, Children's Home Society Records 1920, SWHA (italics mine); Children's Home Society of Minnesota, "The Problem Child," *Minnesota Children's Home Finder*, 22, no. 3–4 (November 1922): 6, SW289, Minnesota Children's Home Society Records, Box 40, Folder 40-8, 1922, SWHA. For same imperative for neglect children in institutions, see "An Outline of Tentative Standards for Child Caring Institutions," 1, CWLA Collection, Box 33, Folder 33, SWHA. For return to normalcy for unwed mothers, see pamphlet "Florence Crittenton Home of Akron," Florence Crittenton Collection, Box 21, Folder 10 Member Homes: Akron, OH 1935–1938, SWHA.

199. Gallagher, 43, 65; Standards for Children's Aid Organizations Engaged in Child-Placing, 10–11, CWLA Collection Box 13, Folder 13:1, SWHA; van Senden Theis and Goodrich, 26.

200. Gesell, "Clinical Phases," 425, 428–429.

201. Van Senden Theis and Goodrich, 27–29, 68.

202. "Study of Virginia Children's Home Society," 44.

203. Ora Pendleton, "A Decade of Experience in Adoption," *Annals of the American Academy of Political and Social Science* 212, no. 1 (November 1, 1940): 190. For a later repudiation of this search for, and expectation of, perfection and a challenge to invite agencies to find homes for "handicapped" children, see Grace Pratt, "What Child Is Suitable for Adoption?" *Minnesota Welfare* (July 1947), CWLA Collection, Box 38, File 38-6, SWHA; Henry Jenkins, "Childhood Innocence and Other Modern Myths," in *The Children's Culture Reader*, ed. Henry Jenkins (New York: New York University Press, 1998), 15; Karen Sanchez-Eppler, "In the Archives of Childhood," in *The Children's Table: Childhood Studies and the Humanities*, ed. Anna M. Duane (Athens: University of Georgia Press, 2013), 215; Ashis Nandy, *Traditions, Tyranny and Utopias: Essays in the Politics of Awareness* (Delhi: Oxford University Press, 1987), 63–64, 67.

204. Brooks and Brooks, 15–16, 44.

205. Lucie K. Browning, "A Private Agency Looks at the End Results of Adoption," *CWLA Bulletin* 21, no. 1 (January 1942): 3, CWLA Collection, Box 89, Folder: Bulletins 1942–1943, SWHA; Eleanor W. Gordon, "There Is a Time in the Affairs of Children . . . ," *CWLA Bulletin* 24, no. 2 (1945): 4–5; Brooks and Brooks, 12–13, 16, 20; Helen G. Taylor, Southern Regional Conference, 1930, *CWLA Bulletin* 17, no. 3 (March 1938): 5, CWLA Collection, Box 89, Folder: Bulletins 1934–1938, SWHA.

206. Smith, "A Study of the Adoption Situation," 11.

207. Herman, *Kinship by Design*, 67; Golden, 31; Children's Home Society of Minnesota, "Children," *Minnesota Children's Home Finder* 23, no. 2 (May 1923): 9, SW289, Box 40, Folder 40-9, Minnesota Children's Home Society Records, 1923, SWHA. For the public's views on eugenics slightly before this period, see Martin S. Pernick, *The Black Stork: Eugenics and the Death of "Defective" Babies in American Medicine and Motion Pictures Since 1915* (Oxford: Oxford University Press, 1996).

208. Prentice, 141–142.

209. Pendleton, "Agency Responsibility in Adoption," 4. The 1940 White House Conference, "Children in a Democracy," put the "handicapped child" on the radar. Six children in every 1000 under 21 years of age were said to be "crippled or seriously handicapped" with polio, tuberculosis, injuries, heart disease, and congenital conditions. Ellis, "The Handicapped Child" (1940), 128, 144–145.

210. Constance Rathbun, "The Adoptive Foster Parent," *CWLA Bulletin*, 23 (November 1944): 7, 12; Gill, "Jurisprudence," 243–244.

211. Licia Carlson, "Rethinking Normalcy, Normalization and Cognitive Disability," in *Science and Other Cultures: Issues in Philosophies of Science and Technology*, ed. Robert Figueroa and Sandra Harding (New York: Routledge, 2003), 158.

212. Ladd-Taylor, *Fixing the Poor*, 174. For continued belief about the heredi-tary nature of feeblemindedness, see McKinley, 7–8; Ryan, "Six Blacks," 257.

213. Carp and Leon-Guerrero, 205, 209–210.

214. Rymph, *Raising Government Children*, Loc. 1606, 1610, 1638, 1771, 1781. For statistics on children and disability in 1946, see "Digest of the Testimony of George J. Hecht, Publisher of Parents' Magazine before the Senate Committee on Education and Labor," 2, CWLA Collection, Box 44, Folder 44-8, SWHA.

215. Indeed, during the war, women headed one in five families while their married or unmarried partners were deployed abroad. Gordon also notes that economic security allowed Black families to apply for and adopt more regularly. Gordon, "Current Trends in Adoption," 4; Rymph, *Raising Government Children*, Loc. 1516, 1559.

216. Americans in the 1940s adopted approximately sixteen thousand children per year.

217. Carp, "Sentimentalization," 18–19; "Study of the Virginia Children's Home Society, 34; Mary Ruth Colby, *Problems and Procedures in Adoption* (Washington, DC: Government Printing Office, 1941), 4; Prentice, xi; Carp and Leon-Guerrero, 209–211; Golden, 30.

218. Prentice, 151.

219. Ladd-Taylor, *Fixing the Poor*, 174; Herman, *Kinship by Design*, 29; Kelso, 308, 310; Workum, 6; Kunzel, *Fallen Women*, 150–153. This shift mirrors a similar change during the interwar period in the understanding of defective delinquency. Rembis, *Defining Deviance*, 58–60, 67. By contrast, while social workers recast white illegitimacy as an individual pathology, they imagined Black illegitimacy as result-ing from cultural pathology. Kunzel, *Fallen Women*, 145, 147, 149, 152, 154–155.

220. Slingerland, 112.

221. Regina G. Kunzel, "The Rise of Gay Rights and the Disavowal of Dis-ability in the United States," in *The Oxford Handbook of Disability History*, ed. M. Rembis, C. Kudlick, and K. E. Nielsen (Oxford: Oxford University Press, 2018), 12.

222. McKinley, 3; Thom, 2; Herman, *Kinship by Design*, 13; Canguilhem, 144. For restriction through selection, see Baynton, *Defectives*, Loc. 460.

Chapter Two

1. Belle Wolkomir, "The Unadoptable Baby Achieves Adoption," *Child Wel-fare League of America* 26, no. 2 (1947): 1.

2. Helen W. Hallinan, "Who Are the Children Available for Adoption?," *Social Casework* 32 (1951): 162.

3. Adoption Committee of Massachusetts Conference of Social Work, "Adop-tions by Child Placing Agencies Questionnaire" (October 11, 1945), I-2, Box 159, File: Adoptions May 1, 1947–June 30, 1947, National Archives.

4. The JCCA gained adoption placement rights in 1938, and rights for cases of abandonment in 1943. "An Experimental Use of the Temporary Home," Child Welfare League of America pamphlet (January 1946), cited in Wolkomir, "The Unadoptable Baby," 6.

5. Harold M. Skeels, "Mental Development of Children in Foster Homes," *Journal of Consulting Psychology* 2 (1938): 33–43; Marie Skodak, *Children in Foster Homes: A Study of Mental Development* (Iowa City, IA: The University, 1939), 1–156; Marie Skodak, "The Mental Development of Adopted Children Whose True Mothers Are Feebleminded," *Child Development* 9 (1938): 303–308; Marie Skodak and Harold M. Skeels, "A Final Follow-Up Study of One Hundred Adopted Children," *Journal of Genetic Psychology* 75 (1949): 85–125; Wolkomir, "The Unadoptable Baby," 1; Belle Wolkomir, "They Are Adoptable," *Better Times: New York City's Welfare News Weekly*, January 31, 1947, 1.

6. Wolkomir, "The Unadoptable Baby," 2.

7. Wolkomir, "They Are Adoptable," 4.

8. Sandra M. Sufian, "As Long as Parents Can Accept Them: Medical Disclosure, Risk and Disability in Twentieth-Century American Adoption Practice," *Bulletin of the History of Medicine* 91, no. 1 (Spring 2017): 106.

9. Ellen Herman, *Kinship by Design: A History of Adoption in the Modern United States* (Chicago: University of Chicago Press, 2008), 122–134.

10. "Brief Summary of Adoption Conference Called by the CWLA in NYC," May 19–21, 1948, 1, 2, CWLA Collection, Box 15, Folder 5, SWHA.

11. "Adoption of Children with Pathology in Their Backgrounds: Report of Workshop Held April 12, 1949" (New York: CWLA, 1949), 1.

12. "Adoption of Children with Pathology in Their Backgrounds: Report of Workshop Held April 12, 1949" (New York: CWLA, 1949), 1; Henrietta L. Gordon, "Adoption: Practices, Procedures and Problems: Report on Workshop Material and Proceedings of the Adoption Conference Held May 19–21, 1948 (1949), 28, CWLA Collection, Box 15, Folder 6; "Brief Summary of Adoption Conference," 3; Sufian, "As Long as Parents," 94–124.

13. "Brief Summary of Adoption Conference," 3.

14. Gordon, "Adoption: Practices," 21, citing Henrietta L. Gordon, "Adoption: Practices, Procedures and Problems," January 1949, in I. Evelyn Smith to Federal Security Agency, Social Security Administration, Children's Bureau Report (April 1949), 1, US Children's Bureau Collection, Box 449, File June 1949–1952, Adoptions, National Archives.

15. Ruth F. Brenner, "Supervision after Adoptive Placement of a Child or Post Placement Counseling," June 6, 1950, 1, CWLA Collection, Box 15, Folder 6, SWHA; David S. Franklin and Fred Massarik, "The Adoption of Children with Medical Conditions: Part I—Process and Outcome," *Child Welfare* 48, no. 8 (October 1969): 460; Alice Lake, "Babies for the Brave," *Saturday Evening Post*, July 31, 1954, 27, 63.

16. E. Wayne Carp and Anna Leon-Guerrero, "When in Doubt, Count: World War II as a Watershed in the History of Adoption," in *Adoption in America: Historical Perspectives*, ed. E. Wayne Carp (Ann Arbor: University of Michigan Press, 2002), 193, 209–210; Vivian Zelizer, *Pricing the Priceless Child: The Changing Social Value of Children*. (Princeton: Princeton University Press, 1985), 189–207; "Adoption of Children with Pathology in their Backgrounds," 11; Marga Vicedo, *The Nature and Nurture of Love: From Imprinting to Attachment in Cold War America* (Chicago: University of Chicago Press, 2013), 40 (Kindle).

17. Vicedo, 24, 27, 28.

18. Browning believed that children with mild impairments were adoptable, but they had to compensate with some other characteristic to be worthy of receiving love from their adoptive parents. Lucie K. Browning, "The Placement of the Child Needing Adoption," *CWLA Bulletin* 23, no. 7 (1944): 13; Rebecca Jo Plant, *Mom: The Transformation of Motherhood in Modern America* (Chicago: University of Chicago Press, 2010), Loc. 1662 (Kindle); Vicedo 39, 234; Jessica Martucci, *Back to the Breast: Natural Motherhood and Breastfeeding in America* (Chicago: University of Chicago Press, 2015), 3, 28, 31, 33, 39–40 (Kindle).

19. Gail Landsman, *Reconstructing Motherhood and Disability in the Age of "Perfect" Babies* (New York: Routledge, 2009), 146; Paul Longmore, "Conspicuous Contribution and American Cultural Dilemmas: Telethon Rituals of Cleansing and Renewal," in *The Body and Physical Difference: Discourses of Disability in the Humanities*, ed. David Mitchell and Sharon L. Snyder (Ann Arbor: University of Michigan Press, 1997), 136.

20. Hallinan, "Who Are the Children?," 162.

21. Viola Bernard, "Application of Psychoanalytic Concepts to Adoption Agency Practice," in *Psychoanalysis and Social Work*, ed. Marcel Heiman (New York: International Universities Press, 1953), 173, CWLA Collection, Box 16, Folder 6, SWHA.

22. Henrietta L. Gordon, "Adoption: Practices, Procedures and Problems: held in NYC under the Auspices of the CWLA: A Report on the Second Workshop Held in NYC under the Auspices of the CWLA" (May 10–12, 1951): 3, CWLA Collection, Box 15, Folder 6, SWHA.

23. Gordon, "Adoption: Practices" (1948), 28.

24. Gordon, "Adoption: Practices" (1948), 27.

25. Gordon, "Adoption: Practices" (1948), 27.

26. Browning, "The Placement of the Child Needing Adoption," 13.

27. For a biography of Black, see http://bankstreet.edu/library/center-for-childrens-literature/irma-black-award/irma-.".-black-biography/.

28. Brenner, "Supervision after Adoptive Placement of a Child or Post Placement Counseling," 1.

29. "Adoption of Children with Pathology in Their Backgrounds," 4.

30. "Adoption of Children with Pathology in Their Backgrounds," 4.

31. "Adoption of Children with Pathology in Their Backgrounds," 3.

32. Tanya Titchkosky, "The Ends of the Body as Pedagogic Possibility," *Review of Education, Pedagogy and Cultural Studies* 34, no. 3–4 (2013): 82–84; Alison Kafer, *Feminist, Queer, Crip* (Bloomington: Indiana University Press, 2013), 2 (Kindle).

33. See "Moppets on the Market: The Problem of Unregulated Adoptions," *Yale Law Journal* (1950): 719; Louise Rainer, "Helping the Child and the Adoptive Parents in the Initial Placement," *Child Welfare* 30, no. 7 (November 1951): 8; Hallinan, "Who Are the Children?," 167.

34. "Adoption of Children with Pathology in Their Backgrounds," 3.

35. Sufian, "As Long as Parents," 110.

36. "Adoption of American Children in the United States" (December 1958), report prepared in reply to request of Chairman of House Judiciary Subcommittee, to regional directors from Clare Golden, specialist on foster family care and adoption, Division of Social Services, US Children's Bureau, Box 889 RG1, File: May 1960, Adoption 1958–1962, 3.

37. "Adoption of Children with Pathology in Their Backgrounds," 4; Sufian, "As Long as Parents," 110.

38. Bernard, "Application of Psychoanalytic Concepts," 185–186.

39. Gordon, "Adoption: Practices" (1951), 30.

40. Helen W. Hallinan, "The Essential Requirements for a Sound Adoption Program," *Catholic Charities Review* (June 1956): 12. CWLA Collection. SWHA. Box 16, Folder 6.

41. Michael Schapiro, *A Study of Adoption Practice*, vol. 1: *Adoption Agencies and the Children They Serve* (New York: CWLA, 1956), 55–56.

42. "Agency Adoption Practices: Abstracts from the Preliminary Report of the Survey of Adoptions of the CWLA" (June 1955), 25, confidential, CWLA Collection, Box 16, Folder 7, SWHA.

43. Elaine Tyler May, *Homeward Bound: Americans in the Cold War Era* (New York: Basic Books, 1988), 35–61.

44. Joseph H. Reid, "Introduction," in Michael Schapiro, *A Study of Adoption Practice*, vol. 1: *Adoption Agencies and the Children They Serve* (New York: Child Welfare League of America, 1956), 31; Barbara Melosh, *Strangers and Kin: The American Way of Adoption* (Cambridge: Harvard University Press, 2002), 105. From 1945 through 1950, adoption petitions increased 40–50 percent. "Moppets on the Market," 716.

45. Clark E. Vincent, "The Adoption Market and the Unwed Mother's Baby," *Marriage and Family Living* 18, no. 2 (May 1956): 124; Clark E. Vincent, "Unwed Mothers and the Adoption Market: Psychological and Familial Factors," *Marriage and Family Living* 22, no. 2 (May 1960): 112; E. Wayne Carp, "The Sealed Adoption Records Controversy in Historical Perspective: The Case of the Children's Home Society of Washington, 1895–1998," *Journal of Sociology and Social Welfare*

19 (May 1992): 42; Carp and Leon-Guerrero, 190–193; "Adoption of American Children in the United States," 5.

46. CWLA memo to all papers, June 25, 1956, 1, CWLA Collection, Box 39, Folder 39:7 Publications, Public Relations, 1929, 1940–1960, SWHA.

47. E. Wayne Carp, *Family Matters: Secrecy and Disclosure in the History of Adoption* (Cambridge, MA: Harvard University Press, 1998), 110; "Moppets on the Market," 718; Virginia Reid, "Black Market Babies," *Women's Home Companion*, December 1944, 31; Martha M. Eliot, "Still More Myths and a Wish: Would-Be Parents Want Any Child Available for Adoption, Anybody Can Place Babies Happily, and Successfully," October 1955, 1, HEW-069-5, CWLA Collection, Box 56, Adoption 1925–1966, SWHA. Cf. Melosh, 108; Herman, *Kinship by Design*, 201; Steven Ruggles, "The Effects of AFDC on American Family Structure, 1940–1990," *Journal of Family History* 22, no. 307 (1997): 313–314.

48. Regina G. Kunzel, *Fallen Women, Problem Girls: Unmarried Mothers and the Professionalization of Social Work, 1890–1945* (New Haven: Yale University Press, 1993), 162.

49. Catherine E. Rymph, "Looking for Fathers in the Postwar US Foster Care System," in *Inventing the Modern American Family: Family Values and Social Changes in 20th Century United States*, ed. Isabel Heinemann (Frankfurt: Campus Verlag, 2012), 179.

50. Herman, *Kinship by Design*, 232–233.

51. Prior to the war, even fewer agencies provided services to birth mothers or adoptive parents of color. Despite Melosh's and Solinger's arguments that postwar adoption was entirely a "white" mandate, primary documents show that there was an overwhelming need for the placement of minority children after the war. CWLA, *Child Care Facilities for Dependent and Neglected Negro Children in Three Cities: New York City, Philadelphia, Cleveland* (New York: CWLA, 1945); Karen Andrea Balcom, *The Traffic in Babies: Cross-Border Adoption, Baby-Selling and the Development of Child Welfare Systems in the United States and Canada, 1930–1960* (Toronto: University of Toronto Press, 2011), 197; "Moppets on the Market," 717; Herman, *Kinship by Design*, 196–197, 199; James N. Gregory, *The Southern Diaspora: How the Great Migrations of Black and White Southerners Transformed America* (Chapel Hill: University of North Carolina Press, 2007).

52. Florence G. Brown, "What Do We Seek in Adoptive Parents?," *Social Casework* 32, no. 4 (1951): 155, 159.

53. Fairweather, 4.

54. Melosh, 105; Karen Andrea Balcom, "The Logic of Exchange: The Child Welfare League of America, the Adoption Resource Exchange Movement and the Indian Adoption Project, 1958–1967," *Adoption and Culture* 1, no. 1 (2008): 8; Herman, *Kinship by Design*, 200–201.

55. Wolkomir, "They are Adoptable," 10; Herman, *Kinship by Design*, 199–200.

56. Michael Schapiro, *A Study of Adoption Practice*, vol. 3: *Adoption of Children with Special Needs* (New York: CWLA, 1957), 42.

57. Balcom, "The Logic of Exchange," 8.

58. Balcom, "The Logic of Exchange," 9; "Adoption Clearance Service," *Child Welfare*, June 1953, 11.

59. Douglas C. Baynton, "Disability and the Justification of Inequality in American History," in *The New Disability History: American Perspectives*, ed. Paul Longmore and Lauri Umansky (New York: New York University Press, 2001), 33, 34, 41, 51.

60. Balcom, "The Logic of Exchange," 9, 16, 36, 42–43; Herman, *Kinship by Design*, 196; Alexandra Minna Stern, *Telling Genes: The Story of Genetic Counseling in America* (Baltimore: Johns Hopkins University Press, 2012), Loc. 1376 (Kindle); Anna Stubblefield, "The Entanglement of Race and Cognitive Dis/ability." *Metaphilosophy* 40, no. 3–4 (July 2009): 533, 540; Anna Stubblefield, "Race, Disability, and the Social Contract," *Southern Journal of Philosophy* 47, no. S1 (2009): 109–110; Balcom, "The Logic of Exchange," 9; Andrew J. Hogan, "Review of Alexandra Minna Stern, *Telling Genes: The Story of Genetic Counseling in America*," *Journal of the History of Medicine and Allied Sciences* 69, no. 4 (2014): 687–689, https://doi.org/10.1093/jhmas/jrt047 (November 1, 2013): 1–3.

61. Bernard, "Application of Psychoanalytic Concepts," 181; Hallinan, "Who Are the Children?," 162, 163.

62. This held true for both African American adopters and white adopters. Herman, *Kinship by Design*, 198–199; Stern, *Telling Genes*, Loc. 1046, 1233–1247 (Kindle); Martucci, 57.

63. Melosh, 37.

64. "Reasons for the Recommendation that a Commission Be Established for the Purpose of Investigation and Study of Adoption Laws and Practices in the Commonwealth," prepared by Patrick A. Tompkins, commissioner, Department of Public Welfare, January 28, 1946, 1, enclosure in letter to Miss Mildred Arnold, director of the Social Service Division of the Children's Bureau, from Mary A. Mason, chairman, Adoption Committee of the Massachusetts Conference of Social Work, February 13, 1946, Box 159, File: Adoptions, May 1, 1947–June 30, 1947, National Archives; Carp, *Family Matters*, 102; Maud Morlock to Mrs. Margaret Mink, director of Social Services of The Cradle, September 25, 1945, 1–3, Box 159, File: Adoptions, January 1946–March 1946.

65. Melosh, 38, 110.

66. Catherine S. Amatruda, "Report of Current Adoption Practices in Connecticut—Independent and Agency Placement," a talk at the annual meeting of the Connecticut Welfare Association, May 1948, 3, Box 449, File: Adoptions, November 1949, National Archives.

67. Maud Morlock to Mrs. Margaret Mink, director of social services of The Cradle, September 25, 1945, 1–3, Box 159. File: Adoptions, January 1946 to March 1946, National Archives.

68. Albert Q. Maisel, "Why You Can't Adopt a Baby," *Woman's Home Companion*, March 1950, 86.

69. Maisel, 86.

70. "Reasons for the Recommendation," 1–3; Charles A. Mosher, editor of *Oberlin News-Tribune*, "Editor Who Used Adoption Service Praises it," in Letters to the Editor, *Cleveland Press*, August 31, 1945, enclosure in letter from Daniel R. Elliott, assistant executive director of Children's Services, Cleveland Ohio, to Maud Morlock, US Children's Bureau, September 20, 1945, 8, Box 159, File: Adoptions, June 1945–October 1945, National Archives.

71. "Moppets on the Market," 724.

72. Amatruda, "Report of Current Adoption Practices," 2; Catherine S. Amatruda and Joseph V. Baldwin, "Current Adoption Practices," *Journal of Pediatrics* 38, no. 2 (February 1951): 209–210.

73. Reid, "Black Market Babies," 31. See also Frederick Brownell, "Why You Can't Adopt a Baby," *Reader's Digest*, September 1948, 58.

74. Reid, "Black Market Babies," 31; Dorothy Barclay, "Adoption Problems," *New York Times*, April 2, 1950, 173.

75. Mr. and Mrs. Wayne Schupp, "Adoption Service Bureau Did Fine Job, Say Parents," letter to the editor, *Cleveland Press*, August 28, 1945, enclosure in letter from Daniel R. Elliott, assistant executive director of Children's Services, Cleveland, Ohio, to Maud Morlock, US Children's Bureau, September 20, 1945, 7, Box 159, File: Adoptions, June 1945–October 1945, National Archives.

76. *Hearings before the Subcommittee to Investigate Juvenile Delinquency of the Committee on the Judiciary*, United States Senate, 84th Congress, 1st Session, November 14 and 15, 1955 (Washington: US Government Printing Office, 1956), 79–80.

77. *Hearings before the Subcommittee to Investigate Juvenile Delinquency*, 159.

78. Rickie Solinger, *Wake Up Little Susie: Single Pregnancy and Race before Roe v. Wade* (New York: Routledge, 2000), 148–186.

79. Katarina Wegar, *Adoption, Identity and Kinship: The Debate over Sealed Birth Records* (New Haven: Yale University Press, 1997), 25.

80. Henrietta Gordon, "Current Trends in Adoption," delivered at the New Jersey State Conference, November 27, 1944, *Child Welfare League of America Bulletin*, February 1945, 3, CWLA Collection, Box 15, Folder 5, Adoption General 1928–1948, SWHA.

81. Donald Brieland, "Foster-Care and Adoption II: Current Research on Adoption," *Social Service Review* 30, no. 3 (1956): 248; Vicedo, 24–28, 37.

82. Brieland, "Foster-Care and Adoption," 248, 257 (in comments).

83. Florence Clothier, "The Psychology of the Adopted Child," *Mental Hygiene* 27 (1943): 224.

84. Weltha M. Kelley, "The Placement of Young Infants for Adoption," *Child Welfare* 29 (July 1949): 14.

85. Browning, "Placement of the Child," 14.

86. Browning, "Placement of the Child," 5; Martucci, 2 (Kindle).

87. Kelley, 14.

88. Kelley, 15.

89. Julia E. Hatch, "Two Early Adoption Placements," *Journal of Social Casework* 29, no. 3 (March 1948): 101.

90. Sylvia Oshlag, "Direct Placement in Adoption," *Journal of Social Casework* 27 (October 1946): 233, CWLA Collection, Box 16, Folder 6, SWHA.

91. Herman, *Kinship by Design*, 134.

92. Oshlag, 230- 238.

93. "Agency Adoption Practices," 35.

94. Therefore, agencies could not adequately determine timetables for successful early placement.

95. Helen Fradkin, "Adoption as the Adoption Agency Sees It," *Jewish Social Service Quarterly* 28 (December 1951): 201, CWLA Collection, Box 16, Folder 6, SWHA.

96. Kafer, 2, 28.

97. Voskine Yanekian, "Teamwork in Developing Criteria for Predictability," in *A Study of Adoption Practice*, vol. 2: *Selected Scientific Papers Presented at the National Conference on Adoption, January 1955*, ed. Michael Schapiro (New York: Child Welfare League of America, 1956), 159.

98. Martin B. Loeb, "Prediction: A Realistic Aspect of Adoption Practice," in *A Study of Adoption Practice*, vol. 2: *Selected Scientific Papers Presented at the National Conference on Adoption, January 1955*, ed. Michael Schapiro (New York: Child Welfare League of America, 1956), 171; Jasbir Puar, "Prognosis Time: Towards a Geopolitics of Affect, Debility and Capacity," *Women and Performance: A Journal of Feminist Theory* 19, no. 2 (2009): 165.

99. Sheldon C. Reed, "The Child's Heritage," in *A Study of Adoption Practice*, vol. 2: *Selected Scientific Papers Presented at the National Conference on Adoption, January 1955*, ed. Michael Schapiro (New York: CWLA, 1955), 39, 43, 44; Stern, *Telling Genes*, Loc. 434.

100. "Agency Adoption Practices," 37.

101. Child Welfare League of America, *Standards for Adoption Service, 1958* (New York: Child Welfare League of America, 1958), 19, CWLA Collection, Box 13, Folder 7, SWHA.

102. Browning, "The Placement of the Child," 6. Pediatric exams included serological (TB) tests, and immunization. Gordon, "Adoption: Practices" (1948), 27; Michael Schapiro, *A Study of Adoption Practice*, vol. 1: *Adoption Agencies and the Children They Serve* (New York: Child Welfare League of America, 1956), 63.

103. Based upon the 1947 CWLA questionnaire during the year ending June 1947 when matching still occurred. Gordon, "Adoption: Practices" (1948), 24–26.

104. "Agency Adoption Practices," 32.

105. Kelley, 15–16.

106. Othilda Krug to Henrietta Gordon, June 16, 1951, 2, CWLA Collection, Box 15, Folder 6, SWHA.

107. "Agency Adoption Practices," 14.

108. Browning, "The Placement of the Child," 6; John Bowlby, *Maternal Care and Mental Health: A Report Prepared on Behalf of the World Health Organization as a Contribution to the United Nations Programme for the Welfare of Homeless Children*, 2nd ed. (Geneva: World Health Organization, 1952); Julia Grant, *Raising Baby by the Book: The Education of American Mothers*. (New Haven: Yale University Press, 1998), 211; letter from Frederic Kapp to Henrietta Gordon, June 25, 1951; letter from Loretta Bender to Henrietta Gordon, June 4, 1951, 6, CWLA Collection, Box 15, Folder 6, SWHA; letter from Othilda Krug to Henrietta Gordon, June 16, 1951, 1–3, CWLA Collection, Box 15, Folder 6, SWHA; letter from Jules Coleman to Henrietta Gordon, June 15, 1951, 1, CWLA Collection, Box 15, Folder 6, SWHA.

109. Gordon, "Adoption: Practices" (1951), 29; Bowlby, 103–104.

110. E. Wayne Carp, "The Sentimentalization of Adoption: A Critical Note on Viviana Zelizer's 'Pricing the Priceless Child,'" *Adoption and Culture* 5 (2017): 10.

111. Plant, Loc. 1664, 1679 (Kindle); Vicedo, 22–39.

112. Carp, *Family Matters*, 111; See also Solinger, *Wake Up Little Susie*.

113. Clothier, "The Psychology of the Adopted Child," 222; Herman, *Kinship by Design*, 265–270.

114. Bernard, "Application of Psychoanalytic Concepts," 175.

115. Louise Raymond, *Adoption . . . and After* (New York: Harper and Brothers, 1955), 87, as quoted in Herman, *Kinship by Design*, 134.

116. The January 1955 conference was a watershed moment in postwar adoption history. Reid, "Introduction," 7–8.

117. Fairweather, 8. Reiterated at the September 14–16, 1955, Conference on Adoption (follow-up). Florence G. Brown, Summary of Conference on Adoption, Chicago, 4. CWLA Collection, Box 16, Folder 11, SWHA.

118. Henrietta Gordon, "Adoption: Practices, Procedures and Problems: A Report of the Second Workshop held in NYC under the Auspices of the CWLA, May 10–12, 1951, 24, CWLA Collection, Box 15, Folder 6, SWHA; Martucci, 56 (Kindle).

119. Hallinan, "Changing Concepts," 114. See also Lela B. Costin, "Implications of Psychological Testing for Adoptive Placements," *Social Casework* (February 1953), as quoted in Bromberg, "Criteria for Improved," 4; Joseph Reid, "Principles, Values and Assumptions Underlying Adoption Practice," *Social Work* 2 (January 1957): 25, quoted in Gill, "Jurisprudence," 277.

120. Bernard, "Application of Psychoanalytic Concepts," 180.

121. Gill, "Jurisprudence," 270, 285–286.

122. Brown, "What Do We Seek in Adoptive Parents?" 155, 158; Bernard, "Application of Psychoanalytic Concepts," 194–195; Robert P. Knight, "Some Problems Involved in Selecting and Rearing Adopted Children," *Bulletin of the Menninger Clinic* 5, no. 3 (May 1941): 67.

123. Alfred Torrie, "The Problems of Placement of Children for Adoption," *Journal of the Royal Sanitary Institute* 71, no. 343 (1951): 344; Gill, "Jurisprudence," 242–243.

124. Knight, 68–69.

125. Abraham Simon, "Social Agency Adoption: A Psycho-sociological Study in Prediction," Ph.D. thesis, Washington University, 1953, 116–117, as quoted in Gill, "Jurisprudence," 246; Dorothy Hutchinson, *In Quest of Foster Parents* (New York: Columbia University Press, 1943), 9–10, as quoted in Gill, "Jurisprudence," 245.

126. Dorothy Barclay, "Adoption Thinking Seen as Too Rigid," *New York Times*, June 17, 1953, 22; Dorothy Barclay, "Adoption Agencies: Pro and Con," *New York Times*, February 17, 1957, SM123.

127. Barclay, "Adoption Thinking," 22.

128. Knight, 68–69, as quoted in Gill, "Jurisprudence," 242–244; Jules Coleman to Henrietta Gordon, June 15, 1951, 1, CWLA Collection, Box 15, Folder 6, SWHA.

129. Henrietta Gordon, "Adoption: Practices, Procedures and Problems" (1949); Herman, *Kinship by Design*, 133, 203; Melosh, 112–113, 120; Brown, "What Do We Seek in Adoptive Parents?" 156; Yanekian, 156–159.

130. Ruth Brenner, *A Follow-up Study of Adoptive Families* (New York: Child Adoption Research Committee), 1951, 13, as quoted in Gill, "Jurisprudence," 284; Plant, Loc. 1679; Vicedo, 28, 32.

131. "Some Principles of Adoption Governing the Practices of Member Agencies of the Child Welfare League of America" affirmed at the Conference on Adoptions held at the league office, May 1948, 3, part of a letter from Leonard Mayo to William Birni on February 23, 1950, CWLA Collection, Box 15, Folder 6, SWHA; Herman, *Kinship by Design*, 232, 234–235.

132. Pamphlet for Adopt-a-Child, 1, CWLA Collection, Box 17, Folder 10, quoted in Herman 238n58.

133. Balcom, "The Logic of Exchange," 13; Herman, *Kinship by Design*, 196, 236–238.

134. Vicedo, 31–35, 233.

135. Janice Brockley, "Rearing the Child Who Never Grew: Ideologies of Parenting and Intellectual Disability in American History," in *Mental Retardation in America: A Historical Reader,* ed. Steven Noll and James W. Trent (New York: New York University Press, 2004), 133, 139, 148; Plant, Loc. 1765.

136. Paul Beaven as quoted in Brockley, "Rearing the Child," 149; Paul Beaven, "The Adoption of Retarded Children," *Child Welfare* 35 (1956): 21.

137. Gill, "Jurisprudence," 275.

138. For the UK, see Sarah Bunt, "A Framework for the Analysis of the Social Processes in the Adoption of Disabled Children," *Journal of Social Work* 14, no. 5 (2014): 530; Loeb, 174.

139. Barclay, "Adoption Problems," 173.

140. Brockley, "Rearing the Child," 130–131, 133.

141. Brockley, "Rearing the Child," 144, 149.

142. Brockley, "Rearing the Child," 130–131, 133.

143. James W. Trent, *Inventing the Feeble Mind: A History of Mental Retardation in the United States* (Berkeley: University of California Press, 1994), 238–239.

144. Brockley, "Rearing the Child," 147; Trent, 231, 237; Ann Fessler, *The Girls Who Went Away: The Hidden History of Women Who Surrendered Children for Adoption in the Decades before Roe v. Wade* (London: Penguin, 2006), 9, 12.

145. Mrs. Austin Melford, "Problems of Placement of Children for Adoption," *Journal of the Royal Sanitary Institute* 71 (1951): 351–356.

146. Melford, 353.

147. Trent, 232–236, 240–241; Nora Ellen Groce, "Parent Advocacy for Disabled Children and the Disability Rights Movement: Similar Movements, Different Trajectories," Institution for Social and Policy Studies, PONPO Working Paper No. 237 and ISPS Working Paper No. 2237 (November 1996), 12.

148. David Oshinsky, *Polio: An American Story, the Crusade that Mobilized the Nation against the 20th Century's Most Feared Disease* (Oxford: Oxford University Press, 2005), 81, 161, 162.

149. Oshinsky, 82–83.

150. Oshinsky, 81–82.

151. For emerging disability policies, see Felicia Kornbluh, "Disability, Antiprofessionalism, and Civil Rights: The National Federation of the Blind and the 'Right to Organize' in the 1950s," *Journal of American History* 97, no. 4 (March 2011): 1032.

152. Bernard, "Application of Psychoanalytic Concepts," 173.

153. Helen Rome Marsh, "Psychologist Can help in planning for baby's adoption," *The Child* (November 1949): 78, as quoted in Schapiro, *A Study of Adoption Practice,* vol. 1, 62; Brieland, "Foster-Care and Adoption," 250; Carp, "The Sealed Adoption Records Controversy," 41; Sufian, "As Long as Parents," 108.

154. Letter from I. Evelyn Smith to Mr. Mac R. Johnson, June 15, 1951, 1–2, US Children's Bureau, US National Archives, RG 102, Box 449, File: Adoptions 1949–1952. For disagreement, see Mildred Arnold, director, social service division, to Joseph C. Neuvirth, president, Chosen Parents League, January 22, 1948, Box 158 Folder: Adoptions January 1948, National Archives.

Chapter Three

1. Patricia Kravik, "Editorial," *Adoption Report: North American Center on Adoption* 1, no. 3 (Fall 1976): 2, CWLA Collection, Box 18, Folder 5, SWHA.

2. Kravik, "Editorial," 2; Allison Carey, *On the Margins of Citizenship: Intellectual Disability and Civil Rights in Twentieth-Century America* (Philadelphia: Temple University Press, 2009), 93; Erving Goffman, *Stigma: Notes on the Management*

of Spoiled Identity (Englewood Cliffs, NJ: Prentice-Hall, 1963); John Gliedman and William Roth, *The Unexpected Minority: Handicapped Children in America* (New York: Harcourt, Brace, Jovanovich, 1980), 25.

3. Kravik, "Editorial," 2.

4. On internal and external risks, see Mary Douglas, *Risk and Blame: Essays in Cultural Theory* (New York: Routledge, 1992), Loc. 358 (Kindle).

5. For fear of risk and acceptable risk, see Mary Douglas and Aaron Wildavsky, *Risk and Culture: An Essay on the Selection of Technological and Environmental Dangers* (Berkeley: University of California Press, 1982), Loc. 28, 53, 61, 96 (Kindle).

6. Paul Longmore, *Telethons: Spectacle, Disability, and the Business of Charity* (Oxford: Oxford University Press, 2016), 230; Daniel J. Wilson, "Crippled Manhood: Infantile Paralysis and the Construction of Masculinity," *Medical Humanities Review* 12, no. 2 (Fall 1998): 15; Michael Rembis, "Athlete First: A Note on Passing, Disability, and Sport," in *Disability and Passing: Blurring the Lines of Identity*, ed. Jeffrey A. Brune and Daniel J. Wilson (Philadelphia: Temple University Press, 2013), 115–116.

7. Amy Fairchild, "The Polio Narratives: Dialogues with FDR," *Bulletin of the History of Medicine* 75, no. 3 (Fall 2001): 493; Daniel J. Wilson, "Fighting Polio like a Man: Intersections of Masculinity, Disability and Aging," in *Gendering Disability*, ed. Bonnie Smith and Beth Hutchinson (New Brunswick: Rutgers University Press, 2004), 119, 121, 130–131.

8. Longmore, *Telethons*, 102–120.

9. Joseph Reid, "Principles, Values and Assumptions Underlying Adoption Practice," *Social Work* 2 (January 1957): 23.

10. Ruddick speaks of love as virtue and attention as capacity; both as parts of maternal thought's conception of achievement. I extend this idea to the capacity of acceptance, analogous to Ruddick's. Sara Ruddick, "Maternal Thinking," *Feminist Studies* 6, no. 2 (Summer 1980): 357–358.

11. Rayna Rapp and Faye Ginsburg, "Enlarging Reproduction, Screening Disability," in ed. Marcia C. Inhorn, *Reproductive Disruptions: Gender, Technology, and Biopolitics in the New Millennium* (New York: Berghahn, 2008), 99, 106.

12. Zitha Turitz, "A New Look at Adoption: Current Developments in the Philosophy and Practice of Adoption," paper presented at CWLA Eastern Regional Conference, February 19, 1965, 11, CWLA Collection, Box 59, Folder: A New Look at Adoption, SWHA; *Guidelines for Adoption Service* (New York: CWLA, 1971), 1, CWLA Collection, Box 61, SWHA.

13. Ruddick, 344.

14. Child Welfare League of America, *Standards for Adoption Service* (New York: Child Welfare League of America, 1958), 6; Turitz, 3; Alfred Kadushin, "A Study of Adoptive Parents of Hard-to-Place Children," *Social Casework* 43 (1962): 227. For caring, relationships, and personhood, see Eva Kittay, "When Caring Is

Just and Justice Is Caring: Justice and Mental Retardation," *Public Culture* 13, no. 3 (2001): 568.

15. CWLA, *Standards for Adoption Service* (1958), 7; Viola Bernard, *Adoption* (New York: Child Welfare League of America, 1964), 98, CWLA Collection, Box 60: Adoption General, Printed Materials, SWHA; *Guidelines for Adoption Service*, 10.

16. "Adoption of Children with Pathology in Their Backgrounds: Report of Workshop Held April 12, 1949" (New York: CWLA, 1949), 1, CWLA Collection, Box 60, Folder Adoption-General, SWHA.

17. Reid, "Principles," as quoted in Julie Berebitsky, *Like Our Very Own: Adoption and the Changing Culture of Motherhood, 1851–1950* (Lawrence: University Press of Kansas, 2000), 163.

18. Bernard, *Adoption*, 71; *Guidelines for Adoption Services*, 10; CWLA, *Standards for Adoption Service* (1958), 43; David S. Franklin and Fred Massarik, "The Adoption of Children with Medical Conditions: Part I—Process and Outcome," *Child Welfare* 48 (1969): 459, 462–463. The American Academy of Pediatrics also promoted expanded adoptability for children with handicaps. Paul Beaven, "Adoption of Handicapped Children," *Pediatrics* 17 (1956): 970–971; Donald G. Tollefson, "What Is New In Adoption," *California Medicine* 78, no. 3 (March 1953): 223.

19. CWLA, *Standards for Adoption Service* (1958), 2; *Guidelines for Adoption Service*, 1.

20. Ruddick, 344; Arlie Hochschild, *The Managed Heart: Commercialization of Human Feeling* (Berkeley: University of California Press, 1983), 170. For changing notions of motherhood in the 1960s and 1970s, see Rebecca Jo Plant, *Mom: The Transformation of Motherhood in Modern America* (Chicago: University of Chicago Press, 2010), Loc. 2211–2239, 2410 (Kindle); Marga Vicedo, *The Nature and Nurture of Love: From Imprinting to Attachment in Cold War America* (Chicago: University of Chicago Press, 2013), 40, 39–41, 233.

21. Rickie Solinger, *Wake Up Little Susie: Single Pregnancy and Race before Roe v. Wade* (New York: Routledge, 2000), 149; Brian Paul Gill, "The Jurisprudence of Good Parenting: The Selection of Adoptive Parents, 1894–1964," Ph.D. diss., University of California, Berkeley, 1997, 311; Ellen Herman, *Kinship by Design: A History of Adoption in the Modern United States* (Chicago: University of Chicago Press, 2008), 240.

22. Nina Bernstein, *The Lost Children of Wilder* (New York: Vintage, 2002), 109.

23. Statement by Elizabeth S. Cole, Director, North American Center on Adoption. Special Project, Child Welfare League of America, Inc., Before the Sub-committee on Children and Youth, United States Senate, July 14, 1975, 4–5, CWLA Collection, Box 18, Folder 5, SWHA; Barbara Pine, "Child Welfare Reform and the Political Process," *Social Service Review* 60 (September 1986): 341. See also Steven Mintz and Susan Kellogg, *Domestic Revolutions: A Social History*

of American Family Life (New York: Free Press, 1988), 209; Bruce Schulman, *The Seventies: The Great Shift in American Culture, Society, and Politics* (Boston: DeCapo, 2002), 171.

24. Alfred Kadushin and Judith A. Martin, eds., *Child Welfare Services*, 4th ed. (London: Pearson, 1988), 539.

25. Zelma Felten, "Adoption Resource Exchanges," *Pediatrics* 23, no. 2 (February 1959), 365–366. Felten served as associate director of the Maas/Engler study in 1959. For community attitudes about the riskiness of adoption in the mid-1950s, see David Kirk, *Shared Fate: A Theory and Method of Adoptive Relationships* (Port Angeles, WA: Ben-Simon, 1984), 25. Trombley noted a parent gap even for "normal, white infants" in 1963 although he backs independent adoptions. William Trombley, "Babies without Homes," *Saturday Evening Post*, February 16, 1963, 16.

26. Anita Colville, "Adoption for the Handicapped Child," in *Readings in Adoption*, ed. I. Evelyn Smith (New York: Philosophical Library, 1963), 201, 203.

27. Franklin and Massarik, "Part I," 459, 462–463; Reid, "Principles," 25.

28. Bernard, *Adoption*, 71–72; Alfred Kadushin, "The Legally Adoptable, Unadopted Child," *Child Welfare* 37, no. 9 (1958): 25.

29. See Herman, *Kinship by Design*, 195–199, 229–246 and E. Wayne Carp, *Family Matters: Secrecy and Disclosure in the History of Adoption* (Cambridge: Harvard University Press, 1998), 168–169.

30. Herman, *Kinship by Design*, 204–215, 229, 246–247, 290. For challenge to transracial placement, see Herman, *Kinship by Design*, 249; Kirk.

31. Other changes include a recognition that birth fathers have rights in adoption, counseling for birth mothers, and postplacement services for adoptive parents. Carp, *Family Matters,* 138–139, 142–143, 147–166.

32. Turitz, 2; Herman, *Kinship by Design*, 196–201.

33. Turitz, 4; Joseph Reid, "Ensuring Adoption for Hard to Place Children," *Child Welfare* 35, no. 3 (1956): 4.

34. David S. Franklin and Fred Massarik, "The Adoption of Children with Medical Conditions: Part III—Discussions and Conclusions," *Child Welfare* 48, no. 10 (1969): 596–597.

35. Herman, *Kinship by Design*, 199–201; Reid, "Ensuring Adoption," 5.

36. I borrow the term "disabling barriers" from Tom Shakespeare, *Disability: The Basics* (New York: Routledge, 2018), chapter 4.

37. Claire Berman, "Parents/Children: Adopting a Multi-handicapped Child," *New York Times*, July 16, 1976, 45; Ann Coyne and Mary Ellen Brown, "Adoption of Children with Developmental Disabilities: A Study of Public and Private Child Welfare Agencies," enclosure in Informational Aids (December 1980), 307–309, CWLA Collection, Box 57, Folder DDAP Reaching Out, 2nd of 2, SWHA.

38. See also Bernice Boehm, "Deterrents to the Adoption of Children in Foster Care," Appendix A: Schedules for Recording Case Material", i, CWLA Collection, Box 60, Folder: Adoption: Parent Selection, SWHA.

39. "Classification of Family for ARENA" (1968), 1, 4. CWLA Collection, Box 18, Folder 4, SWHA.

40. Paul Longmore, "A Note on Language and Social Identity of Disabled People," *American Behavioral Scientist* 28, no. 3 (January/February 1985): 420; Turitz, 3; Reid, "Principles," 23.

41. Vicedo, 40; Bernard, 72; Lucie K. Browning, "The Placement of the Child Needing Adoption: Recent Changes in Practice," *Child Welfare League of America Bulletin* 23, no. 7 (1944): 13; Bowlby.

42. Bernard, 72.

43. Ruth O'Brien, *Crippled Justice: The History of Modern Disability Policy in the Workplace* (Chicago: University of Chicago Press, 2001), 7. For adoption in American culture as itself a form of rehabilitation, see Marina Fedosik, "Orphan and a Member of the Family: Disability and Secrecy in Narratives of Disrupted Eastern European Adoption," *Adoption and Culture: The Interdisciplinary Journal of the Alliance for the Study of Adoption and Culture* 3 (2012): 10, 14–15.

44. See Beatrice Wright, *Physical Disability: A Psychological Approach* (New York: Harper and Brothers, 1960), xviii.

45. O'Brien, 7, 8, 68, 78, 84, 88; Henri-Jacques Stiker, *History of Disability*, trans. William Sayers (Ann Arbor: University of Michigan Press, 1999), 128.

46. O'Brien, 65.

47. Katherine Ott, "The Sum of Its Parts: An Introduction to Modern Histories of Prosthetics," in *Artificial Parts, Practical Lives: Modern Histories of Prosthetics*, ed. Katherine Ott, David Serlin, and Stephen Mihm (New York: New York University Press, 2002), 15; Fairchild, 493; Chloe Silverman, *Understanding Autism: Parents, Doctors, and the History of a Disorder* (Princeton: Princeton University Press, 2012), 108; Bernard, *Adoption*, 78.

48. Wright, 2; O'Brien, 59; Harlan Hahn, "Toward a Politics of Disability: Definitions, Disciplines, and Policies," *Independent Living Institute*, 1985, www.independentliving.org/docs4/hahn2.html.

49. Turitz, 13.

50. Daniel J. Wilson, "Crippled Manhood: Infantile Paralysis and the Construction of Masculinity," *Medical Humanities Review* 12, no. 2 (Fall 1998): 10, 12, 15–16; Rembis, "Athlete First," 113–115; Robert McRuer, *Crip Theory: Cultural Signs of Queerness and Disability* (New York: New York University Press, 2006), 16–18; Anna Waldschmidt, "Who Is Normal? Who Is Deviant? 'Normality' and 'Risk' in Genetic Diagnostics and Counseling," in *Foucault and the Government of Disability*, ed. Shelley Tremain (Ann Arbor: University of Michigan Press, 2005), 191–192, 195–196. Thanks to Aly Patsavas for recommending this path.

51. Dorcas R. Hardy, "Adoption of Children with Special Needs: A National Perspective," *American Psychologist* 39, no. 8 (August 1984): 901; Penny L. Deiner, Nancy J. Wilson, and Donald G. Unger, "Motivation and Characteristics of Families Who Adopt Children with Special Needs: An Empirical Study," *Topics in Early Childhood Special Education* 8, no. 2 (1988): 15–16; Sallie R. Churchill,

Bonnie Carlson, and Lynn Nybell, eds., *No Child Is Unadoptable: A Reader on Adoption of Children with Special Needs* (Beverly Hills: SAGE, 1979).

52. A localized history using specific adoption agency records may be able to explore this issue in more detail. Since this book investigates the macro-dynamics of disability and adoption, its records made it more difficult to examine specifics.

53. Kriste Lindenmeyer, *A Right to Childhood: The US Children's Bureau and Child Welfare, 1912–1946* (Urbana: University of Illinois Press, 1997), 139.

54. Reid, "Principles," 24; Joseph Reid, "Next Steps: Action Called For—Recommendations," in *Children in Need of Parents*, ed. Henry S. Maas and Richard E. Engler Jr. (New York: Columbia University Press, 1959), 379; CWLA, "Supply and Demand in ARENA: An Analysis of the Relation of Characteristics of Children Registered with ARENA and the Characteristics Acceptable to Families Registered" (May 1972), 1, CWLA Collection, Box 18, Folder 4, SWHA; Clayton Hagen, "Placement of the Minority Race Child," in *Frontiers in Adoption: Finding Homes for the "Hard to Place,"* Conference Proceedings of October 1967 (Ann Arbor: NACAC, 1969), 34.

55. Henry S. Maas, "The Successful Adoptive Parent Applicant," *Social Work* 5, no. 1 (January 1960): 14–20, as quoted in Robert E. Young, "From Matching to Making in Adoption: The Interest of Adoptive Applicants in the 'Hard-to-Place' Child," Ph.D. diss., University of Pennsylvania, 1971, 51; Boehm, "Deterrents to the Adoption of Children in Foster Care" (December 1958), 10; Donald Chambers, "Willingness to Adopt Atypical Children," *Child Welfare* 49, no. 5 (May 1970): 272; Robert Lewis, "Adoption and Mental Retardation," *Pediatric Annals* 18, no. 10 (1989): 644; Kravik, "Editorial," 2.

56. Bernice Boehm, "Deterrents to the Adoption of Foster Care," speech at the National Conference on Social Welfare, Morrison Hotel, Chicago, IL (May 15, 1958), 8, CWLA Collection, Box 15, Folder 7, SWHA.

57. Veronica Strong-Boag, "'Children of Adversity': Disabilities and Child Welfare in Canada from the Nineteenth to the Twenty-First Century," *Journal of Family History* 32 (2007): 417.

58. Christopher Unger, Gladys Dwarshuis, and Elizabeth Johnson, *Chaos, Madness and Unpredictability: Placing the Child with Ears like Uncle Harry's, the Spaulding Approach to Adoption* (Chelsea, MI: Spaulding for Children, 1977), 64.

59. Unger, Dwarshuis, and Johnson, 64.

60. Goffman; Gliedman and Roth; Liat Ben-Moshe, "Genealogies of Resistance to Incarceration: Abolition Politics within Deinstitutionalization and Anti-prison Activism in the US," Ph.D. diss., Syracuse University, 2011, 129–135, 155–160.

61. For disability studies perspective on how "special needs" actually reinforces difference, see Longmore, "A Note on Language and Social Identity of Disabled People," 421.

62. Mildred Jacobs and Margaret Kahn, "A Follow-up Study of 'Hard-to-Place' Adopted Children" (unpublished MSS thesis, Graduate Department of Social Work and Social Research, Bryn Mawr College, 1965), as quoted in Young, 3.

63. Statement by Elizabeth S. Cole, 9. The term "hard-to-place" continued to be used, even in NACA reports well into the 1970s. See *Adoption Report: North American Center on Adoption* 1, no. 3 (Fall 1976): 1, CWLA Collection, Box 18, Folder 5, SWHA.

64. For an early example of "special needs," see Esther M. Jacquith, "An Adoption Resource Exchange under Private Auspices," *Child Welfare* (May 1962): 217, CWLA Collection, Box 18, Folder 3, SWHA. See also "Adoption Exchanges, Serving Children in Need of Adoption," California Citizens Adoption Committee (June 1965), 31, CWLA Collection, Box 18, Folder 3, SWHA.

65. Carol Smith, Final Report: Developmental Disabilities Adoption Project: North American Center on Adoption (December 1981): I, 75, CWLA Collection, Box 57 Folder: Developmental Disabilities Adoption Project, 1 of 3, SWHA. See Ronald C. Hughes and Judith S. Rycus, *Child Welfare Services for Children with Developmental Disabilities* (New York: CWLA Press, 1982).

66. Pine, "Child Welfare Reform," 342; Laura Curran, "'Longing to 'Belong': Foster Children in Mid-century Philadelphia (1946–1963)," *Journal of Social History* 42, no. 2 (Winter 2008): 440; Ann Coyne and Mary Ellen Brown, "Developmentally Disabled Children Can Be Adopted," *Child Welfare* 64, no. 6 (November–December 1985): 607; Lewis, 641; Mary Ann Mason, *From Father's Property to Children's Rights* (New York: Columbia University Press, 1994), chap. 4.

67. Kittay, 560.

68. Joseph Shapiro, *No Pity: People with Disabilities Forging a New Civil Rights Movement* (New York: Three Rivers, 1994), 38.

69. Ralph L. Osgood, *The History of Special Education: A Struggle for Equality in American Public Schools* (Westport, CT: Praeger, 2008), 108.

70. Evelyn Hart, "How Retarded Children Can Be Helped," quoted in Janice Brockley, "Rearing the Child Who Never Grew: Ideologies of Parenting and Intellectual Disability in American History," in *Mental Retardation in America: A Historical Reader*, ed. Steven Noll and James W. Trent (New York: New York University Press, 2004), 141–142, 144, 154.

71. Brockley, "Rearing the Child," 147, 155–156.

72. Brockley, "Rearing the Child," 146; Plant, Loc. 1706, 1724.

73. Kadushin, "The Legally Adoptable, Unadopted Child," 25.

74. Mrs. Neville Weeks, "Broadening Concepts of Adoptability and Acceptability in Adoption" (1956), 46, CWLA Collection, Box 16, Folder 6, SWHA.

75. Weeks, 48

76. Colville, "Adoption for the Handicapped Child," 201.

77. Kadushin, "The Legally Adoptable, Unadopted Child," 25.

78. Joseph Goldstein, Anna Freud, and Alfred Solnit, *Beyond the Best Interests of the Child* (New York: Free Press, 1973).

79. Alice Lake, "Babies for the Brave," *Saturday Evening Post*, July 31, 1954, 63, 65.

80. Lake, 26–27.

81. Berman, 45; See also "Three Disabled Children Wait for Adoption," *New York Times*, June 6, 1961, 67; Ruth Carlton, "Talking's Hard, but John, 11, Is Catching On," *Sunday News* (Detroit), May and December, 1975, reproduced in Family Builders by Adoption, *Waiting Child* (April 1977), CWLA Collection, Box 59: NACA, SWHA.

82. Anna Perrott Rose, *Room for One More* (Boston: Houghton Mifflin Company, 1950), 167.

83. Bosley Crowther, "The Screen in Review: 'Room for One More' Starring Cary Grant, Opens at Warner," *New York Times*, January 16, 1952, 21.

84. John Korty, dir., *Who are the DeBolts? And Where Did They Get Nineteen Kids?* Sanrio Communications, 1977.

85. For caring labor, love and disability in the mid-1960s, see Silverman, 108.

86. David S. Franklin and Fred Massarik, "Adoption of Children with Medical Conditions: Part III—Discussions and Conclusions," *Child Welfare* 48, no. 10 (1969): 597–598.

87. Deborah Lupton, *Risk and Everyday Life* (London: SAGE, 2003), Loc. 628 (Kindle).

88. Franklin and Massarik, Part III, 597–598.

89. Elizabeth S. Cole, "Acknowledgement," in Kathryn Wheeler, *Tanya: The Building of a Family through Adoption* (New York: North American Center on Adoption, Child Welfare League of America, 1979), 1.

90. Cole, "Acknowledgement," in Wheeler, 1; Alison Piepmeier, "Saints, Sages, and Victims: Endorsement of and Resistance to Cultural Stereotypes in Memoirs by Parents of Children with Disabilities," *Disability Studies Quarterly* 32, no. 1 (2012): 4, https://dsq-sds.org/article/view/3031.

91. Wheeler, 2.

92. Wheeler, 5.

93. Wheeler, 8.

94. Silverman, 127.

95. Wheeler, 8, 22, 32.

96. Molly Ladd-Taylor and Lauri Umansky, "Introduction," in *"Bad" Mothers: The Politics of Blame in Twentieth-Century America*, ed. Molly Ladd-Taylor and Lauri Umansky (New York: New York University Press, 1998), 16; Katha Pollitt, " 'Fetal Rights': A New Assault on Feminism," *Nation,* March 26, 1990, 409–411; Jane Taylor McDonnell, "On Being the 'Bad' Mother, " in *Bad Mothers: The Politics of Blame in Twentieth-Century America*, ed. Molly Ladd-Taylor and Lauri Umansky (New York: New York University Press, 1998), 227; Katarina Wegar, "In Search of Bad Mothers: Social Constructions of Birth and Adoptive Motherhood," *Women's Studies International Forum* 20, no. 10 (1997): 77–78, 82. See epilogue for more recent accounts of similar accusations; Wheeler, 8.

97. Wheeler, 9–10.

98. Wheeler, 12. See also Janice McLaughlin, Dan Goodley, Emma Clavering, and Pamela Fisher, *Families Raising Disabled Children: Enabling Care and Society Justice* (New York: Palgrave MacMillan. 2008),15; Piepmeier, 13.

99. Wheeler, 12; Rosemarie Garland-Thomson, "The Politics of Staring: Visual Rhetorics of Disability in Popular Photography," in *Disability Studies: Enabling the Humanities*, ed. Sharon L. Snyder, Brenda Jo Brueggemann, and Rosemarie Garland-Thomson (New York: Modern Language Association of America, 2002), 56.

100. Garland-Thomson, "The Politics of Staring," 56.

101. Kirk, 247.

102. Wheeler, 14.

103. Piepmeier, 1, 3.

104. Wheeler, 7.

105. Wheeler, 16.

106. Wheeler, 23.

107. Wheeler, 27.

108. Wheeler, 34.

109. Thank you to Claire Decoteau for raising this point.

110. "A Report of a Conference and Its Impact," foreword to *Frontiers in Adoption: Finding Homes for the "Hard to Place,"* Conference Proceedings of October 1967 (Ann Arbor: NACAC, 1969); David Fanshel, "The Exit of Children from Foster Care," *Child Welfare* 30, no. 2 (1971): 65–81; Arthur Emlen, Janet Lahti, Glen Downs, Alec McKay, and Susan Downs, *Overcoming Barriers to Planning for Children in Foster Care* (Portland: Portland State University, Regional Research Institute for Human Services, 1978).

111. Consistent with the critical appraisal of delivery systems in human services during the 1960s and early 1970s and their role in obstructing services, a call for agencies to self-evaluate their part in the growing problem of these children resulted in changes to casework as well as a niche area of special needs adoptions programs and projects. Katherine Nelson, *On the Frontier of Adoption: A Study of Special Needs Adoptive Families* (New York: CWLA, 1985), 30–32. See also chap. 4.

112. Weeks, 43–44.

113. Weeks, 44.

114. Weeks, 48.

115. Colville, 201, 203.

116. Legalization of these adoptions took place between 1977 and 1980. Nelson, *On the Frontier of Adoption*, 34.

117. Liat Ben-Moshe, "Genealogies of Resistance to Incarceration: Abolition Politics within Deinstitutionalization and Anti-prison Activism in the US," Ph.D. diss., Syracuse: Syracuse University, 2011, 158–159.

118. Nelson, *On the Frontier of Adoption*, 32.

119. Nelson, *On the Frontier of Adoption*, 33–34.

120. Nelson, *On the Frontier of Adoption,* 30–32.

121. For earlier instances of workers' attitudes, see Annual Report, Massachusetts Adoption Resource Exchange (1958), 3, Children's Bureau Collection, Folder: Adoption 1958–1962, Box 889, RG 102, National Archives; Nelson, *On the Frontier of Adoption*, 37.

122. Nelson, *On the Frontier of Adoption*, 32, CWLA 59/Adoption's Frontier, 2 of 2, SWHA.

123. Annual Report, Massachusetts Adoption Resource Exchange, 2; Young, 93.

124. CWLA, Guide for Establishing an Adoption Resource Exchange (year not noted, but likely 1960s), 10, CWLA Collection, Box 18, Folder 2, SWHA; Kadushin, "Study of Adoptive Parents," 231; Muriel McCrea, "The Mix-Match Controversy," in *Frontiers in Adoption: Finding Homes for the "Hard to Place,"* Conference Proceedings of October 1967 (Ann Arbor: NACAC, 1969), 61; Herman, *Kinship by Design*, 236.

125. William Downs, "Is There Life after birth?," *Frontiers in Adoption: Finding Homes for the "Hard to Place,"* Conference Proceedings of October 1967 (Ann Arbor: NACAC, 1969), 14.

126. Eleanor W. Gordon, "There Is a Time in the Affairs of Children," *CWLA Bulletin* 24, no. 2 (1945): 4–5, 7.

127. Turitz, 13.

128. For accounts of foster parents caring for children with disabilities, see Kadushin, "The Legally Adoptable, Unadopted Child," 22; CWLA, *Standards for Adoption Service, Revised Edition, 1968* (New York: CWLA, 1968), 12.

129. Kravik, "Editorial," 2; Churchill, Carlson, and Nybell, 9.

130. Reid, "Principles," 24.

131. Hagen, "Placement of the Minority Race Child," 31; Bernard, *Adoption*, 86, 99; Donald Brieland, *An Experimental Study of the Selection of Adoptive Parents at Intake* (New York: CWLA, 1959), 25.

132. Brieland, *An Experimental Study*, 25, 33.

133. *Guidelines for Adoption Services*, 11; Schulman, 171–189.

134. Joan Cook, "Adoptions of Disabled Children Sought," *New York Times*, January 31, 1976, 40.

135. For single-parent adoptions, see Kadushin, "Single Parent Adoptions," 265–267; Victoria Irwin, "Adoption Process Becoming More Flexible," *Boca Raton News*, December 28, 1980, 3B.

136. Herman, *Kinship by Design*, 204; Kadushin, "Single Parent Adoptions," 263–274.

137. North American Center on Adoption, *The Plight of the Waiting Child: Children in Need of Parents* (New York: CWLA, 1976), 6, 7, 10. The same type of arrangement had been made for Black foster parents in Pennsylvania. See Herman, *Kinship by Design*, 236; Kadushin, "The Legally Adoptable, Unadopted Child," 22–25.

138. Nelson, *On the Frontier of Adoption*, 28. Danny's handicap is not mentioned in the text.

139. Nelson, *On the Frontier of Adoption*, 28; Ann Coyne and Mary Ellen Brown, *Adoption of Children with Developmental Disabilities: A Study of Public and Private Child Welfare Agencies* (New York: CWLA, 1980), 614.

140. Kirk; Clayton Hagen, "A Challenge to the Community," in *Frontiers in Adoption: Finding Homes for the "Hard to Place,"* Conference Proceedings of October 1967 (Ann Arbor: NACAC, 1969), 4. For women and self-realization as individuals during this period, see Plant, Loc. 2207, 2306, 2313, 2413, 2429 (Kindle)

141. Hagen, "A Challenge to the Community," 4.

142. Hagen, "A Challenge to the Community," 5–6; Hagen, "Placement of the Minority Race Child," 30. Separation of parent ego from the child is a condition of attentive love for Ruddick, 358.

143. Quoted in Linda Anne Babb and Rita Laws, *Adopting and Advocating for the Special Needs Child: A Guide for Parents and Professionals* (Westport: Bergen and Garvey, 1997), 14.

144. This letter is distinctive in providing information on adoption by disabled people in the early 1960s. Zelma J. Felten to Adoption Resource Exchanges and State Departments of Public Welfare (November 9, 1961), CWLA Collection, Box 18, Folder 3, SWHA.

145. Anna M. Dixon to CWLA (October 30, 1961), CWLA Collection, Box 18, Folder 3, SWHA.

146. Anna M. Dixon to CWLA.

147. Although there could have been earlier requests similar to this one, I did not find any, suggesting a cultural opportunity for such inquiries to be made (considered even a possibility) during this period, and a disability organization's interest in about adoption for its members.

148. See case of the Cobbs featured in Evan McLeod Wylie, "ARENA Breaks the Adoption Barrier," *Denver Post*, September 27, 1970, 3, CWLA Collection, Box 18, Folder 4, SWHA; Denise Sherer Jacobson, *The Question of David: A Disabled Mother's Journey through Adoption, Family, and Life* (Berkeley: Creative Arts, 1999). Only with the ADA in 1990 was discrimination legally forbidden against disabled applicants. See Madelyn Freundlich and Lisa Peterson, *Adoption and the Americans with Disabilities Act: An Issue Brief* (Washington, DC: CWLA Press, 2000).

149. Young, 102–104; Lewis, 641.

150. David S. Franklin and Fred Massarik, "The Adoption of Children with Medical Conditions: Part II—The Families Today," *Child Welfare* 48, no. 9 (December 1969): 537.

151. Kadushin, "A Study of Adoptive Parents," 227–228, 232–233; Franklin and Massarik, "Part I," 466.

152. Herman, *Kinship by Design*, 204.

153. Judith DeLeon and Judy Westerberg, *Who Adopts Retarded Children?* (Westfield, NJ: Spaulding for Children, 1980), 2, CWLA Collection, Box 58, Folder NAIES, SWHA.

154. By including this observation, they revealed an aesthetic bias of workers when practicing their craft.

155. DeLeon and Westerberg, 7.

156. Henry S. Maas and Richard E. Engler Jr., eds., *Children in Need of Parents* (New York: Columbia University Press, 1959); Kadushin, "A Study of Adoptive Parents"; Franklin and Massarik; DeLeon and Westerberg.

157. Franklin and Massarik, Part I, 461; Part II, 537; Part III, 597.

158. Franklin and Massarik, Part I, 464; Part II, 539; Part III, 599. See also Jessica Martucci, *Back to the Breast: Natural Motherhood and Breastfeeding in America* (Chicago: University of Chicago Press, 2015), 100 (Kindle).

159. Franklin and Massarik, Part III, 599. See also Anita Lightburn, *Study of Mediation of Chronic Illness and Handicap by Special Needs Adoptive Families* (New York: Columbia Teachers College, 1989), 367.

160. Maas and Engler, 377.

161. Franklin and Massarik, Part III, 595, 598.

162. Maas and Engler, 377; Maas, 18.

163. DeLeon and Westerberg, 1–6.

164. Brockley, "Rearing the Child," 151. See epilogue for the twenty-first century examples.

165. Intellectual disability was defined here as an IQ of less than 90. Maas, 16, 18.

166. DeLeon and Westerberg, 1–6.

167. Chambers, 272–279; McCrea, 61.

168. Herman, *Kinship by Design*, 200–201.

169. McCrea argued that having exposure to disability in one's family necessarily enables adoption of a disabled child. On the other hand, she also found that some parents wanted children with a trait that they knew nothing about. McCrea, 61.

170. McCrea, 62.

171. Joseph Davis and Patricia Montgomery, "Adoption Planning for Handicapped Children," *Clinical Pediatrics* 20, no. 4 (1981): 293; Lewis, 638.

172. Davis and Montgomery, 293; Ruddick, 358.

Chapter Four

1. Ralph L. Osgood, *The History of Special Education: A Struggle for Equality in American Public Schools* (Westport, CT: Praeger, 2008), 99.

2. Catherine E. Rymph, "From 'Economic Want' to 'Family Pathology': Foster Family Care, the New Deal and the Emergence of a Public Child Welfare System," *Journal of Policy History* 24, no. 1(2012): 16; Henrietta Gordon, "Long-Time Care," *Child Welfare* 29, no. 1 (1950): 3; Joseph Reid statement in *Children in Need of Parents*, ed. Henry S. Maas and Richard E. Engler Jr. (New York: Columbia University Press, 1959), 379–380; Kathy Barbell and Madelyn Freundlich,

Foster Care Today (Washington, DC: Casey Family Programs National Center for Resource Family Support, 2001), 1–2.

3. Paul Longmore, *Telethons: Spectacle, Disability, and the Business of Charity* (Oxford: Oxford University Press, 2016), 172. For the disparity between parents' desires and children's needs, see Barbara Pine, "Child Welfare Reform and the Political Process," *Social Service Review* 60, no. 3 (1986): 341–342. "Uneven relationship" comes from Cecelia E. Sudia, "Permanency Planning: A Case History of a Children's Bureau Initiative: Including Some Unresolved Issues," presentation at the Community University Symposium, Minneapolis, April 11, 1980, 15, quoted in Pine, "Child Welfare Reform," 341–342.

4. Rymph, "From 'Economic Want,'" 17–18.

5. Barbell and Freundlich, 1–3; Anthony Maluccio and Edith Fein, "Permanency Planning: A Redefinition," *Child Welfare* 62 (May–June 1983): 200.

6. Judith S. Hughes and Ronald C. Rycus, *Child Welfare Services for Children with Developmental Disabilities* (New York: CWLA, 1982), 30–32. For contemporary situation, see epilogue.

7. Henry S. Maas and Richard E. Engler Jr., eds., *Children in Need of Parents*, 374–375; North American Center on Adoption, *The Plight of the Waiting Child: Children in Need of Parents* (New York: CWLA, 1976), 6; Clara J. Swan, "The Adoption Resource Exchange of North America: A New Service for Adoption Agencies," *Juvenile Court Judges Journal* 19, no. 3 (1968): 86; Tim Hacsi, "From Indenture to Family Foster Care: a Brief History of Child Placing. In A *History of Child Welfare*, ed. Eve P. Smith and Lisa A. Merkel-Holguin (New Brunswick: Transaction, 1996), 167.

8. Maas and Engler, 356–362; North American Center on Adoption, *The Plight of the Waiting Child*, 1; David Fanshel, "The Exit of Children from Foster Care," *Child Welfare* 50, no. 2 (1971): 65–81; Alfred Kadushin, "A Study of Adoptive Parents of Hard-to-Place Children," *Social Casework* 43 (May 1962): 227–233.

9. CWLA, *Standards for Adoption Service, Revised Edition, 1978* (New York: CWLA, 1978), 9; CWLA, *Standards for Adoption Services, Revised Edition, 1988* (New York: CWLA, 1988), 3; Stevi Jackson and Sue Scott, "Risk Anxiety and the Social Construction of Childhood," in *Risk and Sociocultural Theory: New Directions and Perspectives*, ed. Deborah Lupton (Cambridge: Cambridge University Press, 1999), 86–87, 91.

10. Edward Schor, "The Foster Care System and Health Status of Foster Children," *Pediatrics* 69 (1982): 526.

11. Joseph Reid, "Ensuring Adoption for Hard to Place Children." *Child Welfare* 35, no. 3 (1956): 6, 8.

12. Reid, " Ensuring Adoption, 6, 8; Gordon, "Long-Time Care," 3–8.

13. See chapter 2.

14. Bernice Boehm, "Deterrents to the Adoption of Children in Foster Care" (December 1958), 8, CWLA Collection, Box 60, Folder: Adoption: Parent Selection.

SWHA; Bernice Boehm, "Deterrents to the Adoption of Foster Care," speech at the National Conference on Social Welfare, Morrison Hotel, Chicago, IL (May 15, 1958), 2, 8, CWLA Collection, Box 15, Folder 7, SWHA.

15. Boehm, "Deterrents" (December 1958), 7–8, 10, 27–29; Boehm, "Deterrents" (May 1958), 5, 23.

16. Joseph Goldstein, Anna Freud, and Alfred Solnit, *Beyond the Best Interests of the Child* (New York: Free Press, 1973), 19.

17. Goldstein, Freud, and Solnit, 18–19, 32.

18. Maluccio and Fein, "Permanency Planning," 197.

19. Anthony Maluccio and Edith Fein, "Family Preservation in Perspective," *Journal of Family Strengths* 6, no. 1 (2002): 1; CWLA, *Standards for Adoption Service, 1958* (New York: CWLA, 1958), 1.

20. Maluccio and Fein, "Family Preservation in Perspective," 1.

21. Laura Curran, "Longing to 'Belong'; Foster Children in Mid-century Philadelphia (1946–1963)," *Journal of Social History* 42, no. 2 (Winter 2008): 427, 430, 432–435, 437, 440.

22. Inspired by John Bowlby's theory of attachment and his work on childhood mourning as well as evidence derived from the study of institutionalized children, the diagnostic category of "attachment disorder" emerged in the 1980s to describe many of these ensuing problems. M. Ainsworth, M. Boston, J. Bowlby, and D. Rosenbluth, "The Effects of Mother-Child Separation: A Follow-Up Study," *British Journal of Medical Psychology* 29, no. 3–4 (1956): 211–247; Inge Bretherton, "The Origins of Attachment Theory: John Bowlby and Mary Ainsworth," *Developmental Psychology* 28 (1992): 759–775.

23. The foster parents who took these children received higher foster care subsidies. Brad Bryant, *Special Foster Care: A History and Rationale* (Verona, VA: People Places, 1980), 18–19, 26–34, 36–39.

24. Social scientists, meanwhile, produced research that showed that individuals gained more skills in community settings than they did in institutions. Similar deinstitutionalization trends released residents from psychiatric and juvenile detention facilities. Deborah S. Metzel, "Historical Social Geography," *Mental Retardation in America: A Historical Reader*, ed. Steven Noll and James W. Trent Jr. (New York: New York University Press, 2004), 432; David J. Rothman and Sheila M. Rothman, "The Litigator as Reformer," in *Mental Retardation in America: A Historical Reader*, ed. Steven Noll and James W. Trent Jr. (New York: New York University Press, 2004), 446; Kim Nielsen. *A Disability History of the United States* (Boston: Beacon, 2012), 164; Allison Carey, *On the Margins of Citizenship: Intellectual Disability and Civil Rights in Twentieth-Century America* (Philadelphia: Temple University Press, 2009), 92; Nina Bernstein, *The Lost Children of Wilder* (New York: Vintage, 2002), 8, 23.

25. Wolf Wolfensberger, *The Principle of Normalization in Human Services* (Toronto: National Institute on Mental Retardation. 1972); Bengt Nirje, "The

Normalisation Principle and Its Human Management Implications," in *Changing Patterns in Residential Services for the Mentally Retarded*, ed. R. Kugel and W. Wolfensberger (Washington, DC: President's Committee on Mental Retardation, 1969); Education for All Act, P.L. 94-142, 89 Stat. 773 at 793 (1975); *Wyatt v. Stickney*, 344 F. Supp. 373 (M.D. Ala. 1972).

26. According to Robert Perske, "The Dignity of Risk," *Mental Retardation* 10, no. 1 (1972): 24, 26, the "mentally retarded" had been subjected to a regime of risk avoidance or minimization via a circumscribed set of community interaction, relationships with the opposite sex, employment and recreation, and even the institutional architecture that housed them. See also Rothman and Rothman, "Litigator," 450; David J. Rothman and Sheila M. Rothman, *The Willowbrook Wars: Bringing the Mentally Disabled into the Community* (New Brunswick: Aldine Transaction, 2009), 48.

27. Thank you to Aly Patsavas for this insight.

28. Betsy Williams, Connie Lavine, and Kathryn Bell, "Working with Handicapped Children and Their Families," prepared for the Developmental Disability Adoption Project, All of Georgia Crippled Children's Clinic in Atlanta, enclosed in Developmental Disability Adoptions Project: Child Assessment Material (no date but probably 1980), 31, 34, CWLA Collection, Box 57, Folder: DDAP; Hughes and Rycus, 37, 39; John Gliedman and William Roth, *The Unexpected Minority: Handicapped Children in America* (New York: Harcourt, Brace, Jovanovich, 1980), pt. 2; Sandra M. Sufian, "As Long as Parents Can Accept Them: Medical Disclosure, Risk, and Disability in Twentieth-Century American Adoption Practice," *Bulletin of the History of Medicine* 91, no. 1 (Spring 2017): 117–119.

29. Clayton Hagen, "A Challenge to the Community," in *Frontiers in Adoption: Finding Homes for the "Hard to Place,"* Conference Proceedings of October 1967 (Ann Arbor: CWLA, 1969), 2; Reid statement in Maas and Engler, 379.

30. Clyde Farrington, "Foster Care Program for Formerly Institutionalized Multiple Handicapped Individuals in Alaska," from monograph no. 1, Model Programs in HEW, Regions IX–X for Developmental Disabilities, December 1977, Informational Aids, 238–239, CWLA Collection. Box 57, Folder: Developmental Disabilities Adoption Project Reaching Out, 2 of 2, SWHA.

31. Farrington, 238–240.

32. Karen Dubinsky, *Babies without Borders: Adoption and Migration across the Americas* (Toronto: University of Toronto Press, 2010), 8, 60.

33. See Maas and Engler.

34. Carey, 109, 115.

35. Mary Jean McDonald, "The Citizens' Committee for Children of New York and the Evolution of Child Advocacy (1945–1972)," *Child Welfare* 74, no. 1 (1995): 297–299. Joyce and Peter Forsythe of Ann Arbor founded COAC in the 1960s. In October 1967, the COAC sponsored the conference "Frontiers in Adoption." McDonald, 300.

36. Christopher Unger, Gladys Dwarshuis, and Elizabeth Johnson, *Chaos, Madness and Unpredictability . . . Placing the Child with Ears like Uncle Harry's, the Spaulding Approach to Adoption* (Chelsea, MI: Spaulding for Children 1977), 4–8.

37. Unger, Dwarshuis, and Johnson, xi.

38. Thank you to Aly Patsavas for raising this.

39. Unger, Dwarshuis, and Johnson, xiv, 6.

40. Unger, Dwarshuis, and Johnson, xi–xii, 65–66.

41. Unger, Dwarshuis, and Johnson, 101.

42. Some media outlets, however, refused to print photographs of children with what was described as profound disability because of their physical appearance. They were trying to protect the viewers from seeing these children. Robert Lewis, "Adoption and Mental Retardation," *Pediatric Annals* 18, no. 10 (1989): 640.

43. Unger, Dwarshuis, and Johnson, 116.

44. Jane Kendall and Carol Smith, *Working Together: The Adoption of Children with Developmental Disabilities* (New York: CWLA, 1980), 4–5.

45. Kathryn Donley, "Opening New Doors: Finding Families for Older and Handicapped Children," *Adoption Report: North American Center on Adoption* 1, no. 3 (Fall 1976): 4.

46. For specificity and disability, see Erik Parens and Adrienne Asch, "The Disability Rights Critique of Prenatal Genetic Testing: Reflections and Recommendations," in *Prenatal Testing and Disability Rights*, ed. Erik Parens and Adrienne Asch (Washington, DC: Georgetown University Press, 2000), 3–43; and Adrienne Asch, "Why I Haven't Changed My Mind about Prenatal Diagnosis: Reflections and Refinements," in *Prenatal Testing and Disability Rights*, ed. Erik Parens and Adrienne Asch (Washington, DC: Georgetown University Press, 2000), 234–258; Joan Rothschild, *The Dream of the Perfect Child* (Bloomington: Indiana University Press, 2005).

47. NACA, Part IV: Program Narrative: Application for Continuation of Funding Developmental Disabilities Adoption Project (July 1979), 3, CWLA Collection, Box 58, Folder DDAP, SWHA.

48. Katherine Nelson, "On Adoption's Frontier," chap. 4, 27 (unpublished), CWLA Collection, Box 59: Adoption's Frontier, 2 of 2, SWHA; David S. Franklin and Fred Massarik, "The Adoption of Children with Medical Conditions: Part III—Discussions and Conclusions," *Child Welfare* 48, no. 10 (1969): 599–600.

49. See Ann Gath, "Mentally Retarded Children in Substitute and Natural Families," *Adoption and Fostering* 7, no. 1 (1983): 35, 37–39.

50. Katherine Nelson, *On the Frontier of Adoption*, 34–36, 85–86.

51. Gliedman and Roth, 95; Longmore, *Telethons*, 172–173, 177, 181–182.

52. CWLA, "Supply and Demand in ARENA" (May 1972), 5, CWLA Collection, Box 18, Folder 4, SWHA.

53. CWLA, "Supply and Demand in ARENA," 9–11; Barbara E. Lewis, ARENA Progress Report #1 (January 1, 1971–June 30, 1971), 2, 5. CWLA Collection, Box 18, Folder 4. SWHA.

54. Patricia Ryan and Bruce L. Warren, *Finding Families for the Children: A Handbook to Assist the Child Welfare Worker in the Placement of Children with a Mental, Emotional or Physical Handicap* (Washington, DC: US Department of Health, Education, and Welfare, 1974), i.

55. "A Proposal of the Child Welfare League of America to Establish a National Adoption Resource Exchange" (April 1966), 1, CWLA Collection, Box 18, Folder 3, SWHA; Adoption Resource Exchange of America (1968) 8, CWLA Collection, Box 18, Folder 3, SWHA; Resume of the Work of the Adoptions Committee, 1954–1957, (April 1957), 1, 3. Children's Bureau Collection, Box 889, File: Adoption 1958–1962, Record Group 102, National Archives.

56. "A Proposal of the Child Welfare League of America to Establish a National Adoption Resource Exchange" (April 1966), 3, CWLA Collection, Box 18, Folder 3, SWHA; National Adoption Project (March 11, 1955), 5–6, CWLA Collection, Box 15, Folder 7, SWHA; Clara Swan, "The Adoption Resource Exchange of North America: A New Service for Adoption Agencies," *Juvenile Court Judges Journal* 19, no. 3 (November 1968): 86; Zelma J. Felten, " Use of Adoption Resource Exchanges," paper given at New England Regional Conference, Boston (March 1958), 1, CWLA Collection, Box 18, Folder 3, SWHA; Reid, "Ensuring Adoption," 6; William Downs, "Is There Life after Birth?" in *Frontiers in Adoption: Finding Homes for the "Hard to Place,"* Conference Proceedings of October 1967 (Ann Arbor: NACAC, 1969), 14.

57. Margaret Jacobs, "Remembering the 'Forgotten Child': The American Indian Child Welfare Crisis of the 1960s and 1970s," *American Indian Quarterly* 37 no. 1–2 (Winter/Spring 2013): 140.

58. Swan, 86.

59. Evan McLeod Wylie, "ARENA breaks the Adoption Barrier," Contemporary, *Denver Post* (September 27, 1970): 3. Reprinted from Reader's Digest. CWLA Collection, Box 18, Folder 4, SWHA.

60. Natalie Jaffe, "National Agency to Aid Adoption: Clearinghouse Planned Here by Child Welfare League," *New York Times*, June 19, 1966, CWLA Collection, Box 16, Folder 2, SWHA; news release, National Adoption Resource Exchange (June 16, 1966), 2, CWLA Collection, Box 16, Folder 2, 2, SWHA; "A Proposal of the Child Welfare League of America to Establish a National Adoption Resource Exchange" (April 1966), 2, CWLA Collection, Box 18, Folder 3, SWHA.

61. Here Reid is speaking of racial prejudice but the logic remains true for all kinds of prejudice. Wylie2. See also Jacobs on Arnold Lyslo and the Indian Adoption Project. Jacobs, 140.

62. Adoption Resource Exchange of North America pamphlet (n.d), back page, CWLA Collection, Box 59, Folder NACA, SWHA.

63. Adoption Resource Exchange of North America pamphlet.

64. The original proposed budget for the national exchange was $82,000 and it was intended to transfer administration to the Children's Bureau after three

years. "A Proposal of the Child Welfare League of America to Establish a National Adoption Resource Exchange" (April 1966), 4–6, CWLA Collection, Box 18, Folder 3, SWHA.

65. Other agencies not on the exchange also adopted this criterion. C. H. Krisheff, "Adoption Agency Services for the Retarded," *Mental Retardation* 15 no. 1 (1977): 38.

66. Procedural Manual and Client Forms: Supplement to Conceptual Design of a National Adoption Exchange. Submitted to Children's Bureau Department of Health and Human Services, Contract 105-79-1102 (September 28, 1982), 77–78, CWLA Collection, Box 58, Folder NAIES, 1981, 1 of 2, SWHA.

67. Statement by Elizabeth S. Cole, director, North American Center on Adoption, Special Project, Child Welfare League of America, Inc., before the Subcommittee on Children and Youth, United States Senate (July 14, 1975): 2, 15, CWLA Collection, Box 18, Folder 5, SWHA.

68. National American Center on Adoption, *Plight of the Waiting Child*, 12.

69. Press Release, North American Center on Adoption (March 1977), 1, CWLA Collection, Box 59, Folder NACA, SWHA; Gilbert Y. Steiner, *The Children's Cause* (Washington, DC: Brookings Institution, 1976), 152.

70. In 1976, Bill Cosby joined Family Builders as its national honorary chairman. Family Builders pamphlet, CWLA Collection, Box 59, North American Center on Adoption folder, SWHA.

71. Final Report submitted to Children's Bureau from NAIES (September 1982), 5, CWLA Collection, Box 58, Folder NAIES 1979–1982, SWHA.

72. Carol E. Smith, Project Description: Developmental Disabilities Adoption Project, North American Center on Adoption, Child Welfare League of America (December 6, 1979), 6, CWLA Collection, Box 56, Folder Developmental Disabilities Adoptions Project, SWHA; Marc Leepson, "Issues in Child Adoption." *Editorial Research Reports 1984* (vol. 2) (Washington, DC: CQ Press), 2, http://library.cqpress.com/xsite/document.php?id=cqresrre1984111600.

73. NAIES, funded through the Children's Bureau of the DHHS, ended on September 30, 1982. Information Resource Services of CWLA to Friends of Waiting Children, January 1983, CWLA Collection, Box 97: Folder: Adoption Policy 1976–1982; Krisheff, 38.

74. "Definitions and Descriptions of Adoption Exchanges" (1982), 1948, CWLA Collection, Box 58, Folder NAIES 1982 2 of 2, SWHA.

75. CWLA/NACA, Addendum to Technical Proposal for the Development and Implementation of a National Adoption Information Exchange System, submitted to Dept. of HEW, Office of Human Development Services by CWLA/NACA (September 19, 1979), A3, CWLA Collection, Box 58, Folder NAIES 1979–1982, SWHA; Procedural Manual and Client Forms: Supplement to Conceptual Design of a National Adoption Exchange. Submitted to Children's Bureau Dept. HHS, Contract 105-79-1102 (September 28, 1982), 35, CWLA Collection, Box 58, Folder NAIES, 1981, 1 of 2, SWHA.

76. Title V of the 1978 Act clarified the 1975 federal definition, Council on Developmental Disabilities For the early history of the DD Act, see "An Interview with Elinor Gollay" and "Celebrating the 50th Anniversary of the Developmental Disabilities Act," both of which are at www.mnddc.org/dd/act/documents /FEDREG/90-DDA-LEGLISLATIVEHISTORY.pdf. See also Ann Coyne and Mary Ellen Brown. "Developmentally Disabled Children Can Be Adopted," *Child Welfare* 64, no. 6 (November/December 1985): 608; Ann Coyne and Elizabeth S. Cole, questionnaire for study on placement of children with developmental disabilities (May 1979), 3, CWLA Collection, Box 57, Developmental Disabilities Adoptions Project, SWHA; Carey, 139; Kendall and Smith, 2; Hughes and Rycus, 16.

77. Carol Smith, Final Report: Developmental Disabilities Adoption Project: North American Center on Adoption (December 1981), I, 1, CWLA Collection, Box 57, Folder: Developmental Disabilities Adoption Project, 1 of 3, SWHA; memo, July 17, 1979 from Elizabeth S. Cole and Gerald Cornez to Advisory Board Members, Subject: renewal of HEW DD adoption project, CWLA Collection, Box 57: DDAP, Folder 1 of 3, SWLA.

78. NACA, Developmental Disabilities Adoption Project (February 15, 1980), insert: letter from Elizabeth S. Cole to Office of Human Development, Developmental Disabilities Office, Dept. of Health, Education and Welfare (September 7, 1979), 1, CWLA Collection, Box 56, Folder DDAP, 1980, SWHA.

79. "Adoption Is an Option," *Giant Steps: The Journal of the New York State Office of Mental Retardation and Developmental Disabilities* (February 1980): 249, enclosed within Informational Aids, Developmental Disabilities Adoption Project, "Reaching Out," CWLA Collection, Box 57, Folder DDAP, 2 of 2, SWHA.

80. The study found that adoption disruption—the phenomenon of ending a placement (before legalization) and returning the child to the agency—occurred less frequently among developmentally disabled children than among other special needs children.

81. Smith, Final Report, 29.

82. Kendall and Smith, 1, 187; NACA, Part IV: Program Narrative: Application, 3, 4; Smith, Final Report, 2, 4; Smith, Project Description, 5, Developmental Disabilities Adoption Project, NACA (December 6, 1979), 5, CWLA Collection, Box 56, Folder: DDAP, SWHA.

83. NACA, Developmental Disabilities Adoption Project, 15.

84. NACA, Part IV: Program Narrative, 6; Program Progress Report: Developmental Disabilities Adoption Project (October 1, 1978–June 30, 1979), Appendix I, 2–3, 5, CWLA Collection, Box 58, Folder DDAP, SWHA.

85. NACA, Part IV: Program Narrative: Application, 3.

86. Kendall and Smith, 3.

87. Smith, Final Report, 25.

88. "Adoption Is an Option," *Giant Steps: The Journal of the New York State Office of Mental Retardation and Developmental Disabilities* (February 1980),

CWLA Collection, Box 57: Developmental Disabilities Adoption Project: Reaching Out, 2 of 2, SWHA; Betsy Cole to Jeanne Hunzeker, Draft Executive Summary of Our HEW Developmental Disabilities Research (January 30, 1981), 5, CWLA Collection, Box 56: DDAP, SWHA; Coyne and Brown, "Developmentally Disabled Children Can Be Adopted," 608.

89. Ann Coyne and Elizabeth S. Cole, Questionnaire for study on placement of children with developmental disabilities (May 1979), 26, 43, 74, CWLA Collection, Box 57, Developmental Disabilities Adoptions Project, SWHA.

90. Ann Coyne and Elizabeth S. Cole, Questionnaire for study on placement of children with developmental disabilities (May 1979), 259, 262, 284, 286, CWLA Collection, Box 57, DDAP, 1981, 2 of 3, SWHA.

91. Smith, Final Report, xi–xii, xix.

92. Smith, Final Report, 14, 16, 18, 25.

93. Smith, Final Report, 35.

94. Kendall and Smith, 4.

95. Together with a similar program in the school of social work, the University of Michigan trained approximately 150 practitioners between 1976 and 1980. David M. Austin, *A History of Social Work Education* (Austin: University of Texas Press, 1986), 28–31.

96. Project CRAFT and the Training Adoption Staff Project, "Values in the Practice of Adoption," in *Training In the Adoption of Children with "Special Needs"* (Ann Arbor: University of Michigan School of Social Work, 1980), 1–4.

97. This changed in 1988 with Title IV-E, US Department of Health and Human Services, Administration for Children and Families, Children's Bureau, Log No. ACYF-PR-88-02.

98. George Seeling, "The Implementation of Subsidized Adoption Problems: A Preliminary Study," *Journal of Family Law* 15 (1977): 739–745.

99. Longmore, *Telethons*, 21, 29, 102, 104–105, 106.

100. CWLA, *Standards for Adoption Service, Revised Edition, 1968* (New York: CWLA, 1968), 72–73, cited in Seeling, 732–733, 740.

101. Sanford N. Katz and Ursula M. Gallagher, "Subsidized Adoption in America." *Family Law Quarterly* 10 (1976): 3; Nelson, *On the Frontier of Adoption*, 26, 162; Franklin and Massarik, Part III, 601n3; Gloria Waldinger, "Subsidized Adoption: How Paid Parents View It," *Social Work* 27, no. 6 (November 1982): 517; Nelson, "On Adoption's Frontier," 3, 518 (unpublished copy), CWLA Collection Box 59: Adoption's Frontier, 2 of 2, SWHA.

102. Katz and Gallagher, 4; Seeling, 734. The act considered children who had an injury at birth with unknown sequelae or a physical disability with a "mental or emotional component which has not yet appeared" as particularly high-risk. A. Klein, "Subsidized Adoptions Cut Costs While Creating Happiness Homes," *Subsidized Adoption in America* 1, no. 1 (1977): 8–9.

103. Chicago and Detroit, two of Nelson's study sites, had long-standing subsidy programs. Another site, Houston, did not and therefore few of her subjects there attained a subsidy. Nelson's study subjects with disabilities included children with cerebral palsy, learning disabilities, visual or hearing impairments, epilepsy, behavioral disorders and intellectual disability. Nelson, *On the Frontier of Adoption*, 49.

104. Coyne and Brown, *Adoption of Children*, 61; Alfred Kadushin and Judith A. Martin, *Child Welfare Services*, 4th ed. (New York: Macmillan, 1988), 538; Katz and Gallagher, 4.

105. Waldinger, 517; Nelson, *On the Frontier of Adoption*, 8, 48.

106. Seeling, 763.

107. Nelson, *On the Frontier of Adoption*, 49–50. For differences in subsidy models, see Seeling, 736.

108. Ryan and Warren, 36; Nelson, *On the Frontier of Adoption*, 88.

109. They averaged $150 for Southern states and $250–$300 for the rest of the country in 1984. Leepson, 4–5.

110. Unger, Dwarshuis, and Johnson, 29.

111. Carey, 152.

112. Kendall and Smith, 10.

113. Kendall and Smith, 11.

114. Katz and Gallagher, 1; Waldinger, 517; Seeling, 859.

115. Nelson, *On the Frontier of Adoption*, 39.

116. Child Abuse Prevention and Treatment and Adoption Reform Act of 1978, PL 95-266 (April 24, 1978): 1, Children's Bureau, "Child Abuse Prevention and Treatment and Adoption Reform Act of 1978, Pub. L. No. 95-266," *Major Federal Legislation Concerned with Child Protection, Child Welfare, and Adoption* (2019), in *Major Legislation Concerned with Child Protection, Child Welfare and Adoption*, 27, https://www.childwelfare.gov/pubpdfs/majorfedlegis.pdf/.

117. Dorcas R. Hardy, "Adoption of Children with Special Needs: A National Perspective," *American Psychologist* 39, no. 8 (1984): 902; Linda Anne Babb and Rita Laws, *Adopting and Advocating for the Special Needs Child: A Guide for Parents and Professionals* (Westport: Bergen and Garvey, 1997), 14. Title XX (1975) of P.L. 93-647 provided federal funds for services needed to promote permanence for children. See Unger, Dwarshuis, and Johnson, 35; Nelson, *On the Frontier of Adoption*, 3. Because of the complexity of its requirements, the Adoption Assistance and Child Welfare Act of 1980 was phased in over three years.

118. Several earlier reform bills that preceded the act in the 1970s that did not pass deeply shaped the 1980 act's component parts. Pine, "Child Welfare Reform," 349; Urban Systems Research and Engineering, *Evaluation of State Activities with Regard to Adoption Disruption: Final Report*, Contract #105-84-8102 Task Order I (Washington, DC: Office of Human Development Services, 1985), 2–11.

119. Judith K. McKenzie, "Adoption of Children with Special Needs," *Future of Children* 3, no. 1 (1993): 2.

120. Pine, "Child Welfare Reform," 354.

121. Pine, "Child Welfare Reform," 355.

122. J. F. Horst, "Adoption Bill Moves Slowly, Unsteadily," *Detroit News*, editorial page, August 10, 1977, CWLA Collection, Box 59: NACA, SWHA; Leepson, 5. For previous attempt in 1977 that meant to use federal dollars for subsidies for disabled children instead of similar money spent on institutionalized care, see Rep. Bill Brodhead (D, MI) to constituent (n.d.), CWLA Collection, Box 59: NACA, SWHA.

123. That same year, California passed the Lanterman Developmental Disabilities Act, which protected the rights of people with developmental disabilities.

124. Hardy, 902.

125. Children's Bureau, "Adoption Assistance and Child Welfare Act of 1980, Pub. L. No. 96-272" in *Major Legislation Concerned with Child Protection, Child Welfare, and Adoption* (Washington, DC: Children's Bureau, 2019), 27, https://www.childwelfare.gov/pubPDFs/majorfedlegis.pdf.

126. Children's Bureau, "Adoption Assistance and Child Welfare Act of 1980."

127. For Pine, "special needs" did not explicitly include Black children, but handicapped and older or sibling groups (who could be Black), Pine, "Child Welfare Reform," 356.

128. States saved about $214 per month per child because of these subsidies. See Penny L. Deiner, Nancy J. Wilson, and Donald G. Unger, "Motivation and Characteristics of Families Who Adopt Children with Special Needs: An Empirical Study," *Topics in Early Childhood Special Education* 8, no. 2 (1988): 17.

129. Hardy, 903.

130. Hardy, 903. See also Robert M. George, Eboni C. Howard, and David Yu, *Adoption, Disruption and Displacement: The Illinois Child Welfare System, 1976–94* (Chicago: Chapin Hall Center for Children at the University of Chicago, 1995), 2, 11, 28; Mary Eschelbach Hansen, "Using Subsidies to Promote the Adoption of Children from Foster Care," *Journal of Family Economic Issues* 28, no. 3 (September 1, 2007): 378.

131. Issued October 8, 1981. National Committee for Adoption, *Model Act for the Adoption of Children with Special Needs: Includes Section-by-Section Comments and Analysis—Model Legislation Series*," 1982, http://eric.ed.gov/?id=ED255292; National Committee for Adoption, *Adoption Factbook: United States Data, Issues, Regulations, and Resources* (November 1985), 171, https://files.eric.ed.gov/fulltext/ED265967/pdf.

132. National Committee for Adoption, *Model Act for the Adoption of Children with Special Needs,* 1–2, 19.

133. See Steiner, 145–149. For same dynamic in Canada, see Veronica Strong-Boag, *Fostering Nation: Canada Confronts Its History of Childhood Disadvantage* (Waterloo: Wilfrid Laurier University Press, 2011), 203; Veronica Strong-Boag, "'Children of Adversity': Disabilities and Child Welfare in Canada from

the Nineteenth to the Twenty-First Century," *Journal of Family History* 32, no. 4 (2007): 426.

Chapter Five

1. Robert Pear, "Many States Fail to Meet Mandates on Child Welfare," *New York Times*, March 17, 1996, 3.

2. Pear, 1.

3. I use the term "special needs" here to maintain the integrity of the phraseology of the period, with the understanding that "special needs" still set apart children with disabilities, rather than embraces difference. Still, the term was operative during this period and used in close to every document dealing with children with disabilities in adoption.

4. By 1977, only 9 percent of all children available for adoption were under the age of one year. CWLA, *Standards for Adoption Service, Revised Edition, 1978* (New York, New York, 1978), 2–3; Pine, "Child Welfare Reform," 342.

5. David Young and Brandt Allen, "Benefit-Cost Analysis in the Social Services: The Example of Adoption Reimbursement," *Social Service Review* 51, no. 2 (1977): 253.

6. Ellen Herman, "Fostering and Foster Care," *The Adoption History Project*, https://pages.uoregon.edu/adoption/topics/fostering.htm. Transnational adoption, including Operation Babylift in the aftermath of the Vietnam War, also took place in the mid-1970s as the foster care system ballooned. Gloria Emerson, "Operation Babylift" (1975), *The Adoption History Project*, https://pages.uoregon.edu/adoption/archive/EmersonOB.htm.

7. Karl Ensign, *Foster Care Summary, 1991* U.S. Department of Health and Human Services, Assistant Secretary for Planning and Evaluation (1991), 1, https://aspe.hhs.gov/basic-report/foster-care-summary-1991.

8. Fred H. Wulczyn, Lijun Chen, and Kristen Brunner Hislop, "Adoption Dynamics and the Adoption and Safe Families Act," *Social Service Review* 80 no. 4 (2006): 584, 604.

9. Judith K. McKenzie, "Adoption of Children with Special Needs," *Future of Children* 1, no. 3 (1993): 2. The American Public Welfare Association estimated a 28.5 percent national increase in the foster care population between 1986 and 1989 (280,000 to 360,000). McKenzie, 5; Barbara Kantrowitz, "Children Lost in the Quagmire," *Newsweek*, May 12, 1991, 64. By 1994, about 400,000 children were in foster homes, while 100,000 children with learning or behavioral disabilities lived in residential care facilities. Richard O'Mara, "Are Orphanages Better for Kids than Welfare?" *Baltimore Sun*, November 27, 1994.

10. Opening statement of Senator Dodd, in *Barriers to Adoption* (1993), Hearings before the Subcommittee on Children, Family, Drugs and Alcoholism of the

Committee on Labor and Human Resources, United States Senate, 103rd Congress, 1st Session, S. Hrg. 103-400, July 15, 1993 (Washington, DC: U.S. Government Printing Office, 1994), 3.

11. Christopher Swann and Michelle Sheran Sylvester, "The Foster Care Crisis: What Caused Caseloads to Grow?," *Demography* 43, no. 2 (May 2006): 309–335.

12. Kantrowitz, 64.

13. Barbara Pine, "Special Families for Special Children: The Adoption of Children with Developmental Disabilities," Ph.D. diss., Brandeis University, Heller School for the Advanced Study of Social Welfare, 1991, 12.

14. Penelope Maza, "Trends in National Data on the Adoption of Children with Handicaps," in *Formed Families: Adoption of Children with Handicaps*, ed. Laraine Masters Glidden (New York: Routledge, 1990), 125, 131.

15. "Adoption in America Surveyed: News Release" (February 14, 1989): 3, Box 97: Folder, CWLA 1988 Adoption Survey CWLA Collection, SWHA.

16. Maza, 136.

17. Social Security, "Compilation of the Social Security Laws: Collection of Data Relating to Adoption and Foster Care," n.d., https://www.ssa.gov/OP_Home/ssact/title04/0479.htm; Children's Defense Fund, *Adoption and Foster Care Analysis and Reporting System (AFCARS): Final Rule* (2016), https://www.childrensdefense.org/wp-content/uploads/2018/08/the-adoption-and-foster-care.pdf; Maza, 120.

18. Edward Schor, "The Foster Care System and Health Status of Foster Children," *Pediatrics* 69 (1982): 524; Pine, "Special Families," 14.

19. Schor, 524; Penny L. Deiner, Nancy J. Wilson, and Donald G. Unger, "Motivation and Characteristics of Families Who Adopt Children with Special Needs: An Empirical Study," *Topics in Early Childhood Special Education* 8, no. 2 (1988): 16, 20; Laraine Masters Glidden, *Parents for Children, Children for Parents: The Adoption Alternative* (Washington, DC: American Association of Mental Retardation, 1989), 41; CWLA, *Standards for Adoption Service, 1988* (New York: CWLA 1988), 5.

20. CWLA, *Standards for Adoption Service* (1988), 5–6.

21. David Fanshel and Eugene B. Shinn, *Children in Foster Care: A Longitudinal Investigation* (New York: Columbia University Press, 1978), 34.

22. Patricia Ryan and Bruce L. Warren, *Finding Families for the Children: A Handbook to Assist the Child Welfare Worker in the Placement of Children with a Mental, Emotional or Physical Handicap* (Washington, DC: US Department of Health, Education, and Welfare, 1974), 37.

23. Child Abuse Prevention, Treatment and Adoption Reform Act of 1978, PL 95-266 (April 24, 1978): 1; Laura Briggs, "Orphaning the Children of Welfare: 'Crack Babies,' Race, and Adoption Reform," in *Outsiders Within: Writing on Transracial Adoption*, ed. Jane Jeong Trenka, Julia Chinyere Oparah, and Sun Yung Shin (Cambridge: South End, 2006), 75; Dorothy Roberts, *Shattered Bonds: The Color of Child Welfare* (New York: Basic Civitas, 2002), 143.

24. Barbara Pine, "Child Welfare Reform and the Political Process," *Social Service Review* 60 (1986): 340; Drew Humphries, *Crack Mothers: Pregnancy, Drugs and the Media* (Columbus: Ohio State University Press, 1999), 127.

25. McKenzie, 2; Roberts, *Shattered Bonds*, 14.

26. Dorothy Roberts, "Adoption Myths and Racial Realities in the United States," in *Outsiders Within: Writing on Transracial Adoption*, ed. Jane Jeong Trenka, Julia Chinyere Oparah, and Sun Yung Shin (Cambridge: South End, 2006), 50-2; Roberts, *Shattered Bonds*, 14.

27. In Chicago and New York City over 80 percent of children in foster care were considered minority children. In New Jersey, Maryland, Louisiana, Delaware, Alabama, North Carolina, and New York, for instance, 45 to 65 percent of children in foster care were Black. New Mexico, Texas, Arizona, Colorado, and New York had high numbers of Hispanic children in foster care, and South Dakota, Oklahoma, Washington, and Nebraska had an overrepresentation of Native American children in foster care. McKenzie, 7-8.

28. Children's Bureau, "Child Abuse Prevention and Treatment Amendments of 1996, Pub. L. No. 104-235," in *Major Federal Legislation Concerned with Child Protection, Child Welfare and Adoption* (2019), 23. https://www.childwelfare.gov/pubpdfs/majorfedlegis.pdf.

29. National Association of Black Social Workers, "National Association of Black Social Workers Position Statement on Transracial Adoptions," September 1972, 1–4; McKenzie, 2; Laura Briggs, *Somebody's Children: The Politics of Transnational and Transracial Adoption* (Durham: Duke University Press, 2012), Loc. 395, 410, 427, 533, 558, 641, 658 (Kindle); Marc Mannes, "Factors and Events Leading to the Passage of the Indian Child Welfare Act," in *A History of Child Welfare*, ed. Eve Smith and Lisa A. Merkel-Holguin (New Brunswick: Transaction, 1996), 259–260.

30. Leah Litman and Matthew L. M. Fletcher, "The Necessity of the Indian Child Welfare Act," *Atlantic*, January 22, 2020, 1–8, https://www.theatlantic.com/ideas/archive/2020/01/fifth-circuit-icwa/605167/.

31. Briggs, *Somebody's Children*, Loc. 840, 896.

32. Patricia Collmeyer, "From 'Operation Brown Baby' to 'Opportunity': The Placement of Children of Color at the Boys and Girls Aid Society of Oregon," in *A History of Child Welfare*, ed. Eve P. Smith and Lisa A. Merkel-Holguin (New Brunswick: Transaction, 1996), 247–249.

33. Litman and Fletcher, 1–8.

34. John Kelly, "Federal Court Ruling on Indian Child Welfare Act Goes in Several Directions," *The Imprint: Youth and Family News*, April 8, 2021, https://imprintnews.org/child-welfare-2/indian-child-welfare-act-ruling-several-directions/53328.

35. Judith K. McKenzie, "Adoption of Children with Special Needs," *Future of Children* 3, no. 1 (Spring 1993): 62.

36. Proposal for National Adoption Information Exchange System (July 9, 1982), 13, CWLA Collection, Box 58, NAIES folder, 2 of 2, SWHA; memo from

Mai Bell Hurley, CWLA, to Adoption Task Force Members, Attachment B: January 6–7, 1986 (January 22, 1986), 6, 9, CWLA Collection, Box 97, Folder: Adoption Task Force 1987–1992, SWHA.

37. Letter to colleague from Exchange Consultant, NAIES (no date but likely 1982) Re: To agencies for kinds of children and families to register interested in those children, 196, CWLA Collection, Box 58, Folder, National Adoption Information Exchange System, 1982, 2 of 2, Procedural Manual and Client Forms: Supplement to Conceptual Design of a National Adoption Exchange, Submitted to Children's Bureau HEW, Contract 105-79-1102, September 28, 1982, SWHA; CWLA, *Standards for Adoption Service* (1988), 5.

38. Burton Sokoloff. "Adoption and Foster Care: The Pediatrician's Role," *Pediatrics in Review* 1 no. 2 (August 1979): 57; Adoption in America Surveyed, News Release (February 14, 1989), 1–2, CWLA Collection, Box 97: Folder: CWLA 1988 Adoption Survey, SWHA.

39. Pine, "Child Welfare Reform," 358n8; Dorcas R. Hardy, "Adoption of Children with Special Needs: A National Perspective," *American Psychologist* 39, no. 8 (August 1984): 901; Ryan and Warren, 7; written statement of Mr. and Mrs. Ashton Avegno, in *Barriers to Adoption* (1985), Hearings before the Committee on Labor and Human Resources, United States Senate, Ninety-Ninth Congress, First Session, S. Hrg. 99-288, June 25 and July 10, 1985 (Washington, DC: U.S. Government Printing Office, 1985, 159; Robert Lewis, "Adoption and Mental Retardation," *Pediatric Annals* 18, no. 10 (October 1989): 637.

40. Opening statement by Senator Dodd, in *Barriers to Adoption* (1993), 1, 4.

41. Pine, "Child Welfare Reform," 342. See *In re Gault,* 287 U.S. 1 (1967) for constitutional protection for children. Pine, 345; American Academy of Pediatrics, Committee on Adoption and Dependent Care, "Adoption of the Hard-to-Place Child," *Pediatrics* 68 no. 4 (October 1981): 598.

42. Sallie R. Churchill, Bonnie Carlson, and Lynn Nybell, *No Child Is Unadoptable: A Reader on Adoption of Children with Special Needs* (Beverly Hills: SAGE, 1979); Final Report Submitted to Children's Bureau from National Adoption Information Exchange System (September 1982): 7, CWLA Collection, Box 58, Folder NAIES 1979–1982, SWHA; Statement by Elizabeth S. Cole, director, North American Center on Adoption, Special Project, Child Welfare League of America, Inc., before the Sub-committee on Children and Youth, United States Senate (July 14, 1975): 9. CWLA Collection, Box 18, Folder 5, SWHA.

43. C. H. Krisheff, "Adoption Agency Services for the Retarded," *Mental Retardation* 15, no. 1 (1977): 38.

44. Testimony of Mrs. Ashton Avegno, in *Barriers to Adoption* (1985), 133.

45. Prepared statement of Mr. and Mrs. Ashton Avegno, in *Barriers to Adoption* (1985), 162.

46. CWLA, no title (1980), A2–A3, CWLA Collection, Box 58: Bibliography on Adoption, 1976–1980, Folder: Adoption Disruptions, SWHA.

47. McKenzie, 7; Richard P. Barth, "Adoption from Foster Care: A Chronicle of the Years after ASFA," in *Intentions and Results: A Look Back at the Adoption and Safe Families Act*, ed. Susan Notkin, Kristen Weber, Olivia A. Golden, and Jennifer Macomber (Washington, DC: Center for the Study of Social Policy; Urban Institute, 2009), 64.

48. Deiner, Wilson, and Unger, 20.

49. Grace Sandness, "Recruitment of Hard-to-Find Families: Ask the De-Bolts," in *Adopting Children with Special Needs*, ed. Patricia Kravik (Riverside, CA: NACAC, 1976), 55.

50. Pine, "Special Families," 9–10.

51. Adoption in America Surveyed: New Release (February 14, 1989): 4, CWLA Collection, Box 97: Folder, CWLA 1988 Adoption Survey, SWHA.

52. Ryan and Warren, 13.

53. Letter from Information Resource Services of CWLA to Friends of Waiting Children (January 1983), CWLA Collection, Box 97, Folder: Adoption Policy, CWLA 1976–1982, SWHA.

54. Letter from Information Resource Services of CWLA to Friends of Waiting Children; Deiner, Wilson, and Unger, 15; Marc Leepson, "Issues in Child Adoption," *Editorial Research Reports 1984* (vol. 2) (Washington, DC: CQ Press), 6, http://library.cqpress.com/xsite/document.php?id=cqresrre1984111600.

55. Richard P. Barth and Marianne Barry, *Adoption and Disruption: Rates, Risks and Responses* (New York: Aldine DeGruyter, 1988), 16.

56. John J. Goldman, "NJ Settlement Oks Adoptions by Gay Couples," *Los Angeles Times*, December 18, 1997, http://articles.latimes.com/1997/dec/18/news/mn-65464.

57. After adopting seven children beginning in the 1960s (an early precedent to be sure), Sandness and her partner received "wistful, frustrated letters from other 'disabled' couples wanting to know how we were able to succeed in adopting our children." Grace Sandness, "Disabled Parents Are Adoptable, Too," in *Adopting Children with Special Needs*, ed. Patricia Kravik (Riverside, CA: NACAC, 1976), 41.

58. CWLA, *Standards for Adoption Service* (1978), 69–70.

59. Jane Zirinsky-Wyatt, "The Prize: Disability, Parenthood, and Adoption," *Women and Therapy* 14, no. 3–4 (July 1993, 49–52.

60. Dottie Blacklock, *Older and Handicapped Children are Adoptable: The Spaulding Approach* (Chelsea, MI: Spaulding for Children, 1975), 21–22.

61. Sandness, "Disabled Parents," 41; Mirim Veni, "Why Should Physically Handicapped People Want to Adopt?," in *Adopting Children with Special Needs*, ed. Patricia Kravik (Riverside, CA: NACAC, 1976), 43. For a social worker's perspective, see Judith DeLeon, "Risk-Taking," in *Adopting Children with Special Needs*, ed. Patricia Kravik (Riverside: NACAC, 1976), 69–70.

62. Garry Abrams, "Parents without Power: Tiffany Callo Lost Her 2 Sons When Social Workers Questioned Whether the Disabled Mother Could Care for

Them. Her Story May Fuel Debate over Family Values, the Right to Be a Parent," *Los Angeles Times*, July 26, 1992, https://www.latimes.com/archives/la-xpm-1992 -07-26-vw-4927-story.html.

63. "Tiffany Callo and the Disability Movement," *The Disability Rag*, March/ April 1988, 20; Jynny Retzinger, "A Mother Remembers," *The Disability Rag*, May/June 1988, 30. Thanks to Richard Scotch for providing me with these articles from his personal Disability Rag archive; National Council on Disability, *Rocking the Cradle: Ensuring the Rights of Parents with Disabilities and Their Children*, ch. 5, "The Child Welfare System: Removal, Reunification, and Termination," 2012, http:// www.ncd.gov/publications/2012/Sep272012.

64. Abrams.

65. Sandness, "Disabled Parents," 40.

66. "The Mom Who Wasn't Sure a Birth Mother Would Choose Her Family," *The Cut*, February 1, 2018, www.thecut.com/article/mom-who-wasnt-sure-a-birth -mother-would-choose-her-family.html.

67. Author conversation with Corbett O'Toole, University of California–Berkeley (April 2014).

68. Adoption of Richardson, 1967, 59 Cal. Rptr. 327, as quoted in Madelyn Freundlich and Lisa Peterson, *Adoption and the Americans with Disabilities Act: An Issue Brief* (Washington, DC: CWLA Press, 2000), 18.

69. Humphries, *Crack Mothers*, 147; Freundlich and Peterson, *Adoption and ADA*, 1, 12, 16.

70. Freundlich and Peterson, *Adoption and ADA*, 4, 10, 11.

71. Ryan and Warren, 33.

72. Letter to Colleague from Exchange Consultant, NAIES (March 1982), referral sent to family for "stretching," 194. CWLA Collection, Box 58: Folder, National Adoption Information Exchange System, 1982, 2 of 2, Procedural Manual and Client Forms: Supplement to Conceptual Design of a National Adoption Exchange, Submitted to Children's Bureau HEW, Contract 105-79-1102, September 28, 1982, SWHA; Blacklock, *Older and Handicapped Children*, 8. See also Ann Coyne, "Memo to Adoption Workers: Who Is a Retarded Child?," in *Adopting Children with Special Needs*, ed. Patricia Kravik (Riverside, CA: NACAC, 1976), 63; Nelson, *On the Frontier of Adoption*, 29–34.

73. For the phrase "disability as inability," see Catherine J. Kudlick, "Disability History: Why We Need Another 'Other,'" *American Historical Review* 108, no. 3 (2003): 769; Marilynn J. Phillips, "Damaged Goods: Oral Narratives of the Experience of Disability in American Culture," *Social Science and Medicine* 30, no. 8 (1990): 851.

74. Eva Brown, "Recruiting Adoptive Parents for Children with Developmental Disabilities," *Child Welfare* 67 no. 2 (March 1, 1988): 125.

75. Blacklock, *Older and Handicapped Children*, 6.

76. Spaulding for Children, *Adapting to the Adoption of Special Children: The Stories of Five Special Families* (Chelsea, MI: Spaulding for Children, 1978), 11.

77. Kravik, *Adopting Children with Special Needs,* 5; Spaulding for Children, *Adapting to Adoption of Special Children,* 9, 22–25. For recruitment practice research on this topic, see Ryan and Warren, 15; Katherine A. Nelson, Parents View Special Needs Adoption: A Study of 177 Families' Experiences, CWLA (May 1982), CWLA Collection, Box 58: Folder: Bibliography on Adoption, SWHA. For a medical discussion of disability and adoptive children, see Deborah A. Frank, John M. Graham Jr., and David W. Smith, "Adoptive Children in a Dysmorphology Clinic: Implications for Evaluation of Children before Adoption," *Pediatrics* 68, no. 5 (1981): 744.

78. Kravik, *Adopting Children with Special Needs,* 10, 22, 28.

79. Blacklock, *Older and Handicapped Children,* 10.

80. Blacklock, *Older and Handicapped Children,* 10.

81. Hardy, 901, 904.

82. Jane S. Wimmer and Sharon Richardson, "Adoption of Children with Developmental Disabilities: Special Report," *Child Welfare* 69, no. 6 (November–December 1990): 568.

83. Wimmer and Richardson, 565–566. For the Lutheran Child and Family Services of Illinois project, see Brown, "Recruiting Adoptive Parents," 123–134.

84. McKenzie, 3.

85. Wimmer and Richardson, 566.

86. Wimmer and Richardson, 569.

87. Barth and Barry, 204.

88. Wimmer and Richardson, 568.

89. The National Exchange: A Question and Answer Update, General Adoption Inquiry Information—Waiting Children on Irving Place, NW (September 28, 1982), 145, CWLA Collection, Box 58: Folder: National Adoption Information Exchange System 1982, 2 of 2, Procedural Manual and Client Forms: Supplement to Conceptual Design of National Adoption Exchange, submitted to Children's Bureau, HEW Contract 105-79-1102, SWHA; letter to colleague from Exchange Consultant, NAIES, Re: To Agencies for Kinds of Children and families to register interested in those children (no date but likely 1982), CWLA Collection, Box 58, Folder: National Adoption Information Exchange System 1982, 2 of 2, Procedural Manual and Client Forms: Supplement to Conceptual Design of National Adoption Exchange, submitted to Children's Bureau, HEW Contract 105-79-1102, September 28, 1982, SWHA; Final Report submitted to Children's Bureau from the National Adoption Information Exchange System. September 1982, 9. CWLA Collection. Box 58, Folder NAIES 1979–1982, SWHA; Christopher Unger, Gladys Dwarshuis, and Elizabeth Johnson, *Chaos, Madness and Unpredictability: Placing the Child with Ears like Uncle Harry's, the Spaulding Approach to Adoption* (Chelsea, MI: Spaulding for Children, 1977), 101.

90. Deiner, Wilson, and Unger, 29.

91. Testimony of Mr. and Mrs. Ashton Avegno, *Barriers to Adoption* (1985), 146.

92. Letter from Linda Knight, in *Barriers to Adoption* (1985), 147–148.

93. American Academy of Pediatrics, Task Force on Pediatric AIDS, "Infants and Children with Acquired Immunodeficiency Syndrome: Placement in Adoption and Foster Care," *Pediatrics* 83, no. 4 (April 1989): 610.

94. See chapter 4.

95. US Senate Committee on Labor and Human Resources, Subcommittee on Child and Human Development, Oversight on Adoption Reform Act (Public Law 95-266): Hearing Before the Subcommittee on Child and Human Development of the Committee on Labor and Human Resources, United States Senate, Ninety-sixth Congress, Second Session, on Oversight on Adoption Reform Act (Public Law 95-266), April 17, 1980. (Washington, DC: US Government Printing Office, 1981).

96. For additional required terms of the agreement, see Barth and Barry, 204, 219.

97. Barth and Barry, 218.

98. Memo, September 26, 1991, to CWLA National Adoption Task Force from Ken Watson and Jean Emery Re: Agenda for meeting November 1–2, 1991, and Minutes, March 1, 1991, 4, CWLA Collection, Box 97, Folder: Adoption Task Force, 1985–1986, SWHA.

99. See chapter 4.

100. Letter from Elizabeth S. Cole to Adoption Advocate, June 5, 1981, CWLA Collection, Box 59: NACA folder, SWHA.

101. Humphries, *Crack Mothers*, 133; McKenzie, 6.

102. ARCH National Resource Center for Respite and Crisis Care Services, *Abuse and Neglect of Children with Disabilities*, Factsheet Number 36, September 1994, in National Council on Disability, "Youth with Disabilities in the Foster Care System: Barriers to Success and Proposed Policy Solutions," (2008), 12, https://ncd.gov/publications/2008/02262008#ExecutiveSummary.

103. Devon Brooks, Richard P. Barth, Alice Bussiere, and Glendora Patterson, "Adoption and Race: Implementing the Multiethnic Placement Act and the Interethnic Adoption Provisions," *Social Work* 44, no. 2 (March 1999): 168.

104. For racialized ideology of colorblindness, see Margaret Jacobs, "Remembering the 'Forgotten Child': The American Indian Child Welfare Crisis of the 1960s and 1970s," *American Indian Quarterly* 37, no. 1–2 (Winter/Spring 2013): 142–143.

105. Brooks et al. 168; Children's Bureau, "Multiethnic Placement Act of 1994, Pub. L. No. 103–382." In *Major Federal Legislation Concerned with Child Protection, Child Welfare, and Adoption* (2019), 24, https://www.childwelfare.gov/pubpdfs/majorfedlegis.pdf. Ortiz and Briggs incorrectly attribute the 1996 MEPA amendment to the Safe Families Act. It was enacted as part of the 1996 Small Business Job Protection Act. Ortiz and Briggs, 50; Children's Bureau, "The Interethnic Provisions of 1996, Pub. L. No. 104-188." In *Major Federal Legislation Concerned with Child Protection, Child Welfare, and Adoption* (2019), 24. https://www.childwelfare.gov/pubpdfs/majorfedlegis.pdf; Laura Briggs and Karen Dubinsky, "Special Issue Introduction: The Politics of History and the History of Politics." *American Indian Quarterly* 37, no. 1–2 (2013): 131; Jacobs, 143.

106. Jacobs, 139.

107. Barth, 64, 66.

108. Roberts, *Shattered Bonds*, 105.

109. Barth, 64.

110. Swann and Sylvester, 310.

111. Roberts, *Shattered Bonds*, 106, 110.

112. Olivia A. Golden, "Testimony on Adoption Promotion Act of 1997," Administration for Children and Families, U.S. Department of Health and Human Services Before the House Committee on Ways and Means, Subcommittee on Human Resources, April 8, 1997; Elizabeth Bartholet, *Nobody's Children: Abuse and Neglect, Foster Drift, and the Adoption Alternative* (Boston: Beacon, 2000); Elizabeth Bartholet, *Family Bonds: Adoption, Infertility and the New World of Child Production* (Boston: Beacon, 1999). Notably, Bartholet has consistently advanced more adoption and less regulation in domestic adoption.

113. Roberts, *Shattered Bonds*, 106–107.

114. Wulczyn, Chen, and Hislop, 584, 594.

115. Wulczyn, Chen, and Hislop, 587, 594, 605. One earlier study is Richard Barth, "Effects of Age and Race on the Odds of Adoption versus Remaining in Long Term Out-of-Home Care," *Child Welfare* 76, no. 2 (1997): 285–308, as cited in Devon Brooks, Sigrid James, and Richard P. Barth, "Preferred Characteristics of Children in Need of Adoption: Is There a Demand for Available Foster Children?," *Social Service Review* 76, no. 4 (December 2002): 577.

116. Barth, 65. Roberts notes that children of color represented only 44 percent of those adopted in 1997. Roberts, "Adoption Myths," 53; Wulczyn, Chen, and Hislop, 586; PL 105-89. Children's Bureau, "Adoption and Safe Families Act of 1997, Pub. L. 105-89," in *Major Federal Legislation Concerned with Child Protection*, 22, https://www.childwelfare.gov/pubpdfs/majorfedlegis.pdf.

117. Barth, 67, 68.

118. Tammy Marie White, "An Evaluation of the Impact of the Adoption and Safe Families Act of 1997 on Permanency-Related Outcomes for Foster Children in Six US States," Ph.D. diss., Department of Social Welfare, University of Pennsylvania, 2003, 21, 40. White suggests that disability data among states is underreported and unreliable, 54.

119. Brooks, James, and Barth, "Preferred Characteristics of Children," 579–580, 598.

Chapter Six

1. Patricia Kravik, "Common Handicaps and Their Implications," in *Adopting Children with Special Needs*, ed. Patricia Kravik (Riverside, CA: NACAC 1976), 67, reprinted from Dottie Blacklock, *Older and Handicapped Children Are Adoptable: The Spaulding Approach* (Chelsea, MI: Spaulding for Children, 1975), 43.

2. Mary Douglas, *Risk Acceptability According to the Social Sciences* (New York: Russell Sage Foundation, 1985), 59–60; Ulrich Beck, Anthony Giddens, and Scott Lash, *Reflexive Modernization: Politics, Tradition and Aesthetics in the Modern Social Order* (Stanford: Stanford University Press, 1994).

3. Thank you to one reviewer for pointing this out.

4. Daryl Michael Scott, *Contempt and Pity: Social Policy and the Image of the Damaged Black Psyche, 1880–1996* (Chapel Hill: University of North Carolina Press, 1997), 187–202; Marilynn J. Phillips, "Damaged Goods: Oral Narratives of the Experience of Disability in American Culture," *Social Science and Medicine* 30, no. 8 (1990): 850.

5. Prepared statement of Mr. and Mrs. Ashton Avegno, in *Barriers to Adoption* (1985), 160.

6. Prepared statement of Mr. and Mrs. Ashton Avegno, in *Barriers to Adoption* (1985), 164. As Herman writes, difference and damage are tightly intertwined. Ellen Herman, *Kinship by Design: A History of Adoption in the Modern United States* (Chicago: University of Chicago Press, 2008), 281.

7. Jim Forderer, "Confessions of a Single Parent," in *Adopting Children with Special Needs*, ed. Patricia Kravik (Riverside, CA: NACAC, 1976), 26–27; Merrily Ripley, "Not all Happy Endings," in *Adopting Children with Special Needs*, ed. Patricia Kravik (Riverside, CA: NACAC, 1976), 36.

8. Herman, *Kinship by Design*, 282.

9. Herman, *Kinship by Design*, 255–256, 265–267, 281; Gunnar Almgren, "Review of David Brodzinsky's *The Psychology of Adoption*," *Social Service Review* 65, no. 3 (1991): 506–508.

10. Jerome Smith, "The Adopted Child Syndrome: A Methodological Perspective," *Families in Society* 82 (2001): 491–497; Herman, *Kinship by Design*, 282, 369n142; David Kirschner, "Understanding Adoptees Who Kill: Dissociation, Patricide, and the Psychodynamics of Adoption," *International Journal of Offender Therapy and Comparative Criminology* 36 (1992): 323–333.

11. Herman, *Kinship by Design*, 267, 282–283.

12. In 1989, Bush described drug use as the "most pressing problem facing the nation," while CBS News noted that 64 percent of the American public agreed with him. Michelle Alexander, *The New Jim Crow* (New York: New Press, 2010), 54.

13. One fourth of all young African American men were behind bars in the early 1990s. Alexander, 55; Stephanie Bush-Baskette, "The War on Drugs and the Incarceration of Mothers," *Journal of Drug Issues* 30 no. 4 (Fall 2000): 919–927.

14. Clarence Lusane, *Pipe Dream Blues: Racism and the War on Drugs* (Boston: South End, 1991), 55, 56, 88. Whereas in 1970 approximately one-third of low-educated Black women were single parents, that number increased to more than 50 percent by 2000. Single female households also increased for white low-educated women but not at as steep a rate (from 8 percent to 18 percent). Bruce Western and Christopher Wildeman, "The Black Family and Mass Incarceration," *Annals*

of the American Academy of Political and Social Science 621 (January 2009): 234, 236; Bush-Baskette, 922.

15. Bush-Baskette, 923.

16. Alexander, 48.

17. Christopher Swann and Michelle Sheran Sylvester, "The Foster Care Crisis: What Caused Caseloads to Grow?," *Demography* 43, no. 2 (May 2006): 309–335.

18. Dorothy Roberts, "Adoption Myths and Racial Realities in the United States," in *Outsiders Within: Writing on Transracial Adoption,* ed. Jane Jeong Trenka, Julia Chinyere Oparah, and Sun Yung (Cambridge: South End, 2006), 52; Laura Briggs, "Orphaning the Children of Welfare: 'Crack Babies,' Race, and Adoption Reform," in *Outsiders Within: Writing on Transracial Adoption,* ed. Jane Jeong Trenka, Julia Chinyere Oparah, and Sun Yung (Cambridge: South End, 2006), 75; Alexander, 56; Gwendolyn Mink, "Ending Single Motherhood," in *The Promise of Welfare Reform: Political Rhetoric and the Reality of Poverty in the Twenty-First Century,* ed. Keith Kilty and Elizabeth Segal (New York: Routledge, 2006), 158.

19. Mink, 158; Tammy Marie White, "An Evaluation of the Impact of the Adoption and Safe Families Act of 1997 on Permanency-Related Outcomes for Foster Children in Six US States," Ph.D. diss., Department of Social Welfare, University of Pennsylvania, 2003, 167.

20. The act also imposed mandatory five-year minimums for drug offenses and enabled the use of the death penalty for serious drug offenses. Western and Wildeman, 236; Swann and Sylvester, 310, 312; Alexander, 52; Lusane, 65.

21. Drew Humphries. "Crack Mothers at 6: Prime-Time News, Crack/Cocaine, and Women," *Violence Against Women* 4, no. 1 (February 1998): 52–54, 57.

22. Ann Fredericks, "The Baby Nobody Wanted," *Ladies' Home Journal,* September 1988, 22–24. See also Jan Sonnenmair and Barbara Maddux, "Mother Love: A Special Woman and Two Babies with Special Needs Make a Family," *Life Magazine,* May 1, 1992, 49.

23. American Academy of Pediatrics, Task Force on Pediatric AIDS, 609.

24. Adoption Agency 1990 Program Activities, CWLA Collection, Box 97: Folder-Adoption Agenda, 1989–1991, SWHA.

25. Michael Cooper, "Living with AIDS Child Is the Easy Part," *New York Times,* Metro section (December 15, 1991), 48L; Sonnenmair and Maddux, 50; Adoption Agency 1990: Program Activities, 1, CWLA Collection, Box 97: Folder: Adoption Agenda 1989–1991, SWHA; minutes: Adoption Task Force Meeting (October 23, 1989), 4, CWLA Collection, Box 97: Folder: Adoption Agenda 1989–1991, SWHA; Drew Humphries, *Crack Mothers: Pregnancy, Drugs and the Media* (Columbus: Ohio State University Press, 1999), 134.

26. In August 1986, *Time* named crack the "issue of the year," and between October 1988 and 1989, the *Washington Post* published 1,565 stories on crack alone. Alexander, 51–52. For follow up, see Jim McDermott, "Some Surprising News

about 'Crack Babies,'" *Huffington Post*, May 25, 2011, https://www.huffingtonpost
.com/rep-jim-mcdermott/some-suprising-news-about_b_562560.html?ncid=engm
odushpmg00000006&ec_carp=533570465950387356.

27. Douglas C. Baynton, "Disability and the Justification of Inequality in America," in *The New Disability History: American Perspectives*, ed. Paul Longmore and Lauri Umansky (New York: New York University Press, 2001), 41; Scott, *Contempt and Pity*, xi–xvii, 12, 146–157, 208n52; Lennard Davis, *Enabling Acts: The Hidden Story of How the Americans with Disabilities Act Gave the Largest US Minority Its Rights* (Boston: Beacon, 2015).

28. Charles Krauthammer, "Crack Babies Forming Biological Underclass," *St. Louis Post-Dispatch*, July 30, 1989, 3B. For fetal alcohol syndrome and welfare, see Michael Dorris, *The Broken Cord* (New York: Harper Collins, 1989), 160, 166.

29. Briggs, "Orphaning the Children of Welfare," 75, 77, 79; Krauthammer, 3B.

30. Krauthammer, 3B.

31. Dorris, 281; G. Thomas Couser, "Raising Adam: Ethnicity, Disability, and the Ethics of Life Writing in Michael Dorris' *The Broken Cord*," *Biography* 21, no. 4 (Fall 1998): 434, 438.

32. Dorris, 158, 168.

33. Fredericks, 22; "Living with AIDS Is the Easy Part," *New York Times*, December 15, 1991, section 1, 48; Dorothy Gilliam, "Giving Life without Giving Birth," *Washington Post* (May 7, 1994): B1.

34. "Little Factory Seconds," *The Disability Rag* (March/April 1989), 26; Jude Lincicome, "Jude's Kids," *Future Reflections: National Federation of the Blind Magazine for Parents and Teachers of Blind Children*, Summer 1991, n.p.; Michele D. Manigault, "Mom by Choice," *Catonsville Times*, May 8, 2002, n.p.

35. Briggs, "Orphaning the Children of Welfare," 81–83. For mother blaming, see Molly Ladd-Taylor and Lauri Umansky, eds., *"Bad" Mothers: The Politics of Blame in Twentieth-Century America* (New York: New York University Press, 1998).

36. Paul Longmore and Lauri Umansky, introduction, "Disability History: From the Margins to the Mainstream," in *The New Disability History: American Perspectives*, ed. Paul Longmore and Lauri Umansky (New York: New York University Press, 2001), 6; Nancy Fraser and Linda Gordon, "Genealogy of Dependency: Tracing a Keyword of the US Welfare State," *Signs* 19, no. 2 (1994): 325–326.

37. Scott, *Contempt and Pity*, 191, 200–201; Fraser and Gordon, 327–328.

38. Molly Ladd-Taylor, *Fixing the Poor: Eugenic Sterilization and Child Welfare in the Twentieth Century* (Baltimore: Johns Hopkins University Press, 2017).

39. Phillips, 851.

40. Daniel Blackie, "Disability, Dependency, and the Family in the Early United States," in *Disability Histories*, ed. Susan Burch and Michael Rembis (Urbana: University of Illinois Press, 2014), Loc. 420 (Kindle); Scott, *Contempt and Pity*, 188; Fraser and Gordon, 309.

41. Fraser and Gordon, 311, 324–325.

42. Eva Feder Kittay, Bruce Jennings, and Angela A. Wasunna, "Dependency, Difference and Global Ethic of Long-term Care," *Journal of Political Philosophy* 13, no. 4 (2005): 443–445, 466, 467, 469; Fraser and Gordon, 331–332.

43. Humphries, *Crack Mothers*, 8, 12; Dorris, 166.

44. Douglas J. Besharov, "Let's Give Crack Babies a Way Out of Addicted Families," *Newsday*, September 3, 1989, http://www.welfareacademy.org/pubs/childwelfare /letsgive-0989.shtml.

45. Humphries, *Crack Mothers*, 13, 16, 128, 140–141.

46. Briggs, "Orphaning the Children of Welfare," 78–79; Ortiz and Briggs, 48; Humphries, 6, 8.

47. Humphries, *Crack Mothers*, 7.

48. Lusane, 56–58; Celia W. Dugger, "A Boy Back from the Brink: When Love and Care Prevail," *New York Times*, September 10, 1992, A1, B2.

49. Humphries, *Crack Mothers*, 139. Such arrests also raised the wider issue of whether mothers could be held legally liable for the health and safety of the fetus.

50. Humphries, *Crack Mothers*, 135–136.

51. Humphries, *Crack Mothers*, 137.

52. Anna Kuzio, *Exploitation of Schemata in Persuasive and Manipulative Discourse in Polish, English, and Russian* (Newcastle upon Tyne, UK: Cambridge Scholars Publishing, 2014), 145.

53. Richard O'Mara, "Are Orphanages Better for Kids than Welfare?," *Baltimore Sun*, November 27, 1994; David Van Biema and Ann Blackman, "The Storm over Orphanages," *Time*, December 12, 1994, 58–62; Jason DeParle, "The 1994 Election: Issues: Momentum Builds for Cutting Back Welfare System," *New York Times*, November 13, 1994; Scott, *Contempt and Pity*, 199.

54. Douglas J. Besharov, "Crack Babies: The Worst Threat Is Mom Herself," *Washington Post*, August 6, 1989; Michele Norris, "Six Year Old Maryland Home Was a Modern Day Opium Den," *Washington Post*, July 30, 1989.

55. Humphries, *Crack Mothers*, 136.

56. In particular, it was very difficult to find Black families to adopt Black disabled children. Answers to questions for Karen and Guenter Lahr, in *Barriers to Adoption* (1985), 22.

57. Gena Corea, *The Mother Machine: Reproductive Technologies from Artificial Insemination to Artificial Wombs* (New York: Harper and Row, 1985), 1. For later critique of Corea and others, see Laura Briggs, "Reproductive Technology: Of Labor and Markets," *Feminist Studies* 36, no. 2 (Summer 2010): 362. See also Sherman Elias and George Annas, *Reproductive Genetics and the Law* (Chicago: Yearbook Medical Publishers, 1987), 222; Jennifer A. Johnson-Hanks, Christine A. Bachrach, S. Philip Morgan, and Hans-Peter Kohler, *Understanding Family Change and Variation: Toward a Theory of Conjunctural Action* (New York: Springer, 2011), 124; Joan Rothschild, *The Dream of the Perfect Child* (Bloomington: Indiana University Press, 2005), 77–79, 148.

58. See Marilyn Strathern, "Introduction: A Question of Context," 17–19, Frances Price, "Beyond Expectation: Clinical Practices and Clinical Concerns," 30, 43, and Sarah Franklin, "Orphaned Embryos," 166–168, in *Technologies of Procreation: Kinship in the Age of Assisted Conception, ed.* Jeanette Edwards, Sarah Franklin, Eric Kirsch, Frances Price, and Marilyn Strathern (Manchester: Manchester University Press, 1993; Susan Lindee, "Intimate Biotechnology," *Isis* 97, no. 3 (September 2006): 539; Briggs, "Reproductive Technology," 359–374; Elias and Annas, 224; Judith Modell, "Last Chance Babies: Interpretations of Parenthood in an In Vitro Fertilization Program," *Medical Anthropology Quarterly* 3, no. 2 (June 1989): 124–125, 135; Jennifer A. Johnson-Hanks, "A Conjunctural History of Assisted Reproduction and Adoption," in *Understanding Family Change and Variation: Toward a Theory of Conjunctural Action*, ed. Jennifer A. Johnson-Hanks, Christine A. Bachrach, S. Philip Morgan, and Hans-Peter Kohler (New York: Springer, 2011), 112; Frances Price, "Beyond Expectation: Clinical Practices and Clinical Concerns," in *Technologies of Procreation: Kinship in the Age of Assisted Conception*, ed. Jeanette Edwards, Sarah Franklin, Frances Price, and Marilyn Strathern (New York: Routledge, 1999), 27; Corea, 54; President's Commission for the Study of Ethical Problems in Medicine and Biomedical and Behavioral Research, *Screening and Counseling for Genetic Conditions* (Washington, DC: US Government Printing Office, 1983), 69–70; Herman, *Kinship by Design*, 4, 7, 15; E. Wayne Carp, *Family Matters: Secrecy and Disclosure in the History of Adoption* (Cambridge, MA: Harvard University Press, 1998); E. Wayne Carp, *Jean Paton and the Struggle to Reform American Adoption* (Ann Arbor: University of Michigan Press, 2014); Margarete Sandelowski, "Compelled to Try: The Never-Enough Quality of Conceptive Technology," *Medical Anthropology Quarterly* 5, no. 1 (1991): 38. For the emphasis on white genetic ties and lesser value placed on Black genetic ties, see Dorothy Roberts, "The Genetic Tie," *University of Chicago Law Review* 62, no. 1 (Winter 1995): 209–273.

59. Memo from Mai Bell Hurley, CWLA, to Adoption Task Force Members, Attachment F: Renewed Client Goals, Barriers and Action Steps (January 22, 1986), 10, CWLA Collection, Box 97, Folder: Adoption Task Force 1987–1992, SWHA.

60. Modell, 130, 134.

61. Burton Sokoloff, "Alternative Methods of Reproduction: Effects on the Child," *Clinical Pediatrics* 26, no. 1 (January 1987): 13.

62. Memo from Mai Bell Hurley (president of CWLA) to Adoption Task Force Members (January 22, 1986), CWLA Collection, Box 97, Folder: Adoption Task Force 1987–1992, 10. SWHA; letter from CWLA to members, Re: Colloquium on Non-traditional Reproductive Technologies (April 24, 1987), CWLA Collection, Box 98: Surrogacy, SWHA; meeting of CWLA Ad Hoc Adoption Task Force (February 22, 1985), New York, 4, CWLA Collection, Box 56, Folder: Adoption Task Force, SWHA; letter from Robert R. Aptekar, director of standards and program development to attendees (April 24, 1987), CWLA Collection, Box 98,

Folder: Surrogacy. SWHA; Sokoloff, "Alternative Methods," 11, 12–13; George J. Annas, testimony presented before the Select Committee on Children, Youth and Families of the US House of Representatives on the *Legal and Ethical Aspects of Regulating the New Reproductive Technologies* (May 21, 1987), 1, CWLA Collection, Box 98, Folder Surrogacy, SWHA.

63. Peter J. Neumann, "Should Health Insurance Cover IVF?: Issues and Options," *Journal of Health Politics, Policy and Law* 22, no. 5 (October 1997): 1225, 1232–1233.

64. Sandelowski, 30, 32, 34; Graham Thompson, *American Culture in the 1980s* (Edinburgh: Edinburgh University Press, 2007), 32–33; Modell, 125–126; Briggs, "Reproductive Technology," 372, 373.

65. Rayna Rapp and Faye Ginsburg, "Enlarging Reproduction, Screening Disability," in *Reproductive Disruptions: Gender, Technology, and Biopolitics in the New Millennium*, ed. Marcia C. Inhorn (New York: Berghahn, 2009), 116–117; Alison Kafer, *Feminist, Queer, Crip* (Bloomington: Indiana University Press, 2013), 34.

66. Perri Klass, "Body and Mind: The Perfect Baby?," *New York Times Magazine*, January 29, 1989, sec. 6, p. 45; Kafer, 6.

67. Mary Douglas, *Risk and Blame: Essays in Cultural Theory* (New York: Routledge, 1992), 30.

68. Kafer, 6, 31. For stigma of "test-tube baby" as "freak," see Modell, 133.

69. Rothschild, 92, 97; Adrienne Asch, "Why I Haven't Changed My Mind about Prenatal Diagnosis: Reflections and Refinements," in *Prenatal Testing and Disability Rights*, ed. Erik Parens and Adrienne Asch (Washington, DC: Georgetown University Press, 2000), 234–258.

70. Gail Landsman, "Does God Give Special Kids to Special Parents? Personhood and the Child with Disabilities as Gift and as Giver," in *Transformative Motherhood: On Giving and Getting in a Consumer Culture*, ed. Linda L. Layne (New York: New York University Press, 1999), 135, 139–141. For the notion of "stratified reproduction," see Faye Ginsburg and Rayna Rapp, "Introduction: Conceiving the New World Order," in *Conceiving the New World Order: The Global Politics of Reproduction*, ed. Faye Ginsburg and Rayna Rapp (Berkeley: University of California Press, 1995), 3; Faye Ginsburg and Rayna Rapp, "Fetal Reflections: Confessions of Two Feminist Anthropologists as Mutual Informants," in *Fetal Subjects, Feminist Positions*, ed. Lynn Morgan and Meredith Michaels (Philadelphia: University of Pennsylvania Press, 1999), 286–287, 291.

71. Karen-Sue Taussig, Rayna Rapp, and Deborah Heath, "Flexible Eugenics: Technologies of the Self in the Age of Genetics," in *Genetic Nature/Culture: Anthropology and Science beyond the Two-Culture Divide*, ed. Alan Goodman, Deborah Heath, and Susan M. Lindee (Berkeley: University of California Press, 2003), 61; Rosemarie Garland-Thomson, *Extraordinary Bodies: Figuring Physical Disability in American Culture and Literature, 20th anniversary ed. (New York: Columbia University Press, 2017*, 8–9.

72. Rosemarie Garland-Thomson coined this term to mean the collective culture's normative, corporeal qualities. See Rosemarie Garland-Thomson, "Integrating Disability, Transforming Feminist Theory," *Feminist Formations* 14, no. 3 (2002): 10.

73. Igor Kopytoff, "Commoditizing Kinship in America," in *Consuming Motherhood*, ed. Janelle S. Taylor, Linda L. Layne, and Danielle Wozniak (New Brunswick: Rutgers University Press, 2004), 272. For similar logic in New Zealand, see Ken R. Daniels, "Adoption and Donor Insemination: Factors Influencing Couples' Choices," *Child Welfare* 73, no. 1 (1994): 7, 9. For adoption as futures trading, Julian Gill-Peterson, "The Value of the Future: The Child as Human Capital and the Neoliberal Labor of Race," *Women's Studies Quarterly* 43, nos.1 & 2 (Spring/Summer, 2015): 188.

74. Patricia Ryan and Bruce L. Warren, *Finding Families for the Children: A Handbook to Assist the Child Welfare Worker in the Placement of Children with a Mental, Emotional or Physical Handicap* (Washington, DC: US Department of Health, Education, and Welfare, 1974), 14; Roberts, "The Genetic Tie," 210, 212, 213, 215.

75. Kafer, 32. Furthermore, the damaged goods stereotype applied not only to adopted children but also to their mothers, as nonnormative mothering—resulting from mothering devalued children or from mothering through adoption or foster care—also took on the association of a type of a delegitimated form of motherhood. Linda L. Layne, "Introduction," *Transformative Motherhood: On Giving and Getting in a Consumer Culture*, ed. Linda L. Layne (New York: New York University Press, 1999), 1–28; Danielle Wozniak, "Gifts and Burdens: The Social and Familial Context of Foster Mothering," in *Transformative Motherhood: On Giving and Getting in a Consumer Culture* (New York: New York University Press, 1999), 89–132.

76. Sandelowski, 33; Barbara Pine, "Special Families for Special Children: The Adoption of Children with Developmental Disabilities," Ph.D. diss., Brandeis University, Heller Graduate School for the Advanced Study in Social Welfare, 1991, 8, 78.

77. Opening statement by Senator Metzenbaum, in *Barriers to Adoption* (1985), 6.

78. Herman, *Kinship by Design* 252.

79. The authors also do not cite any primary sources on which to base their assertions linking the crack baby crisis and Romanian adoption. Ana Teresa Ortiz and Laura Briggs, "The Culture of Poverty, Crack Babies, and Welfare Cheats: The Making of the 'Healthy White Baby Crisis,'" *Social Text* 76, 21, no. 3 (Fall 2003): 39–41, 43.

80. Chris Bell, "Introduction: Doing Representational Detective Work." In *Blackness and Disability: Critical Examinations and Cultural Interventions,* ed. Chris Bell (East Lansing: Michigan State University Press, 2011), 3.

81. Chris Bell, "Introducing White Disability Studies: A Modest Proposal," in *The Disability Studies Reader*, ed. Lennard Davis (New York: Routledge, 2006), 279–280.

82. Kittay, Jennings, and Wasunna, "Dependency, Difference and Global Ethic of Longterm Care," 460.

83. Solangel Maldonado, "Discouraging Racial Preferences in Adoption," *U.C. Davis Law Review* 39 (2006): 1438.

84. "Oh, Baby: Of Corruption and Scandal," *Ukrainian Weekly*, December 31, 1995, http://www.ukrweekly.com/old/archive/1995/539508.shtml.

85. Adoption in America Surveyed: News Release, February 14, 1989, CWLA Collection, Box 97, Folder: CWLA 1988 Adoption Survey, SWHA. The survey was of 151 agencies, including 48 state-wide public agencies.

86. Helga Kuhse and Peter Singer, *Should the Baby Live?: The Problem of Handicapped Infants* (Oxford: Oxford University Press, 1985), 189. For earlier precedent on euthanasia of unfit babies, see Martin S. Pernick, *The Black Stork: Eugenics and the Death of "Defective" Babies in American Medicine and Motion Pictures since 1915* (New York: Oxford University Press, 1996).

87. Kuhse and Singer, 191.

88. Roger Rosenblatt, "The Baby in the Factory," *Time*, February 14, 1983, 90, 94–95.

89. Elias and Annas, 170–173.

90. The hole in her spine closed naturally but she was still intellectually disabled. "Data Update: Baby Jane Doe Turns Nine This Year," *New York Times*, May 17, 1992, 44.

91. Jack Resnik, "The Baby Doe Rules (1984)," *The Embryo Encyclopedia Project*, May 12, 2011, https://embryo.asu.edu/pages/baby-doe-rules-1984.

92. Elias and Annas, 177, 181. For confrontational tactics of antiabortion groups in the 1980s, see Thompson, *American Culture in the 1980s*, 31. See also Children's Bureau, "Child Abuse Amendments of 1984, Pub. L. No. 98-457," in *Major Federal Legislation Concerned with Child Protection, Child Welfare and Adoption* (2019), 26, https://www.childwelfare.gov/pubpdfs/majorfedlegis.pdf.

93. For Elias and Annas's "better off dead" standard to discern what was in the "best interests" of the child in terms of withholding treatment, see Elias and Annas, 184–185. It is within this context and debate that Kuhse and Singer put forward their stance on killing disabled infants. Elias and Annas, 185–186; American Academy of Pediatrics, "Joint Policy Statement: Principles of Treatment of Disabled Infants," *Pediatrics* 73, no. 4 (1984): 559.

94. Reba Michels Hill and Jo Ann Caldwell, "Adoption: An Option for the Imperfect Child," *Pediatrics* 71, no. 4 (April 1983): 664.

95. Hill and Caldwell, 665.

96. Without childcare supports, adoption in some ways served as a solution of re-location, one that then created a "problem" for parents who adopted disabled children. Thanks Aly Patsavas for this insight.

97. Hill and Caldwell, 665.

98. Prepared statement of Mr. and Mrs. Ashton Avegno, in *Barriers to Adoption,* (1985), 163. For similar problematic attitudes of physicians and social workers in relation to preventing children from foster care placement, see Christopher G. Petr and David D. Barney, "Reasonable Efforts for Children with Disabilities: The Parents' Perspective," *Social Work* 39, no. 3 (May 1993): 252.

99. Prepared statement of Lynn G. Gabbard, in *Barriers to Adoption* (1993), 14.

100. Tally Moses, "Stigma and Family," in *The Stigma of Disease and Disability: Understanding Causes and Overcoming Injustices,* ed. Patrick Corrigan (Washington, DC: American Psychological Association, 2014), 248–251.

101. For Canadian cases, see Marie Adams, *Our Son a Stranger: Adoption Breakdown and Its Effects on Parents* (Montreal: McGill-Queens University Press, 2002); Pine, "Special Families," 35.

102. Ryan and Warren, 14.

103. Richard P. Barth and Marianne Barry, *Adoption and Disruption: Rates, Risks and Responses* (New York: Aldine DeGruyter, 1988), 20. See also Douglas, *Risk and Blame.*

104. Pine, "Special Families," 19; George, Howard, and Yu, 12.

105. Susan Partridge, Helaine Hornby, and Thomas McDonald, *Legacies of Loss: Visions of Gain: An Inside Look at Adoption Disruption* (Portland: Center for Research and Advanced Study, University of Southern Maine, 1986), 43. The authors define special needs as over three years of age, with emotional, physical or cognitive disability or hard to place, 32. See also Barth and Barry, 21.

106. Barth and Barry, 21.

107. Urban Systems Research and Engineering, "Evaluation of State Activities with Regard to Adoption Disruption: Final Report Contract #105-84-8102. Task Order I (Washington, DC: Office of Human Development Series, 1985); Trudy Festinger, *Necessary Risk: A Study of Adoptions and Disrupted Adoptive Placements* (Washington, DC: Child Welfare League of America, 1986), 1–2. For drop in disruption due to P.L. 96-272 in Illinois, see George, Howard, and Yu, 11; Alfred Kadushin and Frederick Seidl, "Adoption Failure: A Social Work Postmortem," *Social Work* 16, no. 3 (July 1971): 37.

108. Barth and Barry, 4; Anne Westhues and Joyce S. Cohen, "Preventing Disruptions of Special Needs Adoptions," *Child Welfare* 69, no. 2 (March–April 1990): 142–143; George, Howard, and Yu, 5.

109. Dolores Schmidt, James A. Rosenthal, and Beth Bombeck, "Parents' Views of Adoption Disruption," *Children and Youth Services Review* 10, no. 2 (1988): 119–130; Adams, 106–107.

110. At least thirty journals in psychiatry, psychology, social work, pediatrics, family law, and child welfare featured such studies. Susan MacDonald, Bibliography of current literature on adoption 1976–1980, compiled by NAIES project for publication by Children's Bureau, CWLA Collection, Box 58, Folder: Bibliography

on Adoption, 1976–1980, SWHA. See also David Fanshel and Eugene B. Shinn, *Children in Foster Care: A Longitudinal Investigation* (New York: Columbia University Press, 1978), 20; Barth and Barry, 21; Felstiner, 11; McKenzie, 9. This also occurred among the data in Urban Systems Research and Engineering, ii.

111. Urban Systems Research and Engineering, 5–2; prepared statement of Mr. and Mrs. Ashton Avegno, in *Barriers to Adoption* (1985), 170.

112. Prepared statement of Mr. and Mrs. Ashton Avegno, in *Barriers to Adoption* (1985), 170.

113. Prepared statement of Mr. and Mrs. Ashton Avegno, in *Barriers to Adoption* (1985), 162, 170.

114. George, Howard, and Yu, 4.

115. Partridge, Hornby, and McDonald, v; Barth and Barry, 78. In Arizona, none of the children with physical or mental disabilities disrupted even though almost 40 percent of all adoptive children for FY85 had a disability. See Urban Systems Research and Engineering, 2–4. See also George, Howard, and Yu, 4.

116. Adams, 105; Urban Systems Research and Engineering, iv; Felstiner, 32.

117. Blacklock, *Older and Handicapped Children*, 16; Felstiner, 4; Pine, "Special Families," 154.

118. Barth and Barry, 78. Others worked against this risk = impairment formulation, emphasizing the constellation of family characteristics, agency approaches, and parent perspectives as important for predicting outcomes. Ann Coyne and Mary Ellen Brown, *Adoption of Children with Developmental Disabilities: A Study of Public and Private Child Welfare Agencies* (New York: Child Welfare League of America, 1980), 35; Urban Systems Research and Engineering found similar results, 3–3.

119. Westhues and Cohen, 144.

120. George, Howard, and Yu, 2.

121. Coyne and Brown, *Adoption of Children with Developmental Disabilities,* 59.

122. Barth and Barry, 184; Pine, "Special Families," 101, 106–107.

123. Partridge, Hornby, and McDonald, i–ii, 35, 44–45, 49–50, 52, 54–55; Felstiner, 22–27; Barth and Barry, 93; George, Howard, and Yu report different results for Illinois, showing time in care positively correlated with *lower* disruption rates but higher dissolution rates, suggesting that movement into adoptive placement (from stable fost-adopt scenarios) should be gradual. George, Howard, and Yu, 2, 24, 26, 28.

124. Partridge, Hornby, and McDonald, i–ii, 35, 44–45, 49–50, 52, 54–55; Barth and Barry, 93.

125. [No title], CWLA Collection, Box 58: Bibliography on Adoption, 1976–1980, Folder: Adoption Disruptions 1980, SWHA.

126. McKenzie, 3; Schmidt, Rosenthal, and Bombeck, 128.

127. This study also found that older parents and those with lower incomes were more realistic in their expectations and therefore had a lower percentage of

disruptions. Urban Systems Research and Engineering, iii, iv; Barth and Barry, 74–75; Schmidt, Rosenthal, and Bombeck, 119–130.

128. Westhues and Cohen, 151; Schmidt, Rosenthal, and Bombeck, 126.

129. Adams, 122.

130. James A. Rosenthal, Victor K. Groze, and Herman Curiel, "Race, Social Class and Special Needs Adoption," *Social Work* 35, no. 6 (1990): 532, 534, 536–538. In Illinois, Hispanic children disrupted at higher rates than whites and Blacks but once legally adopted, dissolved at much lower rates. George, Howard, and Yu, 18, 20, 23, 26

131. For components of successful placements, see James A. Rosenthal, Victor K. Groze, and Gloria Duran Aguilar, "Adoption Outcomes for Children with Handicaps," *Child Welfare* 70, no. 6 (1991): 630–631.

132. Barth and Barry, 94, 168.

133. Adams, 113–117. Professionals increasingly recognized the father's role as well. Westhues and Cohen, 149.

134. Pine, "Special Families," 12. For importance of father, see Westhues and Cohen, 144, 149, 151.

135. Partridge, Hornby, and McDonald, 71, 75. The prospect of legal-risk adoptions (placing a child before he is legally freed) for special needs children is also discussed as a way to get around the long waits for placement and therefore a possible way to lower the risk of disruption.

136. Barth and Barry, 191, 194.

137. Prepared statement of Lynn G. Gabbard, in *Barriers to Adoption* (1993), 12–14.

138. Madelyn Freundlich and Lisa Peterson, "Protecting Parents, Children and Agencies by Avoiding Liability in Wrongful Adoption Cases," PowerPoint presentation, Evan Donaldson Adoption Institute; Madelyn Freundlich and Lisa Peterson, "Wrongful Adoption: Litigation/Practice Issues," Evan Donaldson Adoption Institute; Madelyn Freundlich and Lisa Peterson, *Wrongful Adoption: Law, Policy and Practice* (Washington, DC: Child Welfare League of America Press, 1988).

139. Prepared statement of Lynn G. Gabbard, in *Barriers to Adoption* (1993), 12.

140. Ann Kimble Loux, *The Limits of Hope: An Adoptive Mother's Story* (Charlottesville: University Press of Virginia, 1997); Dorris; Adams.

141. Dorris, xviii, 9–10, 14, 79, 109, 113; Couser, "Raising Adam," 422, 425–427, 432–433.

142. Adams, 104. For slightly earlier study discussing parent reporting, see Katherine Nelson, *On the Frontier of Adoption*, 74, 76.

143. Laraine Masters Glidden, "Families Who Adopt Mentally Retarded Children: Who, Why and What Happens," in *Families of Handicapped Persons: Research, Programs and Policy Issues*, ed. James J. Gallagher and Peter M. Vietze (Baltimore: Paul H. Brookes, 1986), 24; Adams, 110–112.

144. Partridge, Hornby, and McDonald, 55–56.

145. Barth and Barry, 210.

146. Ann Kimble Loux, "The Catch that Came with Our Adoption," *Washington Post*, November 23, 1997; prepared statement of Lynn G. Gabbard, in *Barriers to Adoption* (1993), 14.

147. Adams, 113, 127.

148. Statement of Shane Salter, in *Barriers to Adoption* (1993), 8.

149. Westhues and Cohen, 143.

150. Partridge, Hornby, and McDonald, i–ii, 35, 44–45, 49–50, 52, 54–55; Felstiner, 22–27; Sandra M. Sufian, "As Long as Parents Can Accept Them: Medical Disclosure, Risk, and Disability in Twentieth-Century American Adoption Practice," *Bulletin of the History of Medicine* 91, no. 1 (March 2017): 94–124.

151. For studies on components of successful placements, see Glidden, "Families Who Adopt Mentally Retarded Children," 129–142; Laraine Masters Glidden, Veronique N. Valliere, and Sandra L. Herbert, "Adopted Children with Mental Retardation: Positive Family Impact," *Mental Retardation* 26 no. 3 (1988): 119–125.

152. Barth and Barry, cited in Freundlich and Peterson, *Wrongful Adoption*, 8.

153. In 1988, California passed a law that required notification to every family involved in special needs adoption about the difference between adoption subsidies and foster care benefits. Subsidies were usually about one-third of foster care rates, likely leading to a disincentive to adopt. Barth and Barry, 108–110, 111, 113, 204; Schmidt, Rosenthal, and Bombeck, 125.

154. Madelyn DeWoody, "Adoption and Disclosure of Medical and Social History: a Review of the Law." *Child Welfare* 72, no. 3 (May–June 1993): 195.

155. Freundlich and Peterson, *Wrongful Adoption*, 9.

156. Rosenthal, Groze, and Aguilar, 634.

157. Sufian, "As Long as Parents."

158. Pine, "Special Families," 78. Freundlich and Peterson also mention wrongful placement claims by adopted individuals who returned to agencies with complaints that the agency should not have placed them with their adoptive families because of known problems. Freundlich and Peterson, *Wrongful Adoption*, 51.

159. Kittay, Jennings, and Wasunna, "Dependency, Difference and Global Ethic of Long-term Care," 460.

160. Freundlich and Peterson, *Wrongful Adoption*, 71.

161. Freundlich and Peterson, *Wrongful Adoption*, 71–72.

Epilogue

1. Paul Longmore, "Introduction, *Why I Burned My Book and Other Essays on Disability* (Philadelphia: Temple University Press, 2003), 1–2. See also Faye Ginsburg and Rayna Rapp for a similar position in anthropology. Ginsburg and Rapp, "Introduction: Conceiving the New World Order," in *Conceiving the New World*

Order: The Global Politics of Reproduction, ed. Faye Ginsburg and Rayna Rapp (Berkeley: University of California Press, 1995), 12.

2. Barbara Beatty and Julia Grant, "Entering into the Fray: Historians of Childhood and Public Policy," *Journal of the History of Childhood and Youth* 3, no. 1 (Winter 2010): 107–126.

3. Beatty and Grant, 108.

4. Mona Gleason, "In Search of History's Child," *Jeunesse: Young People, Texts, Cultures* 1, no. 2 (Winter 2009): 132; Joy Parr, introduction, in *Histories of Canadian Children and Youth*, ed. Nancy Janovicek and Joy Parr (Don Mills: Oxford University Press, 2003), 1–7; Beatty and Grant, 120.

5. Beatty and Grant, 107.

6. Embryo adoption, for instance, is a relatively newer form of private adoption since the late 1990s. Jo Jones and Paul Placek, *Adoption by the Numbers: A Comprehensive Report of US Adoption Statistics* (National Council for Adoption, 2017), ii–iv, https://indd.adobe.com/view/4ae7a823-4140-4f27-961a-cd9f16a5f362; Kim Phagen-Hansel, "One Million Adoptions Later: Adoption and Safe Families Act at 20," *The Imprint*, November 28, 2018, https://imprintnews.org/adoption/one-million-adoptions-later-adoption-safe-families-act-at-20/32582.

7. Dorothy Roberts, *Shattered Bonds: The Color of Child Welfare* (New York: Basic Civitas, 2002).

8. Michelle Kahan, " 'Put Up' on Platforms: A History of Twentieth Century Adoption Policy in the United States," *Journal of Sociology and Social Welfare* 33, no. 3 (2006): 70.

9. Alison Kafer, *Feminist, Queer, Crip* (Bloomington: Indiana University Press, 2013), 3.

10. Katharine Hill, "Permanency and Placement Planning for Older Youth with Disabilities in Out-of-Home Placement," *Children and Youth Services Review* 34 (2012): 1421.

11. Children's Bureau, "Trends in Foster Care and Adoption: FY 2009–FY 2018," U.S. Department of Health and Human Services, Administration for Children and Families, Administration on Children, Youth and Families, Children's Bureau, http://centerforchildwelfare.fmhi.usf.edu/kb/natres/trends_fostercare_adoption_09thru18.pdf; Cynthia J. Weaver, Diane W. Keller, and Ann H. Loyek, "Children with Disabilities in the Child Welfare System," in *Child Welfare in the Twenty-First Century: A Handbook of Practices, Policies, and Programs, Second Edition*, ed. Gerald Mallon and Peg McCartt Hess (New York: Columbia University Press, 2005), 174, 178; Hill, "Permanency and Placement," 1419.

12. Laurel Leslie, Jeanne Gordon, Lee Meneken, Kamila Premji, Katherine Michaelmore, and William Ganger, "The Physical, Developmental, and Mental Health Needs of Young Children in Child Welfare by Initial Placement Type," *Developmental and Behavioral Pediatrics* 26, no. 3 (June 2005): 177. These statistics are general estimates, however; exact numbers of disabled children over the age of

three because Congress did not require such reporting under the National Child Abuse and Neglect Data System with the reauthorization of Child Abuse Prevention and Treatment Act in 2010. Furthermore, the law does not require reporting on abused disabled children by type of impairment. Children's Bureau, "Risk and Prevention of Maltreatment of Children with Disabilities," January 2018, https://www.childwelfare.gov/pubs/prevenres/focus/.

13. Minli Liao, Sarah Dababnah, and Hyeshin Park, "Relationship between Disabilities and Adoption Outcomes in African American Children," *Journal of Child and Family Studies* 26 (May 2017): 2439; Rosemary J. Avery, "Perceptions and Practice: Agency Efforts for the Hardest-to-Place Children," *Children and Youth Services Review* 22, no. 6 (2000): 407–408; Gleason, 129.

14. National Council on Disability, "Youth with Disabilities in the Foster Care System: Barriers to Success and Proposed Policy Solutions" (2008), 21–22, http://www.ncd.gov/publications/2008/02262008.

15. Hill, "Permanency and Placement," 1419.

16. Children's Bureau, "Trends in Foster Care and Adoption, FY 2010–2019" (2018), https://www.acf.hhs.gov/cb/report/trends-foster-care-adoption-fy-2010-2019-0; Children's Bureau, "Trends in Foster Care and Adoption: FY 2009–FY 2018," 1; Rita Soronen, "Every Child in Foster Care Deserves a Permanent Home and a Loving Family," *Imprint*, December 3, 2019, https://imprintnews.org/child-welfare-2/every-child-in-foster-care-deserves-a-permanent-home-and-a-loving-family/39443.

17. National Council on Disability, "Youth with Disabilities," 14.

18. Dave Thomas Foundation on Adoption, "National Adoptions Attitudes Survey, Research Report," in cooperation with Evan Donaldson Institute (June 2002), 3; National Council on Disability, "Youth with Disabilities," 21; According to policy scholar Michelle Kahan, adoptions may increase if *Roe v. Wade* is overturned because of a likely rise in the number of white "adoptable" children. Kahan, 70.

19. Teresa Wiltz, "New Rules Could Open More Homes to Foster Kids," *Stateline* (Pew Charitable Trusts), December 5, 2018, www.pewtrusts.org/en/research-and-analysis/blogs/stateline/2018/12/05/new-rules-could-open-more-homes-to-foster-kids.

20. Administration for Children and Families, "Budget for Foster Care and Permanency, HHS FY 2018 Budget in Brief—ACF—Mandatory," https://www.hhs.gov/about/budget/fy2018/budget-in-brief/acf/mandatory/index.html; Administration for Children and Families, "Foster Care: 2020 Budget Request," https://www.acf.hhs.gov/olab/fy-2020-budget-request. In 2006, $22 billion was spent. "Facts on Foster Care in America," ABC News, May 30, 2006, www.abcnews.go.com/Primetime/FosterCare/story?id=2017991; Sandra Bass, Margie K. Shields, and Richard E. Behrman, "Children, Families, and Foster Care: Analysis and Recommendations," *The Future of Children* 14, no. 1 (Winter 2004): 8–9.

21. "President Clinton Announces First Adoption Bonus Awards to States, Unveils Report that Shows Administration Strategy Is Working," September 24, 1999, http://www.hhs.gov/news/press/1999pres/990924b.

22. Richard P. Barth, "Adoption from Foster Care: A Chronicle of the Years after ASFA," in *Intentions and Results: A Look Back at the Adoption and Safe Families Act*, ed. Susan Notkin, Kristen Weber, Olivia A. Golden, and Jennifer Macomber (Washington, DC: Center for the Study of Social Policy; Urban Institute, 2009), 64–69; Mary Eschelbach Hansen, "State-Designated Special Needs, Post-adoption Support, and State Fiscal Stress," *Children and Youth Services Review 29, no. 11 (November 2007): 1411–1425.*

23. New laws have changed the ways the federal government allocates subsidies to the states, for example. In 1998, the Promoting Safe and Stable Families Program (PSSF) became the name of the 1993 Family Preservation and Support Services Program. It was reauthorized through ASFA and kept the 1993 provisions intact but added time-limited family reunification services for children in foster care and adoption support and promotion services. The PSSF has been reauthorized five times, the latest in 2016 under the name the Child and Family Services Improvement and Innovation Act. *The Promoting Safe and Stable Families Program: Background and Content*, 2011, https://www.casey.org/media/PromotingSafeand StableFamilies.pdf; For changes to Title IV-E of the Social Security Act, see the Preventing Sex Trafficking and Strengthening Families Act.

24. John Kelly, "A Complete Guide to the Family First Prevention Services Act," *Imprint*, February 25, 2018, https://imprintnews.org/finance-reform/chronicles -complete-guide-family-first-prevention-services-act/30043.

25. National Conference of State Legislatures, "Family First Prevention Services Act," April 1, 2020, https://www.ncsl.org/research/human-services/family-first -prevention-services-act-ffpsa.

26. Roberts, *Shattered Bonds*.

27. Ashley Provencher, Nicholas Kahn, and Mary Eschelbach Hansen, "Adoption Policy and the Well-Being of Adopted Children in the United States," *Child Welfare* 95, no. 1 (2017): 28.

28. Soronen, 2019.

29. Children's Bureau, "Risk and Prevention of Maltreatment of Children"; Elizabeth Lightfoot, Katharine Hill, and Traci LaLiberte, "Prevalence of Children with Disabilities in the Child Welfare System and Out of Home Placement: An Examination of Administrative Records," *Children and Youth Services Review* 33 (2011): 2069.

30. Weaver, Keller, and Loyek, 177; Hill, "Permanency and Placement," 1418– 1424.

31. Blace Nalavany, Scott Ryan, Jeanne Howard, and Susan Livingston Smith, "Pre-adoptive Child Sexual Abuse as a Predictor of Moves in Care, Adoption Disruptions, and Inconsistent Adoptive Parent Commitment," *Child Abuse and*

Neglect 32, no. 12 (2008): 1087; Susan Livingston Smith, Jeanne Howard, Phillip Garnier, and Scott Ryan, "Where Are We Now: A Post-ASFA Examination of Adoption Disruption," *Adoption Quarterly* 9, no. 4 (2006): 37–38.

32. Avery, "Perceptions and Practice," 410–411.

33. Avery, "Perceptions and Practice," 415.

34. Avery, "Perceptions and Practice," 414.

35. Avery, "Perceptions and Practice," 415.

36. Patricia Harris, *Loving the "Unadoptable"* (Bloomington, IN: AuthorHouse Publishing, 2008), 65.

37. Liao, Dababnah and Park, 2438.

38. Christie Petrenko, Michelle Alto, Andrea Hart, Sarah Freeze, and Lynn Cole, "'I'm Doing My Part, I Just Need Help from the Community': Intervention Implications of Foster and Adoptive Parents' Experiences Raising Children and Young Adults with FASD," *Journal of Family Nursing* 25, no. 2 (2019): 327.

39. Petrenko et al., 327.

40. Ralph James Savarese, *Reasonable People: A Memoir of Autism and Adoption* (New York: Other Press, 2007), 181.

41. Robyn Powell, "For Parents around the Country, Having a Disability Can Mean Losing Custody of Their Kids," *Rewire News*, March 12, 2018, https://rewire.news/article/2018/03/12/parents-around-country-disability-can-mean-losing-custody-kids/.

42. Powell.

43. Powell.

44. Abbie Goldberg, "Stigmas about Adoption Remain, and Hurt Families," *Psychology Today*, May 21, 2012.

45. Goldberg, "Stigmas about Adoption Remain," 2; Abbie Goldberg, Lori Kinkler, and Denise Hines, "Perception and Internalization of Adoption Stigma among Gay, Lesbian, and Heterosexual Adoptive Parents," *Journal of GLBT Family Studies* 7 (2011): 133.

46. Signe Howell, "Changes in Moral Values about the Family: Adoption Legislation in Norway and the U.S.," *Social Analysis* 50 (2006): 150.

47. Ashley Fetters, "When 'You're Adopted' Is Used as an Insult," *Atlantic*, July 25, 2019, www.theatlantic.com/family/archive/2019/07/youre-adopted-insult/594667.

48. Allan Fisher, "Still 'Not Quite as Good as Having Your Own'?: Toward a Sociology of Adoption," *Annual Review of Sociology* 29 (2003): 344, 353.

49. Goldberg, Kinkler, and Hines, "Perception and Internalization of Adoption Stigma," 136, 151.

50. Thomas Couser, "The Empire of the 'Normal': A Forum on Disability and Self-Representation," *American Quarterly* 52, no. 2 (June 2000): 305.

51. E.g., Mia Mingus's *Leaving Evidence*, https://leavingevidence.wordpress.com, and Lydia X. Z. Brown, "Adoption and Inappropriate Questions," *Autistic Hoya*, February 3, 2013, https://www.autistichoya.com/2013/02/adoption-and-inappropriate-questions.html.

52. Couser, "The Empire of the 'Normal,'" 305.

53. Denise Sherer Jacobson, *The Question of David: A Disabled Mother's Journey through Adoption, Family and Life* (Berkeley: Creative Arts, 1999).

54. Jacobson, *Question of David*, 23.

55. Jacobson, *Question of David*, 146.

56. Jacobson, *Question of David*, 11, 121, 140; Deborah Marks, "Dimensions of Oppression: Theorising the Embodied Subject," *Disability and Society* 14, no. 5 (1999): 615.

57. Jacobson, *Question of David*, 37, 63–64, 82, 188.

58. Jacobson, *Question of David*, 38.

59. Jacobson, *Question of David*, 39.

60. Savarese, *Reasonable People*, 77.

61. Savarese, *Reasonable People*, 82, 116.

62. Savarese, *Reasonable People*, 251, 433.

63. Savarese, *Reasonable People*, 64.

64. Savarese, *Reasonable People*, 80, 171.

65. Savarese, *Reasonable People*, 67.

66. Savarese, *Reasonable People*, 264.

67. Savarese, *Reasonable People*, 309.

68. Maria Thompson Corley, "Deej: A Non-verbal Autistic Man Raises His Voice for Inclusion," *Medium*, September 20, 2017, https://medium.com/@maria thompsoncorley/deej-a-non-verbal-autistic-man-raises-his-voice-for-inclusion -ce4de0d22a8c; Imade Borha, "DJ 'Deej' Savarese Pursues Freedom as a Non-speaking Autistic Man in New Documentary," *Frederick News Post*, October 16, 2017, 3.

69. Kate Fishman, "'Deej' Highlights Interdependence, Challenges Assumptions," *Oberlin Review*, October 6, 2017.

70. DJ Savarese, "Cultural Commentary: Communicate with Me," *Disability Studies Quarterly* 30, no. 1 (2010), https://dsq-sds.org/article/view/1051/1237; Craig A. Foster, "Deej-a Vu: Documentary Revisits Facilitated Communication pseudoscience," *Behavioral Interventions* 34 (2019): 577–586.

71. Patrick Ryan, "How New Is the 'New' Social Study of Childhood? The Myth of a Paradigm Shift," *Journal of Interdisciplinary History* 38, no. 14 (Spring 2008): 555.

72. Jonathan Karsh, dir., *My Flesh and Blood* (Docurama, 2004). For user reviews, see https://www.imdb.com/title/tt0342804/.

73. See Chapter 4.

74. Kari Wagner-Peck, *Not Always Happy: An Unusual Parenting Journey* (Las Vegas: Central Recovery Press, 2017), xi.

75. Adrienne Asch and David Wasserman, "Where Is the Sin in Synecdoche? Prenatal Testing and the Parent-Child Relationship," in *Quality of Life and Human Difference: Genetic Testing, Health Care, and Disability*, ed. David Wasserman, Jerome Bickenbach, and Robert Wachbroit (Cambridge: Cambridge University

Press, 2005), 172–216; Adrienne Asch, "Prenatal Diagnosis and Selective Abortion: A Challenge to Practice and Policy," *American Journal of Public Health* 89, no. 11 (1999): 1649–1657.

76. Wagner-Peck, 4.

77. Wagner-Peck, 19.

78. Wagner-Peck, 5–6, 17.

79. *A Typical* Son, atypicalson.com; Wagner-Peck, 93, 117, 133.

80. Harris.

81. Harris, 33.

82. Harris, 63.

83. Kristin Berry, *Born Broken: An Adoptive Journey* (Green Forest, AR: New Leaf, 2017), 151.

84. Berry, *Born Broken*, 97, 121.

85. Berry, *Born Broken*, 45, 63.

86. Berry, *Born Broken*, 64, 102.

87. Here Berry makes a call to her religion. Berry, *Born Broken*, 156.

88. Couser, "The Empire of the 'Normal,'" 309.

89. Jennifer Poss Taylor, *Forfeiting All Sanity: A Mother's Story of Raising a Child with Fetal Alcohol Syndrome* (Mustang, OK: Tate Publishing, 2010), 50, 52.

90. Poss Taylor, 127.

91. Gleason, 128; Ryan, "How New," 566, 576.

92. Leslie Wind, Devon Brooks, and Richard P. Barth, "Influences of Risk History and Adoption Preparation on Post-adoption Services Use in US Adoptions," *Family Relations* 56 (October 2007): 385.

93. Petrenko et al., 326.

94. Thank you to Sue Schweik for having this conversation with me, September 20, 2015. Article 23 of the UN's Convention on the Rights of Persons with Disabilities makes a commitment to eliminate discrimination relating to marriage, family, and personal relations. The rights the CRPD commits to, however, center on adult concerns about forming a family rather than access to family by children. https://www.ohchr.org/EN/HRBodies/CRPD/Pages/ConventionRightsPersonsWithDisabilities.aspx#23. The Convention on the Rights of the Child (1989) states that a child *should* grow up in a family that nurtures her development and it. protects the adoptive family but does not give children the explicit right to access family. https://www.unicef.org/sites/default/files/2019-04/UN-Convention-Rights-Child-text.pdf.

95. 1930 Children's Charter, White House Conference on Child Health and Protection, 1930, US Children's Bureau File, National Archives.

96. Petrenko et al., 314–347.

97. Petrenko et al., 328–329.

98. Petrenko et al., 332.

99. Avery, "Perceptions and Practice," 418.

100. Avery, "Perceptions and Practice," 413.

101. Weaver, Keller, and Loyek, 176.

102. Hill, "Permanency and Placement," 1418–1419, 1422.

103. Hill, "Permanency and Placement," 1419–1421.

104. Avery, "Perceptions and Practice," 408, 411.

105. Weaver, Keller, and Loyek, 173.

106. Avery, "Perceptions and Practice," 417; Wind, Brooks, and Barth, 387.

107. Avery, "Perceptions and Practice," 415.

108. Provencher, Kahn, and Hansen, 43.

109. Petrenko et al., 330.

110. Hill, "Permanency and Placement," 1419.

111. Elissa Madden, Amy Chanmugam, Ruth G. McRoy, Laura Kaufman, Susan Ayers-Lopez, Mary Boo, and Kathleen Ledesma, "The Impact of Formal and Informal Respite Care on Foster, Adoptive, and Kinship Parents Caring for Children Involved in the Child Welfare System," *Child Adolescent Social Work* 33 (2016): 524.

112. Petrenko et al., 332.

113. Katharine Hill and Fintan Moore, "The Postadoption Needs of Adoptive Parents of Children with Disabilities," *Journal of Family Social Work* 18 (2015): 178.

114. Liao, Dababnah, and Park, 2447.

115. Hill, "Permanency and Placement," 1423; Petrenko et al., 330.

116. Bass, Shields, and Behrman, 5–7.

117. Provencher, Kahn, and Hansen, "Adoption Policy," 46.

118. Leslie et al., 177.

119. Bass, Shields, and Behrman, 19; "Facts on Foster Care in America," ABC News, May 30, 2006, www.abcnews.go.com/Primetime/FosterCare/story?id=2017991.

120. Robert McRuer, "The Then and There of Crip Futurity," review of *Feminist, Queer, Crip* by Alison Kafer, *GLQ: A Journal of Lesbian and Gay Studies* 20, no. 4 (2014): 532.

121. National Council on Disability, "Youth with Disabilities," 7.

122. National Council on Disability, "Youth with Disabilities," 22. Coordination might also relieve the amount of time foster and adoptive parents report they spend making and attending all the necessary medical appointments for their disabled children, depending upon their needs. Jason Brown and Susan Rodger, "Children with Disabilities: Problems Faced by Foster Parents," *Children and Youth Services Review* 31 (2009): 44.

123. Hill, "Permanency and Placement," 1419.

124. Hill, "Permanency and Placement," 1419.

125. For a review, see Madelyn Freundlich, "Adoption Research: An Assessment of Empirical Contributions to the Advancement of Adoption Practice," *Journal of Social Distress and the Homeless* 11, no. 2 (April 2002): 143–166.

126. Petrenko et al., 316.

127. Dan Goodley, "Dis/entangling Critical Disability Studies," in *Culture—Theory—Disability: Encounters between Disability Studies and Cultural Studies*, ed.

Anne Waldschmidt, Berressem Hanjo, and Moritz Ingwersen (Bielefeld: Transcript, 2017), 83; Carolyn Kagan et al., *Critical Community Psychology: Critical Action and Social Change* (Oxford: Wiley-Blackwell, 2011); Marks, 611.

128. Brodzinsky notes the difference between placement outcomes for children with disabilities who have "predictable manifestations," like physical and developmental impairments and chronic medical conditions, and those who have unpredictable ones, like emotional or behavioral problems. The latter have a higher rate of adoption dissolutions and disruptions than the former. According to Brodzinsky, placement disruption rates for these adoptions range from 10 to 20 percent, but the study he cites is old, even for the time his article was published. David M. Brodzinsky and Ellen Pinderhughes, "Parenting and Child Developing in Adoptive Families," in *Handbook of Parenting: Children and Parenting*, ed. Marc H. Bornstein (Mahwah, NJ: Erlbaum, 2002), 293.

129. See chapter 3.

130. Wind, Brooks, and Barth, 379.

131. Goldberg, Kinkler, and Hines, 134.

132. Brodzinsky and Pinderhughes, "Parenting and Child Developing in Adoptive Families," 282–285; David M. Brodzinsky, Daniel W. Smith, and Anne B. Brodzinsky, *Children's Adjustment to Adoption: Developmental and Clinical Issues* (Thousand Oaks, CA: SAGE, 1998), 51–64.

133. Evan Donaldson Adoption Institute, Keeping the Promise, 5; Katarina Wegar, "Adoption, Family Ideology, and Social Stigma: Bias in Community Attitudes, Adoption Research, and Practice," *Family Relations* 49, no. 4 (October 2000): 363; Fisher, 356.

134. Evan Donaldson Adoption Institute, Keeping the Promise, 15; Doreen Arcus and Patrick Chambers, "Childhood Risks Associated with Adoption," in *Family Influences on Childhood Behavior and Development: Evidence-Based Prevention and Treatment Approaches*, ed. Thomas Gullotta and Gary Balu `(New York: Routledge, 2008), 117–142; Freundlich, "Adoption Research," 152–154.

135. Deborah Siegel and Jessice Strolin-Goltzman, "Adoption Competency and Trauma-Informed Practices with Adoptive Families," *Families in Society: The Journal of Contemporary Social Services* 98, no. 3 (2017): 167; Fisher, 336.

136. Wegar, "Adoption, Family Ideology," 364, 366.

137. See Anna Waldschmidt, "Disability Goes Cultural: The Cultural Model of Disability as an Analytic Tool," in *Culture—Theory—Disability: Encounters between Disability Studies and Cultural Studies*, ed. Anne Waldschmidt (Bielefeld: Transcript, 2017), 19–28. For critique of this type of research by an adoptive father, see Savarese, *Reasonable People*, 198–199, 202–203.

138. Evan Donaldson Institute, 15–19; and Appendix III, 91–99; Jesús Palacios, "The Ecology of Adoption," in *International Advances in Adoption Research for Practice*, ed. Gretchen M. Wrobel and Elsbeth Neil (Oxford: Wiley-Blackwell, 2009), 71–94.

139. Wegar, "Adoption, Family Ideology," 364; Marks, 619; Samuel Perry, "Adoption in the United States: A Critical Synthesis of Literature and Directions for Sociological Research" (unpublished paper, 2013), 16–18, doi: 10.13140 /RG.2.2.12929.25448/1.

140. Petrenko et al., 316, 336; Ryan, "How New," 555.

141. For patient-engaged research and community based participatory research, see J. R. Kirwan et al., "Emerging Guidelines for Patient Engagement in Research," *Value in Health* 20 (2017): 482; Lori Frank, Laura Forsythe, Lauren Ellis, Suzanne Schrandt, Sue Sheridan, Jason Gerson, Kristen Konopka, and Sarah Daugherty, "Conceptual and Practical Foundations of Patient Engagement in Research at the Patient-Centered Outcomes Research Institute," *Quality of Life Research* 24, no. 5 (2015): 1035; S. Cashman et al., "The Power and the Promise: Working with Communities to Analyze Data, Interpret Findings, and Get to Outcomes," *American Journal of Public Health* 98, no. 8 (August 2008): 1407–1414.

142. So too is an analysis of adoption science that critically examines the field's conception of disability risk, my next project.

143. Waldschmidt, "Disability Goes Cultural," 26.

144. Waldschmidt, "Disability Goes Cultural," 26.

145. For parenting strategies that are "outside of the box," see Petrenko et al., 323.

146. Goodley, 84.

147. For this question, see Andrew Solomon, *Far from the Tree: Parents, Children, and the Search for Identity* (New York: Scribner, 2013).

148. Sue Schweik, "Disability and the Normal Body of the (Native) Citizen," *Social Research* 78, no. 2 (Summer 2011): 417–442.

Appendix Two

1. As quoted in Allison Carey, On the Margins of Citizenship: Intellectual Disability and Civil Rights in Twentieth-Century America (Philadelphia: Temple University Press, 2009), 154; Chloe Silverman, *Understanding Autism: Parents, Doctors, and the History of a Disorder* (Princeton: Princeton University Press, 2012), 106.

2. Deborah S. Metzel, "Historical Social Geography" in *Mental Retardation in America: A Historical Reader*, eds. Steven Noll and James W. Trent Jr. (New York: New York University Press, 2004), 438.

3. Public Law 95-602, 95th Congress, November 6, 1978, 50–51, https://www .govinfo.gov/link/statute/92/2982.

4. McKenzie, 2.

Index

alcoholism, 200–202, 221–22; barriers to
adoption, 166, 175, 178–79; behavioral
issues, 196, 202, 217–20, 224; belonging, 220; best interest, 204, 210, 344n93;
Black people, 194–99, 204; boarder baby
crisis, 202–3; casework assessment, 203,
217–18, 222–23; Child Welfare League
of America (CWLA), 198–99, 203, 205;
class, 201, 218–19; "defectives," 200,
205, 207; deinstitutionalization, 168,
172, 192; dependency, 196, 199–204;
disability risk, 194, 206; drugs, 194–
204, 207–8, 221–22, 337n12, 338n20;
emotional issues, 196, 201, 208, 213–23;
euthanasia, 210; exclusionary practices,
31, 64; fathers, 195, 210; foster care, 193–
209, 212, 215–22; futurity, 206, 210; gender, 199, 202, 219; genetics, 205–8; Ginsburg on, 7; handicapped children, 207,
209–11, 216–17; historical perspective
on, 3–4, 7, 10, 17–20, 227–28, 237, 252–
53; imperfect children, 213–24; importance of, 252–53; inherent risk, 194–96;
intellectual issues, 211, 216–18, 224;
legal issues, 201, 203, 208, 211, 214–15,
221, 224; limits of, 3, 193–225, 227–28;
love, 200, 206, 213–14, 217, 220; matching, 205; "mental retardation," 221;
moral issues, 200–201, 204, 208; mothers,
197–204, 207, 210, 219, 221, 340n49,
343n75; neglect, 194, 197, 203, 212–13,
218, 222; normality, 199, 202, 207, 212,
225; orphans, 203; overcoming, 133,
141–42, 150, 161–62; pathological issues,
196, 208; people of color, 194, 199–200,
207–8; perfectionism, 20, 193–95, 204–25;
possibility of, 161–62; prejudice, 19,
162, 166, 195; psychiatrists, 195–96, 218,
345n10; psychologists, 194–96, 201, 208,
214, 222, 345n110; racial issues, 194–201,
208; Rapp on, 7; reform, 201; rehabilitation, 201–4, 209, 211, 219; reproductive
technologies, 204–9; special needs, 194–
99, 208–9, 215–21, 229, 231, 240–47, 253,
347n135, 348n153; stigma, 194–96, 201,
204, 214, 221, 224; trauma, 194–96, 209,
213, 218, 222
Indian Adoption Project, 92, 146, 171
Indian Child Welfare Act (ICWA), 14,
171–72, 189

Individuals with Disabilities Education Act
(IDEA), 247–48
inferiority, 7–8, 17, 31, 199
infertility, 12, 77, 124, 205–6, 218
injuries, 170, 220–21, 325n102
insanity, 38–39, 47, 49
instability, 46, 65, 70, 193, 196, 245, 248
Institute for Juvenile Research, 55
insurance, 5, 92, 153, 156–57, 186, 216, 223,
240
intellectual issues: barriers to adoption, 166,
172–73, 177; cognitive status, 53–57 (see
also cognitive status); exclusionary practices, 37, 40, 43, 55; historical perspective on, 14, 19, 249, 256–58; inclusion,
211, 216–18, 224; insanity, 38–39, 47, 49;
mental hygiene, 44, 52, 261–65; "mental
retardation," 50 (see also "mental retardation"); overcoming, 112, 114–15, 125,
128, 130–35, 139–40, 145, 148; psychosis,
47, 51–53, 70, 261–62; risk equivalence,
71, 73, 89, 92–95
intelligence: barriers to adoption, 169, 177;
exclusionary practices, 43, 46, 48, 50–51,
54–58, 61, 65, 67–68; heredity, 11, 54, 57,
73, 75, 87, 95; IQ tests, 46, 48, 53–57, 60,
66, 68, 75, 87, 120, 137, 151; normality, 43,
46, 50–51, 54–55, 57, 61, 67, 83, 86, 131,
169; overcoming, 111, 114, 120, 131; risk
equivalence, 83, 86–87, 91; shifts in understanding, 56; suitability, 43, 51, 55, 262
Interethnic Placement Provisions Act, 189
Interstate Compact for the Protection of
Children, 146
IQ tests: Binet-Simon, 55; exclusionary
practices, 46, 48, 53–57, 60, 66, 68;
Gesell on, 54; intelligence, 46, 48, 53–57,
60, 66, 68, 75, 87, 120, 137, 151; Jenkins
on, 55–56; Kuhlmann-Binet, 55; "mental
retardation," 151; overcoming, 120, 137,
151; psychologists, 53–57, 87, 120; risk
equivalence, 75, 87; score categorization,
56; shifts in understanding, 56; Stanford-
Binet, 55; Thompson on, 51, 57
isolation, 141, 214, 220, 239, 241

Jacobson, Denise, 235–36
Janis family, 123
Jenkins, Henry, 63
Jenkins, R. L., 55–56